Dental and Oral Tissues
An Introduction

Dental and Oral Tissues
An Introduction

3rd Edition

LETTY MOSS-SALENTIJN, D.D.S., Ph.D.

Professor
School of Dental and Oral Surgery
Columbia University

MARLENE HENDRICKS-KLYVERT, R.D.H. Ed.D.

Associate Professor
School of Dental and Oral Surgery
Columbia University

Illustrations by
MARSHA DOHRMANN

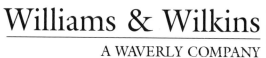

Williams & Wilkins
A WAVERLY COMPANY

BALTIMORE • PHILADELPHIA • LONDON • PARIS • BANGKOK
HONG KONG • MUNICH • SYDNEY • TOKYO • WROCLAW

Williams & Wilkins
351 West Camden Street
Baltimore, Maryland 21201-2436 USA

Rose Tree Corporate Center
1400 North Providence Road
Building II, Suite 5025
Media, Pennsylvania 19063-2043 USA

Library of Congress Cataloging in Publication Data

Moss-Salentijn, Letty
    Dental and oral tissues: an introduction / Letty Moss-Salentijn,
Marlene Hendricks-Klyvert; illustrations by Marsha Dohrmann.—3rd ed.
      p.   cm.
    Includes bibliographical references.
    ISBN 0-8121-1320-9
    1. Mouth—Histology. 2. Teeth—Histology. 3. Embryology, Human.
4. Dental auxiliary personnel. I. Hendricks-Klyvert, Marlene.
II. Title.
    [DNLM: 1. Dental Auxiliaries. 2. Mouth–anatomy & histology.
3. Mouth—embryology.   WU 101 M913d]
RK280.M62   1990
611'.31—dc20
DNLM/DLC
for Library of Congress   89—13713
                                 CIP

1st Edition, 1980
2nd Edition, 1985
3rd Edition, 1990

PRINTED IN THE UNITED STATES OF AMERICA

Print number: 5   4   3

For Melvin

Preface

In this third edition, we have made many small changes throughout the text and in some of the illustrations, reflecting not only advances made during the past 5 years, but also helpful suggestions and comments from colleagues and students.

Although it is difficult to resist the common tendency to write a much more expanded and comprehensive text, we have tried as much as possible to preserve the original format of the book: that of a simple, clinically oriented **introduction** to dental and oral tissues.

The greatest emphasis of the text's material is on topics that, from a clinical standpoint, require more detailed knowledge, such as the various properties of the oral mucosa (oral diagnosis, local anesthesia, full mouth impressions), surface characteristics of enamel (sealants, bonding), and the fine structure of the dentogingival attachment (prophylaxis, curettage). Wherever possible, we emphasize the immediate, practical application of this information.

We have attempted to write this text in plain language, intentionally avoiding, as much as warranted, the introduction of unnecessary terms. We believe that students often tend to lose themselves in memorizing nomenclature, which does not really add to their understanding, and they therefore miss the critical, much needed information being presented.

The intent of this text is to provide students with an introduction to orofacial histology and embryology, which may be supplemented or enhanced by lectures, slides, and when possible, laboratory exercises. It is our hope that this text will provide the students with a morphologic basis for their future work in clinical dentistry.

Once again, we acknowledge with gratitude the capable and professional assistance of the editorial staff and the production staff of Lea & Febiger. We have further been particularly fortunate in securing the artistic assistance of Marsha Dohrmann and the professional photographic support of Mr. Alfred Lammé.*

Finally, we thank our colleagues, who have graciously supplied

Technical note: The "original magnifications," listed with each of the photographs of microscopic material, represent the ratio between the size of the photographic image on the original negative and the size of the microscopic specimen itself, and should be used only as an appropriate indication, because they do not reflect subsequent magnifications and/or reductions in the final reproduction of the photographs.

us with unpublished photographic materials or have given us permission to use previously published illustrations. Specific acknowledgements are given in the text.

New York, New York   Letty Moss-Salentijn
                                                       Marlene Hendricks-Klyvert

Contents

Basic Tissues: Nondental Tissues in the Orofacial Region

1

Introduction

The oral cavity is a complex environment in which the teeth are but one of the components. It is our intention to introduce to you, in this book, both the nondental and the dental components of the mouth, a study that requires careful observations. It is therefore a good idea to start with an exercise in *observation.* This can be done alone, standing in front of a mirror, or in cooperation with a partner. In either case, good lighting is essential.

EXERCISE IN OBSERVATION

With the mouth opened wide, identify and compare what you see with the aid of the diagram (Fig. 1–1).

Stick out your *tongue,* move it to the left, to the right and back. Notice how the shape of the tongue alters during these movements. When you move your *lips* from a wide smile to a pout, you will notice how their lengths change.

Now place the tip of your tongue in your *cheeks* and see the bulge on the outside.

With your fingers feel, gently, the *hard palate.* It has a ribbed surface.

Going backward your fingers move from the hard palate to the *soft palate.* Remove the fingers immediately when there is an indication of *choking.* The palate is extremely sensitive.

Stick out your tongue and say "Aaah." If you still have your tonsils, you may see them between two folds on either side of the passage way *(fauces)* between the oral cavity and the pharynx.

Next take the lower lip between both thumbs and index fingers and gently pull it downward and forward. You now have a good look at the space between the teeth and jaws on one side and the lips and cheeks on the other. This space is called the *vestibule.*

The *oral cavity proper* is the space enclosed by the two arches formed by the teeth and jaws.

Gently move the lip up and down and notice that the lips and

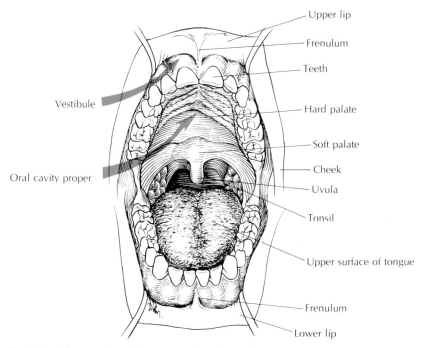

Upper lip

Frenulum

Teeth

Vestibule

Hard palate

Soft palate

Cheek

Oral cavity proper

Uvula

Tonsil

Upper surface of tongue

Frenulum

Lower lip

Fig. 1–1. Diagram of a wide open mouth. The two large arrows indicate the vestibule (the space between lips/cheeks and teeth/jaws) and the oral cavity proper (the space enclosed by the two dental arches). Attachment bands (or frenula) run between the lips and the dental arches. A similar frenulum is present between the underside of the tongue and the inside of the lower jaw. It is, however, not visible in this diagram, since it can be seen only when the tongue is lifted.

cheeks themselves are soft and moveable, but that the covering of the jaws is not moveable.

Repeat this part of the exercise for the upper lip, pulling it gently forward and upward.

Lift up the tongue and place the tip on the hard palate. Inspect the area underneath the tongue. This is the *sublingual* area.

The attachment band between the underside of the tongue and the inside of the lower jaw is called a *frenulum.* Similar frenula are also present between the inside of the lower lip and the lower jaw and the inside of the upper lip and the upper jaw.

Finally, identify and count the *teeth.* A complete *dentition* in an adult has 32 teeth, 16 in each jaw (Fig. 1–2).

Ideally you should find in each jaw 4 *incisors,* 2 *canines,* 4 *premolars* and 6 *molars.* Try to identify, in case of missing teeth, which teeth are missing. Also notice any excess (supernumerary) teeth, if present.

The "milk" dentition *(primary or deciduous dentition)* of a child

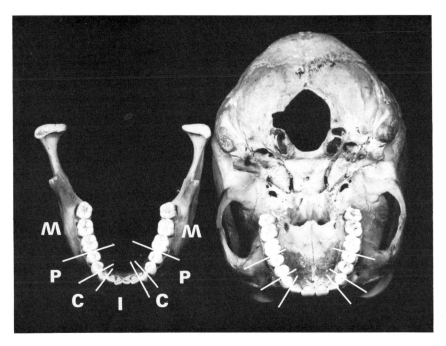

Fig. 1–2.   The complete (permanent) dentition of an adult, shown in a human skull. The separate lower jaw is at the left, seen from above, while the rest of the skull, with the upper jaw, is seen from below, at the right. In each jaw there are 4 incisors (I), 2 canines (C), 4 premolars (P), and 6 molars (M).

consists of 20 teeth. These teeth, 4 *incisors,* 2 *canines* and 4 *molars* in each jaw, are eventually lost and replaced by the adult *(secondary* or *permanent)* dentition.

Review of Observations

In the foregoing exercise you should have noted the following:

The oral cavity has a pink-red lining, the *oral mucosa,* which covers all surfaces, except the teeth. This lining is kept moist by a watery fluid, *saliva.*

There are many regional differences in the oral mucosa; the texture of the surface of the tongue, for instance, is quite different from that of the sublingual area.

Chapters 2 and 3 will deal extensively with the structure of the oral mucosa.

The various parts of the oral cavity have different textures and characteristics. There are hard immoveable structures, such as the teeth, the jaw bones (to which the teeth are attached), and the hard palate. There are also soft, moveable, yielding structures, such as the tongue, lips, cheeks, soft palate and sublingual area.

Even in a small space, like the oral cavity, there are many different components, specialized and adapted for different functional needs.

ORGANIZATION OF THE BODY

The human body's smallest unit of organization is a *cell*. Groups of similarly specialized cells, and their products, form *tissues*. The tissues of the human body, separately or in combination, form *organs*. Groups of organs, related to a specific function, may be combined in *organ systems*. A coordinated series of organ systems is an *organism*.

The patient, who will seek your professional services, is an organism.

The oral cavity is the gateway to two major systems: the *digestive* and the *respiratory* systems. The oral cavity is involved in many activities, some related to digestion (chewing, tasting, swallowing) and others related to respiration and speech. The organs *inside* the oral cavity are the teeth and the tongue.

TEETH. The shapes of teeth and their hardness are well suited for the breaking up and grinding down of food into particles small enough to be swallowed.

TONGUE. The tongue assists in the chewing process by redistributing the food particles in the oral cavity. It is further involved in the initiation of the swallowing process, and it is essential for speech. On the top surface, the tongue carries a large number of small taste organs, the *taste buds.*

Organs that are not located inside the oral cavity, but are associated with it and important to its functions are the salivary glands and the tonsils.

SALIVARY GLANDS. The salivary glands produce saliva, which is carried via ducts into the oral cavity. Saliva contains enzymes that start the breakdown process of the chewed food particles.

TONSILS. The oral cavity is a major entrance point for foreign matter into the body. Tonsils form a ring of defensive tissue in the passage from the oral cavity to the pharynx.

In the following chapters you will be familiarized with the appearance of the specialized cells and tissues, which form the organs and organ systems of the oral cavity and its related parts. This study of cells and tissues, at the microscopic level, is called *histology.*

Part I of this book, Chapters 2 through 7, is devoted to the "basic tissues" of the human body, illustrated with examples of the nondental tissues of the oral cavity. Thus, you will be able to study the histology of the oral mucosa, salivary glands, blood vessels, muscles, nerves and skeletal elements.

In Part II of this book, Chapters 8 through 14, the material from Part I is applied and expanded in the study of the tissues of the tooth itself and the tissues immediately surrounding the tooth, the *periodontium*.

2

Basic Tissues and Cells

BASIC TISSUES

As we noted in Chapter 1, a cell is the smallest unit of organization of a living organism. It is capable of prolonged, independent existence and self-renewal as long as it is in a suitable environment.

At the beginning of human development the future organism consists of 'one cell. This cell multiplies and different groups of its descendants become specialized for different specific functions. Such cell specialization is called *differentiation.* As the result of differentiation many different tissues develop in the human body, which may be classified into four *basic tissue* types: epithelium, connective tissue, muscle tissue and nervous tissue. Each of these basic tissue types is further subdivided into several variations. These will be discussed in the appropriate chapters.

Epithelium

Epithelium consists exclusively of cells. These cells form a surface covering. Any surface of the human body that is in contact with the outside world is covered with this tissue type. This includes the lining of the oral cavity, the digestive tract and the respiratory tract, since the contents of these tracts are in *open* connection with the outside world and are thus technically considered as being outside the body.

The further specializations of epithelia depend on their location in the body and their function in that location. An epithelium may *protect* the underlying tissues against mechanical damage or drying. An epithelium may also be *resorptive* (in the digestive tract) or *secretory* (glandular cells, derived from epithelium).

Connective Tissue

Connective tissue consists of cells and large amounts of *intercellular* (between cells) *substance,* produced by the cells. The nature of the intercellular substance may vary according to the nature of the connective tissue. In general, this type of tissue connects and supports other tissue types, as the name would suggest.

Connective tissue occurs in a wide spectrum: connective tissue proper, bone, cartilage, bone marrow, and lymphoid tissue.

Muscle Tissue

Muscle tissue consists predominantly of cells. In this tissue type the cells have become specialized in contraction. They have an extensive and highly efficient *contractile* apparatus *intracellularly* (inside the cells).

Various types of muscle tissue, with different contractile properties, are present in the human body: striated, smooth and cardiac muscle.

Nervous Tissue

This tissue type consists predominantly of cells. Most of these cells have specialized in *communication,* the transmission of a message from one cell to the next, sometimes over large distances in the body.

Various types of nerve cells, with different properties, may be found. This tissue is organized in a concentrated form in the *central nervous system* (brain and spinal cord) and in a dispersed form throughout the body in the *peripheral nervous system* (nerves and ganglia).

STRUCTURE OF AN INDIVIDUAL CELL

A cell is capable of performing a variety of functions, necessary both for its own survival and for that of the organism. While there are structural differences between the various cell types, they all have some structures in common.

1. *Cell membrane,* a surface covering, which surrounds the cell contents: cytoplasm and organelles. While the cell membrane is not impressive microscopically, it is a complex structure, which serves as the interface between the cell contents and the environment of the cell.

(a) It serves as a "gatekeeper" in that it *regulates the movement* of molecules and ions into and out of the cell.

(b) Regions of the membrane surface are specialized for recognition of outside substances, such as hormones. When these substances are recognized, the membrane gives a signal to the cell, stimulating it to provide an appropriate response.

(c) Other specialized membrane regions allow the cell to communicate with or to attach itself to other cells.

2. *Cytoplasm*, a fluid medium which surrounds the organelles of the cell. It is composed of a *cytoskeleton:* a complex 3-dimensional meshwork of fibrillar components (microfilaments, intermediate filaments and microtubules) and a *cytoplasmic matrix*: the fluid which occupies all spaces not occupied by either the cytoskeleton or some free polyribosome complexes.

3. *Organelles,* metabolically active, internal organs of the cell. They carry out specific essential functions. Organelles are to the cell what organs are to the human body. Important organelles, that are common to nearly all cell types, are nucleus, endoplasmic reticulum, Golgi complex, mitochondria and lysosomes (Fig. 2–1).

Before we start with a description of the cell components, we should clarify at what *level of observation* these structures are visible. Table 2–1 should be used as a guideline for the ensuing presentation.

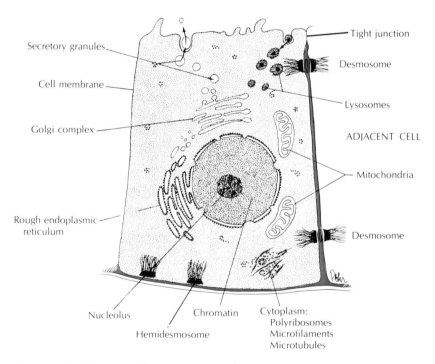

Fig. 2–1. The ultrastructural appearance of a "theoretical cell." The cell membrane and the various organelles inside the cytoplasm are indicated. Some of these organelles are involved in synthetic activities (rough endoplasmic reticulum, Golgi complex), some in digestive activities (lysosomes), and others in energy generation (mitochondria). The cell may be attached to neighboring cells by one or several types of cell junctions. Desmosomes and a tight junction are illustrated in this diagram. The cell is attached to a noncellular surface by hemidesmosomes.

Table 2–1. Microscopic Levels of Organization

Object	Size of Object	Limits of Observation	Method of Observation
		_____ 100 μm	The unaided eye
Cell Nucleus	5-100 μm		The light microscope
Mitochondria	.5–5 μm		
Lysosomes	.25–.5 μm (only visible with special stains)		
		.2 μm (200 nm 2000 Å)	
Ribosomes	12–15 nm (120–150 Å)		
Microfilaments	6–7 nm (60–70 Å)		The electron microscope
Microtubules	20–27 nm (200–270 Å)		
Cell membrane	8–10 nm (80–100 Å)		
		1 nm (10 Å)	

1 mm (1 millimeter) = 0.001 m (meter)
1 μm (1 micrometer) = 0.001 mm
1 nm (1 nanometer) = 0.001 μm
1 Å (1 Ångstrom unit) = 0.1 nm (somewhat older unit of measurement)

In routinely stained and fixed specimens, studied with the light microscope, the nucleus, nucleolus and a mass of cytoplasm are visible. The other cellular components may be seen only after special fixation and staining techniques and/or with the electron microscope.

Membranes

In the architecture of a cell, membranes are important structures:

a *cell membrane* surrounds the contents of the cell and significant components of the organelles are membranous as well. These membranes are thin sheets, not commonly visible with the light microscope. They consist of two layers of lipid molecules, into which globular masses of protein are inserted. Different proteins may be found in different parts of a membrane, reflecting the different functions or metabolic activities in the membrane. On the outer surface of a cell membrane, complex carbohydrates may be attached to such proteins, giving the cell a carbohydrate-rich surface coat (Fig. 2–2).

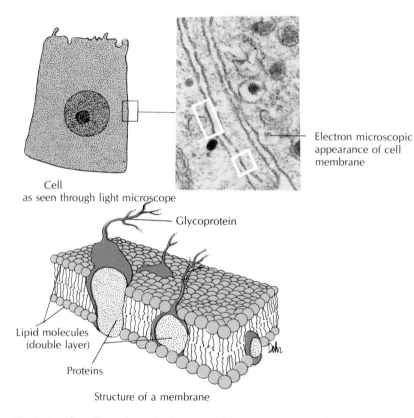

Electron microscopic appearance of cell membrane

Cell
as seen through light microscope

Glycoprotein

Lipid molecules
(double layer)

Proteins

Structure of a membrane

Fig. 2–2. The cell membrane is shown in this figure at several levels of magnification. Light microscopically (upper left) the membrane may not be visible as a separate entity. Electron microscopically (upper right) a cell membrane appears as a complex of two darkly staining lines, running parallel with each other, about 3 nm apart. × 100,000. (Courtesy of Dr. E.A. Nuñez.) The third illustration represents one of the proposed models for the structure of a cell membrane: a double layer of lipid molecules, facing each other. Inserted in these layers are globular protein masses, some of which have glycoproteins, protruding from the outside surface of the membrane.

Cytoskeleton

The cytoskeleton is the fibrillar component of the cytoplasm. It is a three-dimensional structural framework, composed of at least three different groups of delicate structures.

MICROTUBULES. Microtubules are delicate tubes, 20 to 27 nm in diameter. One of their principal functions is the *maintenance of cell shape.* Microtubules also play a role in *cell shape changes,* because they can be rapidly taken apart and reassembled in a different direction. Finally, they appear to participate in the *movements of particles* in a cell, in a manner, that is not yet clearly understood. Microtubules are prominently present in cells undergoing cell division or major alterations in cell shape.

MICROFILAMENTS. Microfilaments are threadlike strands, 6 to 7 nm in diameter. They are composed of *actin.* As will be seen in Chapter 6, this protein is present in large amounts in muscle cells and is involved in the process of *contraction.* Actin filaments interacting with myosin molecules produce contraction.

In non-muscle cells microfilaments are responsible for the contractility of the cell, movements of the cell membrane and movements of the cell as a whole, relative to its environment.

INTERMEDIATE FILAMENTS. These filaments are thicker, threadlike strands, 8 to 10 nm in diameter. The chemical composition of the intermediate filaments varies according to what basic tissue type the cell belongs to. There is at least one unique class of intermediate filaments for each basic tissue type: one for epithelia, one for connective tissues, one for muscle tissue and two for different cells of the nervous tissue.

These filaments probably have a supportive, "skeletal" function inside the cells.

CELL FUNCTIONS

A summary outline of some of the major functions of a cell and the role played by the organelles in these functions will be given in this section. Please remember that, because of the differentiations that led to the development of different tissues and organs, each group of cells has its own distinct appearance, in which certain organelles may be prominent and others barely present. There is no such thing as the "theoretical cell" (Fig. 2–1), in which all organelles are equally well represented.

Synthetic Activities in a Cell

Figure 2–3 is a diagram of the organelles involved in synthetic activities of a cell.

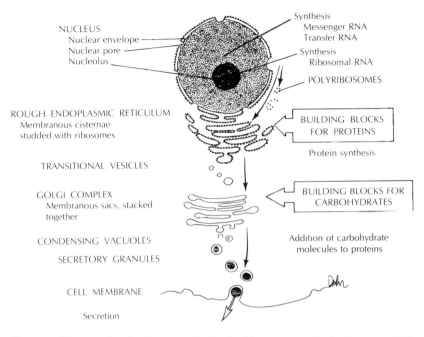

Fig. 2–3. Diagram, showing the organelles involved in protein synthesis. Messenger RNA molecules, copies of short segments of the genetic code, are synthesized in the nucleus and transported into the cytoplasm. There they form a complex with the ribosomes, produced originally in the nucleolus. The ribosomes appear ultrastructurally as darkly staining, small granules. Groups of them, polyribosomes, are scattered in the cytoplasm. These are responsible for the synthesis of proteins, which will be used inside the cell itself. Other ribosomes are attached to the surfaces of the rough endoplasmic reticulum, where they will be responsible for the synthesis of proteins, which will be released outside the cell.

Proteins are assembled into the sacs of the rough endoplasmic reticulum and are transported from there by transitional vesicles to the Golgi complex. Here carbohydrates are assembled and attached to some of the newly synthesized proteins. The product, inside the sacs of the Golgi complex, is then pinched off in small condensing vacuoles and moved in secretory vesicles or granules to the cell membrane. At the cell membrane, the membranes of these vesicles become fused to the cell membrane itself. The product inside the vesicles is then released outside the cell.

NUCLEUS. The nucleus is usually the most readily visible structure inside the cell. In this separate compartment, surrounded by its own membrane, the genetic material of the cell is stored. This material is more acid than the compounds and structures in the cytoplasm, and as a result, the nucleus shows up prominently in stained, histologic sections.

The nucleus serves as the archives of the cell. The genetic material—deoxyribonucleic acid (DNA)—is stored here in long, coiled strands or *chromosomes.* The human nucleus contains 46 chromosomes. They are only visible during cell divisions, when they become tightly coiled. Between divisions the nuclear contents (chromosomes and other materials) are granular and clumped, and they are collectively called *chromatin* (Fig. 2–4, A).

The nucleus is surrounded by a double membrane: the *nuclear envelope.* There are small "openings" in this envelope, which permit selective communication between the contents of the nucleus and the cytoplasmic contents. These "openings" are the nuclear pores.

In the nucleus the following materials are produced: *messenger RNA* (ribonucleic acid), which are copies of short segments of DNA, the genetic code; *transfer RNA,* which are molecules capable of transporting specific amino acid units, the building blocks necessary for protein synthesis. Finally, the *nucleolus,* a small distinct component of the nucleus, produces *ribosomal RNA,* which is one of the structural components of a ribosome.

POLYRIBOSOMES AND ROUGH ENDOPLASMIC RETICULUM. The various RNA structures leave the nucleus and enter the cytoplasm. Ribosomal RNA is organized into distinct structures, the *ribosomes,* which are visible electron microscopically as dark granules. They may be free in the cytoplasm, or attached to an organelle consisting of a connecting membranous system of tubes and flattened sacs (cisternae), the *endoplasmic reticulum* (Fig. 2–4, B).

The endoplasmic reticulum is continuous with the outer membrane of the nuclear envelope, but it is not directly connected with the cell membrane. The presence of ribosomes, studding the outer surfaces of the endoplasmic reticulum membranes, gives it the name *rough* (granular) endoplasmic reticulum. This is in contrast to a *smooth* endoplasmic reticulum, found in some cell types (liver cells, striated muscle cells), the function of which is beyond the scope of this book.

Messenger RNA is somewhat similar to a tape that is run through the ribosomes. During this movement the ribosomes act as read-out units of the genetic code. As each segment of the code is read in sequence, transfer RNA molecules, carrying specific *amino acids* (building blocks of proteins) move to the ribosomal surface. Here the amino acids are released by the transfer RNA and become incorporated in the protein that is assembled on the ribosome. Thus, the sequential read-out of the message of messenger RNA leads to the sequential addition of amino acids to the forming protein.

Protein synthesis takes place both at the polyribosomes and at the surface of the rough endoplasmic reticulum. The *polyribosomes,* a group of ribosomes attached to a strand of messenger RNA, synthesize proteins for use inside the *cell* itself. They include components of organellar membranes and cell membrane.

The ribosomes at the surfaces of the *rough endoplasmic reticulum* assemble proteins destined for incorporation in the cell membrane

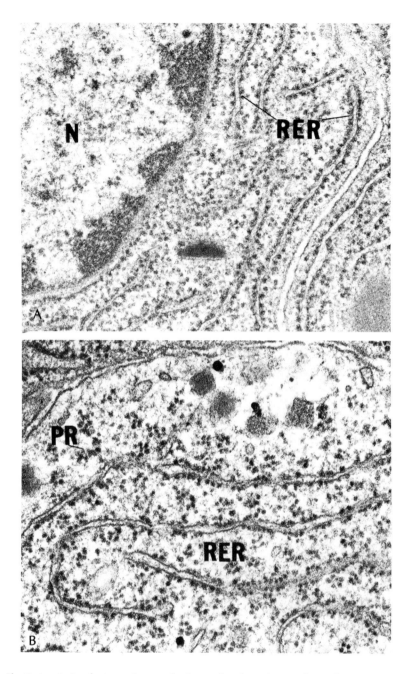

Fig. 2–4. *A,* An electron micrograph of a section through part of a nucleus (N). Darkly staining clumps of chromatin are arranged largely at the periphery of the nucleus. Notice the continuity of the double membrane around the nucleus with the sectioned, flattened sacs of rough endoplasmic reticulum (RER). The dark granules attached to these sacs are ribosomes. × 100,000. (Courtesy Dr. E.A. Nuñez.)

B, Electron micrograph of ribosomes, studding the outside surfaces of the rough endoplasmic reticulum (RER). Some polyribosomes (PR) are visible in the adjacent cytoplasm. × 100,000. (Courtesy Dr. E.A. Nuñez.)

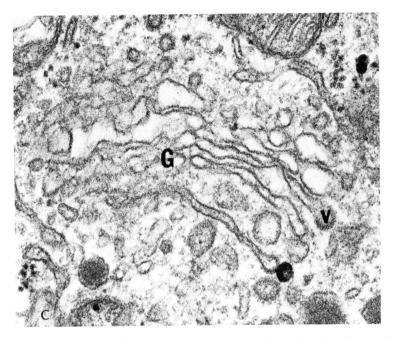

Fig. 2–4. *(Continued)*   C, Electron micrograph of a Golgi complex (G). The complex consists of a series of flattened sacs, stacked together and slightly distended at the edges, where a vesicle can be seen budding off (V). × 120,000. (Courtesy Dr. E.A. Nuñez.)

and, importantly, for export outside the cell. The newly assembled proteins are deposited directly in the internal spaces of the endoplasmic reticulum. The size of the endoplasmic reticulum is positively correlated with the volume of proteins that is synthesized by the cell.

TRANSITIONAL VESICLES. Transitional vesicles are small membranous sacs, filled with the newly formed proteins. They are pinched off from the ribosome-free areas of the rough endoplasmic reticulum and shuttle the proteins to the next organelle, the *Golgi complex.*

GOLGI COMPLEX. The Golgi complex is composed of a stack of curved, flattened membranous sacs (Fig. 2–4, C). It has a central role in organizing the synthetic and digestive activities of the cell, as well as in processing and recycling of membranes of the cellular organelles and membrane-bound vesicles. In the Golgi complex newly formed proteins are concentrated, chemically modified and packaged for export out of the cell or insertion into membranes. Large carbohydrate molecules are synthesized and attached to the proteins here.

From the Golgi complex small membrane-bound vesicles pinch off, forming secretory granules.

SECRETORY GRANULES. These granules attach themselves to the inside of the cell membrane, which then opens up and allows the newly formed proteins and protein-carbohydrate complexes to be discharged outside the cell.

Energy Generation

MITOCHONDRIA. In order to perform all its functions, a cell needs energy. Cells possess their own mobile powerhouses, the *mitochondria* (Fig. 2–5). These are organelles concerned principally with the generation of energy. A mitochondrion has a smooth outer membrane and an inner membrane, folded in pleats (cristae). Between these pleats, and attached to them, are a large number of respiratory enzymes, capable of utilizing oxygen and the final breakdown products of the food we eat (amino acids, glucose and fatty acids), and generating energy in the process.

In addition to having an energy generating function, mitochondria may play a role in the calcification of the hard tissues of the body, by serving as a temporary storage place for the calcium and phosphate ions needed for the formation of the mineral phase of these tissues.

Digestive Activities in a Cell

In order to maintain a tissue, old components constantly have to be removed and replaced by new ones. Similarly, parts of organelles inside a cell have to be replaced regularly. This is called *turnover.* All cells are involved to some degree in the turnover of both *intracellular* (inside the cell) and *extracellular* (outside the cell) components (Fig. 2–6).

The organelle responsible for the breakdown of intracellular and/ or extracellular waste is the *lysosome.* Primary lysosomes are membranous sacs, filled with digestive enzymes. Enzymes are proteinaceous substances that have been produced by a specially differentiated region of the endoplasmic reticulum and transported to a Golgi complex. The lysosomes form by pinching off the Golgi complex. If the membrane of a lysosome is disrupted, its powerful contents, when spilled in the cytoplasm, are quite capable of digesting the cell itself. If the contents of a lysosome are inadvertently released outside the cell, they can cause some tissue damage.

Lysosomes generally function inside the cell. When extracellular material must be broken down, it is engulfed by the cell membrane in a process called *phagocytosis,* and a membranous sac is formed around it. Intracellular material is surrounded directly by a membrane.

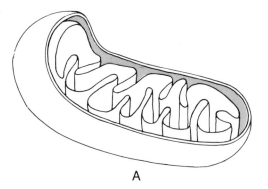

A

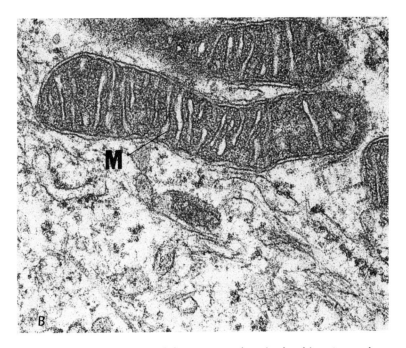

Fig. 2–5. *A,* Simplified diagram of the structure of a mitochondrion. A smooth outer membrane surrounds an inner membrane, which is thrown into folds. Part of the mitochondrion has been cut away to reveal its internal structure. *B,* An electron micrograph of a sectioned mitochondrion (M) reveals the outer membrane and the folds of the inner membrane. Between these folds the dark granular contents of the mitochondrion are visible. The contents include enzymes, attached to the surfaces of the inner membrane, DNA and RNA strands. × 80,000. (Courtesy Dr. E.A. Nuñez.)

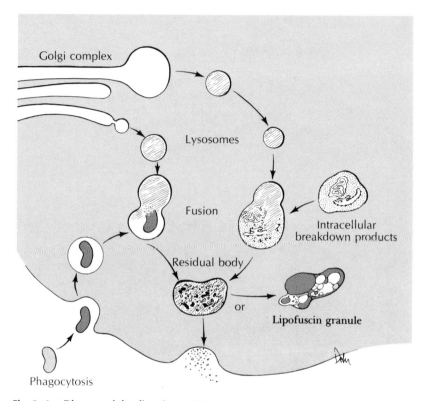

Fig. 2–6. Diagram of the digestive activities of a cell. Lysosomes, containing enzymes, are pinched off from the Golgi complex. Extracellular materials are engulfed by the cell (phagocytosis) and surrounded by a vesicle consisting of a piece of pinched off cell membrane. Intracellular materials, which must be broken down, are surrounded directly by a membrane. Both types of membranous vesicles fuse with lysosomes. The lysosomal enzymes break down the materials inside the fused membranous sac. After the completion of the breakdown process, this membranous sac, now a residual body, may release its contents outside the cell or it may be retained as a lipofuscin granule inside the cell.

These membranous sacs or vacuoles fuse with the primary lysosomes, forming *secondary lysosomes,* and their contents mix with the lysosomal enzymes. The enzymes proceed to digest the contents. The vacuole with the digested material becomes a *residual body,* which may either discharge the digested materials outside the cell or become a remnant (lipofuscin granule) inside the cell. Many such remnants are found in older cells.

While all cells are capable of *some* digestive activity, some cells become particularly specialized in digestion. Among these are *macrophages* (Chap. 4) and *osteoclasts* (Chap. 5).

CELL JUNCTIONS

Because cells in the human body generally are *not* isolated units, but elements of a tissue, junctions between adjacent cells are commonly found. Various types of junctions have been identified. Their structure depends on the function they have to perform.

DESMOSOMES. Desmosomes are patch-like attachments between neighboring cells (Fig. 2–7). They provide purely *mechanical* attachments and might be compared with a pair of suction cups, stuck together. In these attachments the cell membranes of two adjacent cells come closer, but not completely, together. The distance

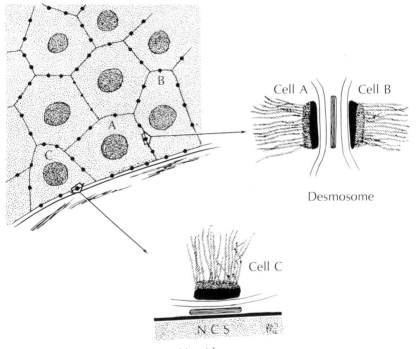

Fig. 2–7. **Desmosomes and hemidesmosomes provide mechanical attachments between neighboring cells and between cells and noncellular surfaces. In this diagram several cells of an epithelium are illustrated. The dots between these cells represent desmosomes. One such desmosome (between cells A and B) is enlarged to show ultrastructural detail. Each cell membrane is represented by two dark, parallel lines. In a desmosome, these membranes come so close together that their glycoprotein-rich surface coats touch, forming a dense line, midway between the two cell membranes. Tonofibrils loop in and out of the attachment plaques, adjacent to the cell membranes. A hemidesmosome is a mechanical attachment between a cell (C) and a noncellular surface (NCS). In such junctions only one cell membrane is present, its glycoprotein-rich coat compressed into a dense line midway in the space between the cell and the noncellular surface. Tonofibrils loop in and out of the attachment plaque adjacent to the cell membrane.**

between the two membranes in these junctions is 15 to 20 nm. The carbohydrate-rich surface coats of the membranes may touch each other in the middle of this space, producing a thin, dense adhesion line when viewed with the electron microscope. The cytoplasm near the cell membranes in the areas of the desmosomes is composed of a dense feltwork of filaments, forming an attachment plaque. Tonofibrils (bundles of intermediate filaments) form hairpin loops in these plaques. The tonofibrils do *not cross over* from one cell to the next. Desmosomes probably are attachment sites, not only *externally,* for adjacent cells, but also *internally* for the supportive intermediate filaments inside these cells.

HEMIDESMOSOMES. Desmosomes are attachments formed by *two* neighboring cells. Certain cells, facing a *noncellular* surface, may form attachments against such a surface. Since this surface itself cannot produce the other half of the attachment, only one half of a desmosome, or a *hemidesmosome,* results. Compare the structure of such a half-attachment with that of a desmosome (Fig. 2–7).

TIGHT JUNCTIONS. Tight junctions are junctions between adjacent cells, in which the membranes of these cells are actually *fused* together, leaving no space between the cells (Fig. 2–8). Such junctions constitute barriers against (extracellular) movement of ions and molecules through the areas between the cells. Tight junctions are therefore found in areas where a *seal* is required. In order to be an effective seal, a tight junction is not just a round patch like a desmosome, but a belt going along the entire circumference of a cell. Such junctions are present frequently in transporting epithelia, where the integrity of the epithelial lining is essential, as in the ducts of the salivary glands.

GAP JUNCTIONS. Gap junctions are patch-like junctions where cell membranes of adjacent cells come close together. In such junctions the space between adjacent membranes is only 2 nm wide (Fig. 2–8). Small tubular channels run through both cell membranes inside this junction. Through these channels free exchange of small molecules is possible between the cytoplasmic components of the adjacent cells. A low resistance to ion flow (electric coupling) exists as well in these junctions. This allows for communication between the cells and for coordination of their activities. Such communication is essential in certain stages of embryologic development and during activities that require coordination of many cells, such as smooth muscle contractions.

CELL DIVISION (MITOSIS)

In an individual organism cell division or *mitosis* is necessary to *increase* the numbers of cells during growth, and to *replace* dying cells during and after growth.

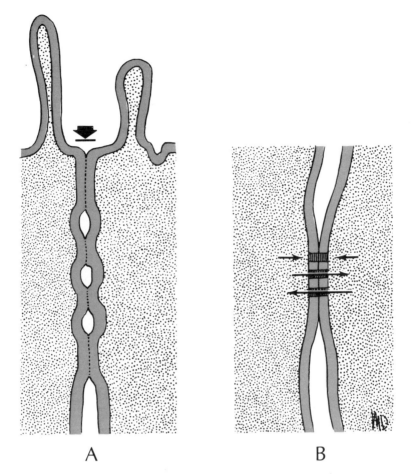

A   B

Fig. 2–8.   A, Diagram of a tight junction. The cell membranes of two adjacent cells (each illustrated by a grey band) are fused together in several places. Such a junction runs all around the circumference of a cell, in belt-like fashion, providing an effective seal. Thus, it prevents the movement of any substance, in the direction of the arrow, into the intercellular spaces. B, Diagram of a gap junction. In this type of junction, the two cell membranes come very close together, without fusing. Several channels (gaps) through both cell membranes provide passageways for free transport of small molecules and ion flow in the directions of the arrows.

During mitosis a duplication of all cell structures must occur (Fig. 2–9). The most critical duplication is that of the structures in the nucleus. As stated before, the nucleus contains the genetic material, stored in 46 chromosomes. All cells with nuclei have the same basic information in their chromosomes. An exact duplication of these structures is necessary to give the two resulting daughter cells at the end of the mitosis the identical genetic material.

During mitosis the chromosomes become visible and move toward

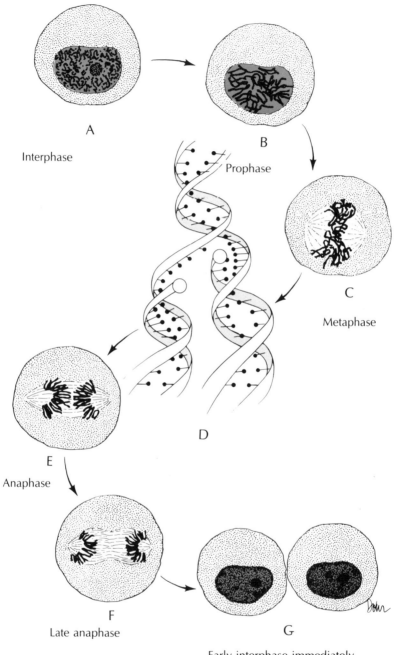

A

Interphase

B

Prophase

C

Metaphase

D

E

Anaphase

F

Late anaphase

G

Early interphase immediately
after telophase

the equatorial plane of the nucleus. The nuclear envelope disappears. Each chromosome consists of two strands of DNA, twisted around each other. During chromosome duplication, which takes place next, the two strands slowly separate. Each strand builds an exact replica of the other strand. We now have two identical chromosomes. One is pulled toward one nuclear pole, the other is pulled toward the opposite pole.

This same process occurs simultaneously in all 46 chromosomes. While the chromosomes are duplicating, in the equatorial plane, a spindle-shaped structure of microtubules is formed. The duplicated chromosomes move apart to the opposite nuclear poles *along* the microtubules. As the cytoplasm undergoes division, two new nuclear envelopes are formed, each enclosing 46 chromosomes.

FINAL NOTE

The ultrastructural information supplied in this chapter has been adapted as much as possible to the needs of the following chapters. As you study those chapters, continue to review this material, wherever reference is made to it.

The primary objective of this textbook is to provide an understanding of the dental and oral tissues at a level that is *clinically useful.* We will refer to ultrastructural aspects of these tissues only when they appear to contribute to a better understanding of the material. Emphatically, this text does not attempt to provide a comprehensive ultrastructural description of the dental and oral tissues.

Fig. 2–9. Diagrammatic illustration of the changes in the appearance of a cell during cell division. *A,* Between cell divisions no chromosomes are visible in the nucleus of a cell. Some diffuse chromatin and a nucleolus are shown. *B,* At the beginning of a cell division the chromosomes become very tightly coiled and may be seen as strands in the nucleus. *C,* All chromosomes (dark lines) move to the equatorial plane of the nucleus. A spindle-shaped arrangement of microtubules appears (light lines). The nuclear membrane disappears. *D,* In the equatorial plane, the two strands of DNA, present in each chromosome, become separated. On each separate DNA strand, a duplicate copy of the second strand is formed. In the illustration, the growing ends of the duplicate strands are at the two points marked with an open circle. All chromosomes are duplicated in this way. *E,* One of each of all duplicated sets of chromosomes is now pulled along the microtubular frame in opposite directions. *F,* In this stage, 46 chromosomes are present at each of the 2 opposite poles of the microtubular spindle. *G,* The spindle disappears. Both groups of chromosomes are surrounded by a nuclear membrane. Once the two nuclei are thus formed, the cytoplasm undergoes division and two "daughter cells" are formed, essentially similar to the original "mother cell."

SELECTED READING LIST

Allison, A.: Lysosomes and disease. Sci. Am., *217:*62, 1967.

Capaldi, R.A.: A dynamic model of cell membranes. Sci. Am., *230:*26, 1974.

DeDuve, C., and Wattiaux, R.: Function of lysosomes. Ann. Rev. Physiol., *28:*435, 1966.

Fawcett, D.W.: *The Cell.* 2nd Ed. Philadelphia, W.B. Saunders Co., 1981.

Fawcett, D.W.: *Bloom and Fawcett: A Textbook of Histology.* 11th Ed. Philadelphia, W.B. Saunders Co., 1986.

Francke, W.W.: Structure, biochemistry, and functions of the nuclear envelope. Int. Rev. Cytol., *Suppl.4:*72, 1974.

Goodenough, D.A., and Revel, J.P.: A fine structural analysis of intercellular junctions in the mouse liver. J. Cell. Biol., *45:*272, 1970.

Holtzman, E., and Novikoff, A.B.: *Cells and Organelles.* 2nd Ed. New York, Holt, Rinehart and Winston, 1976.

Hopkins, C.R.: *Structure and Function of Cells.* Philadelphia, W.B. Saunders Co., 1978.

Lazarides, E.: Intermediate filaments as mechanical integrators of cellular space. Nature, *283:*249, 1980.

Lentz, T.: *Cell Fine Structure. An Atlas of Drawings of Whole Cell Structure.* Philadelphia, W.B. Saunders Co., 1971.

Mazia, D.: The cell cycle. Sci. Am., *230:*54, 1974.

Nagle, R.B.: Intermediate filaments: a review of the basic biology. Am. J. Surg. Pathol., *23(Suppl. 1):*4, 1988.

Neutra, M., and Leblond, C.P.: The Golgi apparatus. Sci. Am., *220:*100, 1969.

Olmsted, J.B., and Borisy, G.B.: Microtubules. Ann. Rev. Biochem., *42:*507, 1973.

Peracchia, C.: Gap junction structure and function. Trends Biochem. Sci., Feb., 1977.

Porter, K.R., and Bonneville, M.A.: *Fine Structure of Cells and Tissues.* 4th Ed. Philadelphia, Lea & Febiger, 1973.

Singer, S.J.: Molecular organization of membranes. Ann. Rev. Biochem., *43:*805, 1974.

Singer, S.J., and Nicolson, G.L.: The fluid mosaic model of the structure of cell membranes. Science, *175:*720, 1972.

Whaley, W.G.: *The Golgi Apparatus.* New York, Springer-Verlag, 1975.

3

Oral Mucosa—Epithelium

In Chapter 1 we found that there are variations in appearance, structure, and texture of the various parts of the oral cavity. We shall now study more precisely the appearance of the *lining* of the oral cavity, the *oral mucosa.*

Inspect, once more, the area of the oral vestibule by gently pulling the lower lip downward and forward. Compare your observations with the structures indicated in Figure 3–1. Using this figure as a guide, locate the following in your own mouth: *interdental papillae,* bulges of oral mucosa between adjacent teeth; *free gingiva,* a strip about 1.5 mm wide along the free edge of the gingiva; *free gingival line,* the borderline between free and attached gingiva; *attached gingiva,* the gingiva directly overlying the bone of the jaw; *mucogingival line,* the borderline between attached gingiva and alveolar mucosa; *alveolar mucosa,* the mucosa covering the floor of the vestibule; and *labial mucosa,* the mucosa covering the inside of the lip.

Compare the color and texture of the *attached gingiva* with those of the *alveolar* and *labial mucosae.* Which is redder? Which looks moister? Notice the relatively sharp lines between free and attached gingivae (the *free gingival line)* and between attached gingiva and alveolar mucosa (the *mucogingival line).*

Now, move the lip gently up and down and see to what extent the mucosa may be moved.

Ideally, you should have noticed that the *attached gingiva* is generally lighter and pinker in color than the *alveolar* and *labial mucosae.* If the gingiva is healthy, it may have a slightly pitted, "orange peel" appearance. The alveolar and labial mucosae look somewhat moister than the gingiva. When the lip is pulled, the alveolar and labial mucosae are moved along, but the motion stops at the mucogingival line.

The attached gingiva is strongly tied to the underlying tissue—the bone of the jaw. It is difficult to compress the attached gingiva and it cannot be shifted from left to right or up and down, relative to the underlying bony structures. On the other hand, the labial mucosa

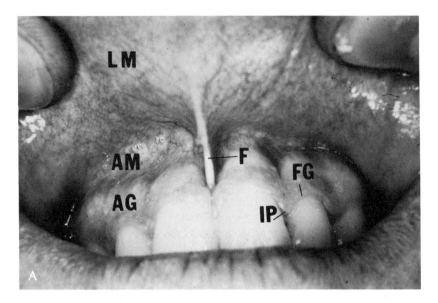

Fig. 3–1. Part of the oral vestibule is shown in this photograph. The upper front teeth and a frenulum (F) are prominently visible. IP = interdental papilla; FG = free gingiva; AG = attached gingiva; AM = alveolar mucosa; LM = labial mucosa. (Courtesy Dr. E.V. Zegarelli.)

may be compressed readily. When released it jumps back. The labial mucosa may be easily shifted back and forth over the underlying tissues, that is, muscles and salivary glands.

You have just seen good examples of two types of oral mucosa—the attached gingiva is an example of *masticatory mucosa;* labial and alveolar mucosae both are examples of *lining mucosa.*

Actually, we distinguish *three* types of mucosae in the oral cavity (Fig. 3–2): (1) *lining mucosa,* the lining of lips, cheeks, soft palate and sublingual area; (2) *masticatory mucosa,* the lining of attached gingiva and of hard palate; and (3) *specialized mucosa,* the lining of the top surface of the tongue, which carries specialized papillae, some with *taste buds.*

Clinically, the distinction between lining and masticatory mucosae is important. Let us illustrate this with the following exercise.

Place your fingers in the oral vestibule, between upper jaw and upper lip. Now, with the finger in place, vigorously move the lip in all directions. You will notice that the only stable region is that of the attached gingiva. Repeat this exercise by placing your finger against the inner surface of the lower jaw, behind the incisors. With the finger in place, move the tongue in all directions. Again, you will find that the only stable region is that of the attached gingiva. Select as many areas of the oral cavity as possible, to repeat this

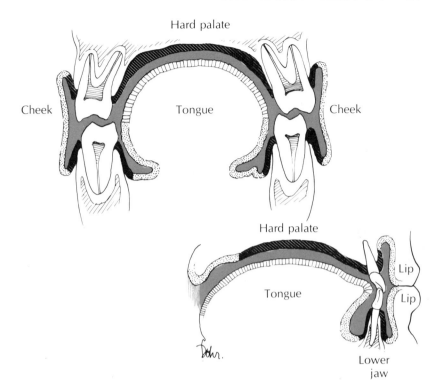

Fig. 3–2. Two diagrams showing the distribution of the three types of mucosa in the oral cavity. The top figure represents a section from side to side through the tissues of the mouth, while the bottom figure illustrates a midline section from back to front. The stippled areas are covered with lining mucosa. The darkly hatched areas are covered with masticatory mucosa. The top of the tongue is covered with specialized mucosa.

exercise. You will find that only the *attached gingivae* and the *lining of the hard palate,* the areas covered with *masticatory mucosa,* are stable.

A full denture, or any other prosthetic device, which rests on an area of oral mucosa, needs a stable surface for optimal functioning. A successful denture therefore, should not only fit well, it should also be supported exclusively by masticatory mucosa. If it does extend further, onto areas of lining mucosa, it will become unseated during the movements of the soft tissues. This distinction is so important that in the first impression taken for the construction of a prosthesis, the lines separating lining and masticatory mucosae are indicated as a guide for subsequent procedures.

GENERAL STRUCTURE OF THE ORAL MUCOSA

The oral mucosa consists of *two basic tissues—epithelium* superficially and an underlying, supporting layer of *connective tissue.*

A cut through the thickness of the oral mucosa reveals structural features that are in many ways similar to those of the skin (Fig. 3–3):

1. The superficial layer of the oral mucosa is the *oral epithelium.* In the skin it is the *epidermis* (epithelium).

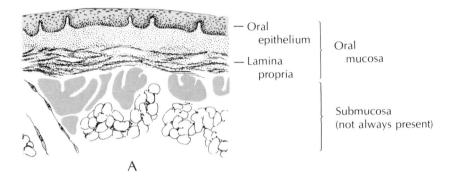

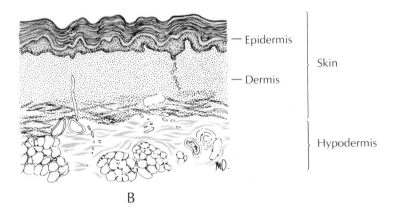

Fig. 3–3.   In these two diagrams, a comparison is made between the appearances of sections through oral mucosa (A) and skin (B). The oral epithelium and the epidermis are the superficial epithelial layers. The lamina propria and the dermis are the highly organized connective tissue layers underneath the epithelial layers. The submucosa (not always present) and the hypodermis are somewhat more loosely organized connective tissue layers, located between oral mucosa or skin and the underlying tissues (muscles, bones).

2. The supporting connective tissue layer in the oral mucosa is the *lamina propria:* in the skin it is the *dermis.*

3. Underneath the oral mucosa in some areas a *submucosa* (connective tissue) is found; comparable to the *hypodermis* underneath the skin.

Despite a general structural similarity, a major functional difference between skin and oral mucosa is that the skin has great significance in the protection against loss of tissue fluids and in the maintenance of body temperature, while the oral mucosa has mainly a role in mechanical protection. Further, skin and oral mucosa have some uniquely different specializations, such as hairs, nails and sweat glands in the skin; salivary glands and tonsillar tissues in the oral mucosa.

The oral epithelium forms a mechanical barrier, protecting the underlying tissues. The connective tissue provides mechanical support, because of its structural density and arrangement, but it also carries the vital supply systems to the region: the blood vessels and nerves.

While a more complete listing of the *regional differences* between lining, masticatory and specialized mucosae may be found at the end of Chapter 4, we should note here the *principal characteristics* of each of these oral mucosa types (Fig. 3–4). Specific details of the tissues listed in this brief outline, will then follow.

LINING MUCOSA. The epithelial layer of this type of mucosa usually consists of *nonkeratinized,* stratified squamous epithelium (this Chapter). The interface between epithelium and connective tissue is gently undulated. Relatively few, short and broad connective tissue extensions *(papillae)* project into the epithelial layer. A lining mucosa is generally compressible and moveable, relative to the underlying tissue, a characteristic that is due to the presence of a *submucosa* between lamina propria and that underlying tissue (usually muscle tissue).

MASTICATORY MUCOSA. The epithelial layer of this type of mucosa usually consists of *keratinized* stratified squamous epithelium. The interface between epithelium and connective tissue is strongly interdigitated: many tall, narrow connective tissue papillae project into the epithelium. Alternating with these are usually as many tall, thin epithelial extensions *(rete pegs),* projecting into the underlying connective tissue. A submucosa is usually absent. The lamina propria is tied strongly and directly to the underlying tissue (generally bone). A masticatory mucosa is largely resistant to compression and immoveable, relative to the underlying tissue. This is a mechanically strong lining, capable of withstanding masticatory loading.

SPECIALIZED MUCOSA. This type of mucosa is found on

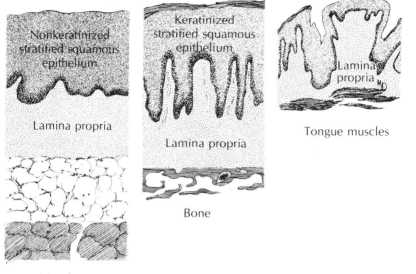

LINING MUCOSA   MASTICATORY MUCOSA   SPECIALIZED MUCOSA

Fig. 3–4. Diagram of the general characteristics of the three types of oral mucosae. Highlighted are the differences in epithelial thickness, degree of epithelial keratinization, thickness of lamina propria, shapes of connective tissue papillae and presence or absence of a submucosa.

the top surface of the tongue *only*, and it forms distinct specializations: *lingual papillae*, some of which carry *taste buds.* The connective tissue forms the cores of these extensive and specialized lingual papillae. The overlying stratified squamous epithelium varies in thickness and in degree of keratinization. There is *no* submucosa; the specialized mucosa is tied directly to the underlying muscles of the tongue. This makes the specialized mucosa immoveable relative to these muscles and allows it to conform precisely to the muscle movements. The three different types of oral mucosa are illustrated schematically in their most general form in Figure 3–4.

EPITHELIUM

Despite the existence of many different types of epithelium, all types have in common the following characteristic: epithelium consists of a layer of cells in close contact with each other over a large part of their cell surfaces, with little intercellular space.

Epithelia may be *classified* according to their *function* as (1) a protective barrier (examples: epidermis, oral epithelium), (2) a group of secretory cells (example: epithelium of salivary glands), (3) a group of resorbing cells (example: gut epithelium), and (4) a group of cells with special sensory function (example: taste cells).

Another, more frequently used classification of epithelia is based on two *morphologic characteristics:*

1. The *shapes* of the *most superficial cells* of an epithelium. We distinguish 3 shapes (Fig. 3–5): flat *(squamous),* cuboidal, and columnar.

2. The *number of cell layers* in an epithelium. An epithelium may consist of *one* cell layer (a *simple* epithelium) or of *several* cell layers (a *stratified* epithelium).

Using combinations of these distinguishing morphologic characteristics, six different types of epithelium may be described: simple squamous, simple cuboidal, simple columnar, stratified squamous, stratified cuboidal and stratified columnar. Add to these combinations some intermediate forms, as well as some surface specializations, and you will have some appreciation of the variations in epithelial tissues. The various differences in epithelial cells are related to their different functions in different locations of the body.

ORAL EPITHELIUM

Oral epithelium of the oral mucosa and epidermis of the skin are examples of *stratified squamous epithelia.*

The main functions of such epithelia are *protective.* They form protective barriers against mechanical insults, bacterial invasions and, in the case of the epidermis, loss of tissue fluids.

Stratified squamous epithelia consist of constantly renewing cell populations. Under normal conditions the rate of cell loss from the superficial layers of the epithelia matches the rate of new cell production by mitosis in the deepest layers of these epithelia. In the process of aging each cell moves slowly up from the deepest *(basal)* layer to the more superficial layers, where it finally becomes detached. Thus, in a certain time span, an epithelium may be entirely replaced by a new cell generation. This time span, or *turnover time,* has been studied for some regions of the human epidermis and oral epithelium. Turnover times in the epidermis range from 12 to 75 days. Turnover times for the oral epithelium of the cheek (buccal epithelium) range from 5 to 16 days. The turnover times for the epithelium of the hard palate and the sublingual epithelium are slightly longer, but still shorter than for the epidermis.

Since the superficial cells of the oral epithelium are readily detached, it is relatively simple to remove some of them from your own mouth and study them with the light microscope (see Appendix 1 for instructions on the use of the microscope).

Move the tip of your tongue or a cotton swab over the inside of

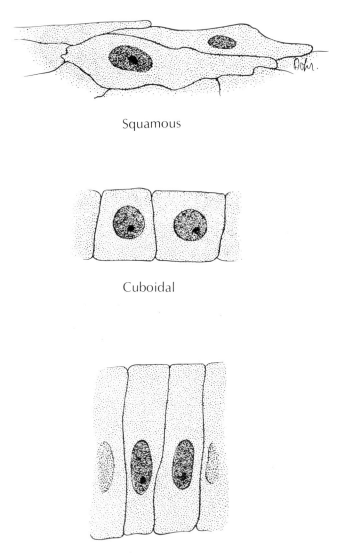

Squamous

Cuboidal

Columnar

Fig. 3–5. Principal morphologic characteristics of epithelial cells: squamous cells (flat), cuboidal cells and columnar cells. While the cuboidal and columnar cells are shown here in one cell layer (simple epithelium), the squamous cells are illustrated in an arrangement of several cell layers, stacked together (stratified epithelium).

your cheek. Then touch the center of a glass slide *lightly* with tongue tip or cotton swab. Place an even smaller and thinner glass cover *(cover glass)* over the area of the glass slide you just touched. The preparation is now ready for study under the microscope. For better visibility of the structures you want to study under the microscope, the area with the material from the oral cavity may be stained with a histologic dye, such as methylene blue.

Under the microscope, your preparation will show several flattened structures. These are detached superficial cells from the oral epithelium. These cells are predominantly flat and pancake-shaped and have given the epithelium its classification: *squamous.* The cells clearly show how closely they have been compressed against their neighboring cells prior to being moved to your glass slide. They actually have little depressions on their surfaces. If the cells are properly stained, you may see an ovoid to rounded nucleus, roughly in the center of the cells, and variable numbers of bacteria, visible as tiny, darkly stained dots, on the cell surfaces. The latter are members of the normal bacterial population of the mouth. In addition, you may see inside the cells dark, rounded structures, that are smaller than the nucleus, but several times larger than the bacteria. These are *keratohyaline granules* (see: parakeratinized epithelium) (Fig. 3–6).

Depending on their location, stratified squamous epithelia may or may not become cornified *(keratinized)* in their superficial layers. We distinguish three forms of stratified squamous epithelia.

1. (Ortho)*keratinized* stratified squamous epithelium. This is found in the skin and in some parts of the masticatory and specialized mucosae. The keratinization is effective for mechanical protection, but it acts especially to provide a barrier against fluid loss. If present in the oral cavity, this type of stratified squamous epithelium is the *least* frequently found of these three.

2. *Nonkeratinized* stratified squamous epithelium. This is found in the mouth, in most areas of the lining mucosa. It acts as a cushion, protecting against mechanical damage, and as a selective barrier.

3. *Parakeratinized* stratified squamous epithelium. This is an intermediate form between orthokeratinized and nonkeratinized epithelia. It is found in the mouth: in most of the masticatory mucosa and in some of the specialized mucosa.

Layers in Stratified Squamous Epithelia

As stated previously, cell divisions occur in the basal layers of the stratified squamous epithelia, while the cells in the superficial layers become detached and are lost. On its journey from the basal layer to the most superficial layer, an epithelial cell undergoes definite

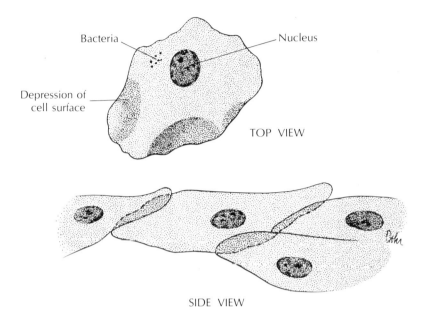

Fig. 3–6. Diagram of the appearance of a nonkeratinized, squamous epithelial cell, following its removal from the oral cavity and the histologic preparation, described in the text. In the flat, pancake-shaped cell a nucleus is usually visible as are occasionally some bacteria on the cell surface. Where the cell was compressed against neighboring epithelial cells, depressions of the cell surface are present. The bottom diagram illustrates how several epithelial cells may be pressed together to create such depressions on their surfaces.

maturational changes, and since all its neighbors at the same vertical level undergo the same changes, there are morphologically distinct zones or *layers* in a stratified squamous epithelium. These layers, in order are (Fig. 3–7):

BASAL LAYER (deepest). This layer consists of one single cell layer. The cells are cuboidal in shape. The primary role of this layer is cell division and thus epithelial renewal.

PRICKLE CELL LAYER. The prickle cell layer is several cell layers thick. This name is given because the cells in it, which are polygonal in shape, have a "spiky" appearance. This appearance is the result of the histologic fixation, which frequently causes shrinkage of the cells.

A cell may shrink in all areas where junctions with neighboring cells are absent. However, where cell junctions (desmosomes) are present, the cell membranes are prevented from pulling away during cell shrinkage. At those sites spikes are formed. The primary role of the cells in this layer is to form attachments with their neighbors and thus preserve the structural integrity of the epithelium.

In the three different types of stratified squamous epithelia, the

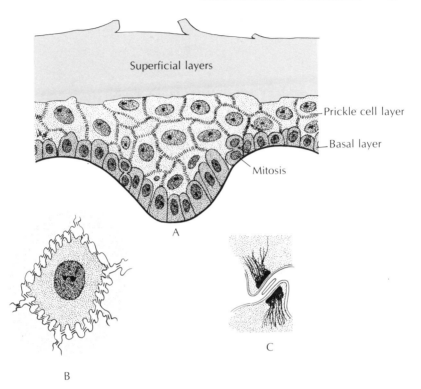

Fig. 3–7. *A,* Histologic appearance of the deeper layers of the three types of stratified squamous epithelia. Thicknesses of such layers may vary locally, but generally both are present. The superficial layers, which are different in the three types of epithelia, have been left blank in this diagram. The basal layer is the deepest layer, adjacent to the connective tissue. These cells stain darkly and undergo continued mitoses. Some mitoses are indicated here. The prickle cell layer, above the basal layer, consists of polygonal cells. *B,* A single cell of the prickle cell layer is shown. The spikes on the cell surface make contact with similar spikes on the neighboring cell surfaces. These contacts consist of desmosomes, one of which is illustrated in *C.* The desmosomes themselves are not visible with the light microscope, but the spikes, produced by fixation shrinkage, indicate the desmosome locations.

two layers just described are always present. They account for about one half to two thirds of the total epithelial thickness, and they have approximately the same appearance in these three types. All three epithelia, furthermore, have a well-developed *internal,* intracellular support system of *tonofibrils,* a cytoskeleton that is suitable for their mechanical functions. These tonofibrils are well organized *bundles* of 10-nm thick intermediate *keratin* filaments. They run inside the cytoplasm of the epithelial cells and attach into the attachment plaques of the desmosomes.

In their more *superficial* layers, the three forms of stratified squamous epithelia exhibit a distinctly *different* appearance, which will be described next.

Orthokeratinized Epithelium

This type of epithelium (Fig. 3–8) consists of a basal layer (deepest), a prickle cell layer, a granular layer and a keratinized layer.

GRANULAR LAYER. The granular layer is located superficial to the prickle cell layer. This layer is usually two to four cell layers thick. The epithelial cells are flattened in shape and are filled with darkly staining *keratohyaline granules.* These granules consist of a chemical precursor of *keratin.* The most superficial cells in this layer contain the largest concentrations of keratohyaline granules. The nuclei in those cells are somewhat flat and dark, showing signs of degeneration. The cells in the granular layer also contain vesicles, called *lamellar granules,* whose lipid contents are released in the intercellular spaces, where they help form a water-tight barrier (remember that protection against loss of tissue fluids is one of the functions of a keratinized stratified squamous epithelium).

KERATINIZED LAYER. This layer is the superficial layer. Functionally, it is the principal barrier layer. There is an abrupt transition between the preceding granular layer and this layer.

The *cells* in the keratinized layer have the shapes of flattened discs or *squames.* They are responsible for the name of this type of epithelium. The cells are no longer vital. *No nuclei* are present and most other organelles have been broken down by lysosomal action as well. The contents of the keratohyaline granules have formed a complex

---

Fig. 3–8. *A,* Diagram of the characteristic superficial layers in the orthokeratinized, stratified squamous epithelium. No detail is shown in the basal and prickle cell layers, which have been illustrated in Figure 3–7. The cells of the granular layer are flattened. As they move more superficially, they are filled gradually with keratohyaline granules. These darkly staining granules are responsible for the name of this layer. The superficialmost cells in this layer contain most granules. The keratinized layer is the most superficial layer of this type of epithelium. It consists of very flat cells, which have lost their organelles. Light microscopically, no nuclei are visible in this layer. These nonvital cells are completely filled with keratin. The top cells of the keratinized layer are detached and lost. The bottom drawing is an enlarged detail, showing one cell from the granular layer and one cell from the keratinized layer. The transition between these 2 layers is as abrupt as the illustration shows. *B,* Histologic section of epidermis from a human fingertip. The various layers of keratinized, stratified squamous epithelium are illustrated. B = basal cell layer; P = prickle cell layer; G = granular layer; K = keratinized layer. Original magnification × 100.

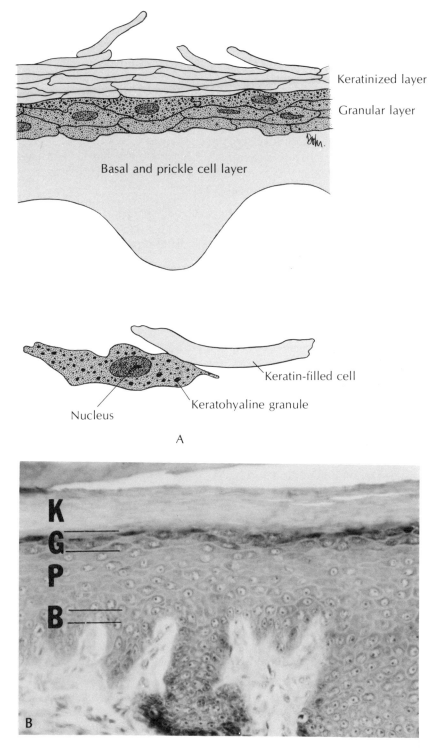

Keratinized layer

Granular layer

Basal and prickle cell layer

Keratin-filled cell

Keratohyaline granule

Nucleus

A

K

G

P

B

B

with the tonofibrils. This complex, *keratin,* now fills the cells in this layer. The superficial-most cells become detached and are lost.

The *intercellular spaces* between these keratin squames are filled with lipid (from the lamellar granules). The keratinized layer resembles a brick wall, in which the keratin squames resemble the bricks and the intercellular lipid the mortar.

The thickness of this type of epithelium is variable. Areas of the body that are not normally subjected to a great deal of wear have a thin epithelium and a thin keratinized layer. Other areas have thicker epithelia. Especially thick epithelia with thick keratinized layers are found on the palm, sole and calluses.

Nonkeratinized Epithelium

The following layers are present in nonkeratinized epithelium (Fig. 3–9): (1) basal layer (deepest) and (2) prickle cell layer.

In this type of epithelium there are no further *distinctly* recognizable layers above the prickle cell layer. These cells undergo a gradual increase in size as they move closer to the surface of the epithelium. Because this increase in size is *not* accompanied by an increase in the number of organelles, the enlarged cells look *emptier.* Fluid-filled sacs, or *vacuoles,* form inside the cells and push the cytoplasm toward the cell periphery. In the largest, most superficial cells the cytoplasm remains only as a thin layer next to the cell membrane. The rest of these cells is filled with fluid.

There are several layers of such fluid-filled cells. They act as cushions and are firmly attached to each other, protecting the underlying tissues against mechanical damage.

Parakeratinized Epithelium

In this form of stratified squamous epithelium keratinization does occur, but with less of the widespread destruction of cellular organelles seen in orthokeratinization (Fig. 3–9, C).

As seen with the light microscope, parakeratinization differs from orthokeratinization in the following:

1. In parakeratinization a granular layer either does *not* form at all or remains indistinct. In either case some small keratohyaline granules may be seen in the cells closest to the keratinized layer.

2. The keratinized layer in parakeratinized epithelium contains cells in which the nuclei still may be visible. Parakeratinized cells are no longer vital, however, and their nuclei are shrunken and degenerated. These cells are gradually detached and lost.

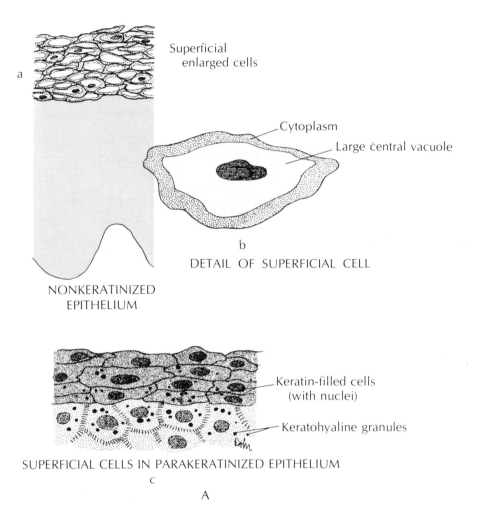

Superficial
enlarged cells

a

Cytoplasm

Large central vacuole

b

DETAIL OF SUPERFICIAL CELL

NONKERATINIZED
EPITHELIUM

Keratin-filled cells
(with nuclei)

Keratohyaline granules

SUPERFICIAL CELLS IN PARAKERATINIZED EPITHELIUM

c

A

Fig. 3–9. *A*, Diagram of a nonkeratinized, stratified squamous epithelium, a. No detail is shown in the basal and prickle cell layers, which have been illustrated in Figure 3–7. The superficial layer in this type of epithelium consists of gradually enlarging cells, with fluid accumulating in a centrally located space or vacuole. The nuclei remain present in these cells. The superficial-most cells are detached readily (see Fig. 3–6). In b, one of the superficial cells is shown. Its cytoplasm has been pushed toward the periphery of the cell, while the central part, fluid-filled in life, looks empty. The bottom diagram, c, shows the superficial layers of a parakeratinized, stratified squamous epithelium. In these layers, the cells are gradually filled with keratin. However, few keratohyaline granules are formed, so that there is no distinct granular layer. In addition, the nuclei and other organelles remain present in the cytoplasm of the keratin-filled superficial-most cells. As in the other types of epithelium, the superficial cells are eventually lost.

(Continued p. 42.)

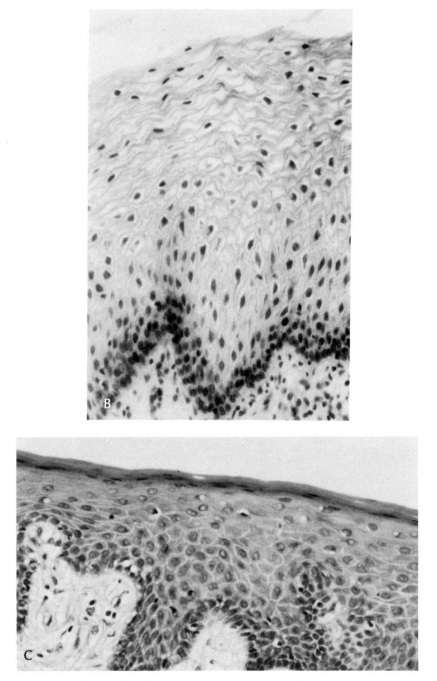

Fig. 3–9. (Continued) B, A thick layer of nonkeratinizing, stratified squamous epithelium from the inside of a human lip, in histologic section. The superficial cells look empty and some have collapsed, owing to the loss of the central fluid during the histologic tissue preparation. Original magnification × 100. C, Parakeratinized, stratified squamous epithelium from human attached gingiva, in histologic section. Compare this photograph with Figure 3–8 B. In this epithelium, no distinct granular layer is present, and the nuclei in the keratinized layer are still visible. Original magnification × 100.

Other Cell Types in Oral Epithelium

In addition to the epithelial cells, already described, the oral epithelium contains several other cell types. These cells have few or no desmosomal attachments to the surrounding epithelial cells. Following fixation, they shrink away from the surrounding cells and leave an empty, clear space around them.

NON-EPITHELIAL RESIDENT CELLS. There are three types of non-epithelial cells that normally reside and perpetuate themselves in the oral epithelial, and epidermal, territories. These are: melanocytes, Langerhans cells and Merkel cells.

Among these, the *melanocytes* are most conspicuous. They are located in the basal layers of the epithelium, where they comprise approximately one-seventh of the total basal cell population. Some may be found in the underlying connective tissue. These cells have long extensions protruding between the surrounding epithelial cells (Fig. 3–10). They are responsible for the production of pigment, *melanin.* Melanin is stored in the cell in the form of specific granules. These granules, visible with the light microscope as intracellular brown dots, are transferred from the melanocytes to the basal epi-

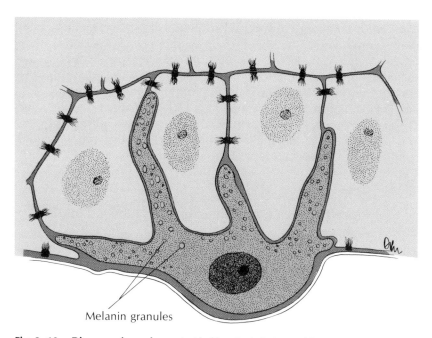

Melanin granules

Fig. 3–10. Diagram of a melanocyte (darkly stippled), located between the basal cells of oral epithelium. Few or no desmosomes are present between these two different cell types. Melanin granules, produced by the melanocytes, are visible in the cytoplasm of these cells and are responsible for the pigmentation of the epithelium.

thelial cells.' In the more superficial epithelial layers the melanin granules are broken down by lysosomal action.

The presence of melanin in the basal layers of oral epithelium and epidermis is responsible for the brown color component of oral mucosa and skin. The difference in intensity of brown skin color between different racial groups is *not* due to a difference in the number of melanocytes, but to a difference in the *rate of melanin production,* the *size of the pigment granules* and the *length of time of their preservation.*

If clinically visible pigmentation is present in the oral cavity, it is found most frequently in the attached gingiva, the lips, the buccal mucosa and the soft palate. Pigmentation in the oral cavity does not *necessarily* coincide with pigmentation of the skin.

Langerhans cells are located in the more superficial layers of the epithelium. They resemble the melanocytes in shape, but functionally and developmentally they are an altogether different group of cells. They have specific immune receptors on their cell membranes, and as antigen-presenting cells they are part of the body's immune defense system.

Merkel cells are cells that are associated with nerve terminals inside the epithelium. They are usually located in the basal layer. Unlike the melanocytes and the Langerhans cells, Merkel cells are descendants of highly specialized epithelial cells. They do have some desmosomal connections with their neighbors.

INFLAMMATORY CELLS. Certain cell types, commonly associated with inflammation, may transiently "immigrate" into the oral epithelium. This immigrant population includes lymphocytes, monocytes, neutrophilic granulocytes and, occasionally, mast cells. These cells do *not* commonly live and perpetuate themselves in the oral epithelium, as do the epithelial cells and the non-epithelial resident cells. These cell types will be discussed further in Chapters 4 and 6.

Interface Between Oral Epithelium and Lamina Propria

The interface between the oral epithelium and the underlying connective tissue is not smooth and straight, but corrugated. Where the two tissue types interdigitate, the epithelial extensions are called (epithelial) *rete pegs* and the connective tissue extensions *connective tissue papillae* (Fig. 3–11).

This corrugated arrangement is useful for two reasons:

1. It increases the surface area over which the two tissue types are in contact with each other. This in turn increases the *strength of the junction* between the two tissues. Areas that are subjected to a great deal of mechanical loading, such as the areas of the masticatory

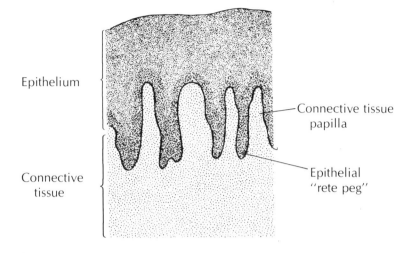

Fig. 3-11. Diagram of a corrugated interface between epithelium and underlying connective tissue. Epithelial "rete pegs" alternate with connective tissue papillae.

mucosa, have many thin, tall connective tissue papillae, interdigitating with many long epithelial rete pegs. The lining mucosa, on the other hand, has fewer and much shorter connective tissue papillae and wide, blunt epithelial extensions in between.

2. It decreases the distance between vascular supply and the epithelial cells. Epithelium does *not* have its own vascular supply. All blood vessels that carry the nutrients for the epithelial cells remain inside the connective tissue. Blood vessels in the connective tissue papillae can carry more nutrients closer to more epithelial cells than can blood vessels that are located underneath a straight epithelium-connective tissue interface (Fig. 3–12).

Basement Membrane at the Epithelium-Connective Tissue Interface

Between the basal cell layer of the oral epithelium and the underlying connective tissue, a sheet-like border structure is present: the *basement membrane* (Fig. 3–13).

The basement membrane is a noncellular structure, produced in part by the basal epithelial cells and in part by the connective tissue cells. In the light microscope this structure is barely visible, having a thickness of only 1 to 2 μm. In the electron microscope more details are visible within the basement membrane.

The basement membrane is composed by *two* layers or *laminae:*

1. A *basal lamina,* a thin, amorphous layer of 20 to 70 nm thick. It appears as a thin, dark line in electron micrographs, parallel to

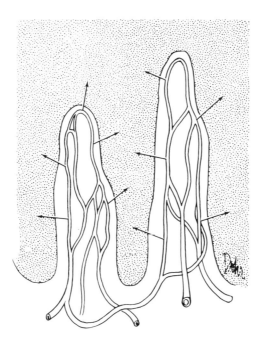

Blood vessels in
connective tissue papillae

Fig. 3–12. Epithelium does not have its own blood vessels. A rich blood vessel supply in the tall connective tissue papillae, penetrating deeply into the epithelium, is capable of supplying many epithelial cells over short distances *(arrows).*

the basal cell membranes of the basal epithelial cells. The principal component of the basal lamina is a unique type of collagen (Type IV collagen; Chap. 4), that is produced by the basal epithelial cells. The epithelial cells form hemidesmosome attachments to the basal lamina (Chap. 2).

2. A *reticular lamina,* considerably thicker than the basal lamina. The reticular lamina consists mainly of delicate collagen fibers (Type III collagen; Chap. 4), produced by the connective tissue cells.

Specialized Mucosa—The Tongue

The top surface of the tongue is covered with specialized mucosa. This mucosa is characterized by the presence of numerous *lingual papillae,* some of which have a *mechanical function* (remember that the tongue assists in the process of chewing), while others carry the specialized taste organs, or *taste buds.*

The distribution of these papillae is best seen by inspection of your

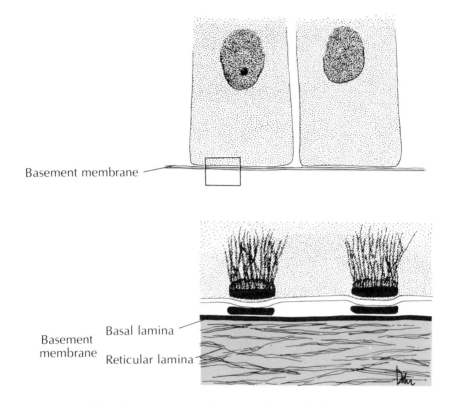

Basement membrane

Basement membrane   Basal lamina

Reticular lamina

Fig. 3–13. Light-microscopic (top) and electron-microscopic (bottom) appearances of this basement membrane, which is found between epithelium and the underlying connective tissue. Light-microscopically, the basement membrane is a very delicate, band-like structure, which is barely visible. Electron-microscopically, the basement membrane consists of a thin, darkly staining basal lamina and a much wider reticular lamina. Hemidesmosomal attachments (visible with the electron microscope only) are present between the epithelial cells and the basal lamina, which is a noncellular surface.

own tongue, in front of a mirror, and by comparison of your findings with Figure 3–14.

When inspecting the tongue, the part you see most readily is the *body* of the tongue. The body of the tongue comprises two-thirds of the tongue's length and lies horizontally in the oral cavity. Further back, near the throat, the tongue curves downward and becomes vertical. This vertical part of the tongue, comprising one third of its length, is the *root* or *base* of the tongue. The body of the tongue carries all types of lingual papillae, while the base of the tongue is covered with tonsillar tissue (Chap. 6).

We distinguish four types of lingual papillae (Figs. 3–15 and 3–16): filiform papillae, fungiform papillae, vallate papillae and foliate papillae. For the distribution of these papillae see Fig. 3–14.

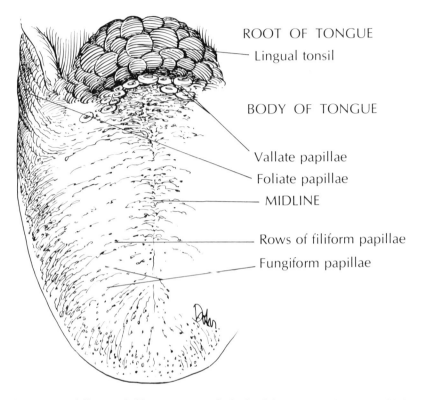

ROOT OF TONGUE
Lingual tonsil

BODY OF TONGUE

Vallate papillae
Foliate papillae
MIDLINE

Rows of filiform papillae
Fungiform papillae

Fig. 3–14.   A fully extended human tongue. The body of the tongue makes up two thirds of its length, from the tip backward. It is covered with filiform papillae. Interspersed among these are occasional fungiform papillae. The root of the tongue makes up one third of its length. It is covered with tonsillar tissue. At the border between body and root of the tongue is a V-shaped row of vallate papillae. At about the same level, a few foliate papillae are present along the edges at the sides of the tongue.

All lingual papillae consist of large, specialized connective tissue papillae, covered with orthokeratinized or parakeratinized stratified squamous epithelium. The basic structure of a (specialized) connective tissue papilla is that of a conical mountain (or a ridge, in the case of foliate papillae). This is the *primary papilla*. On top of the primary papilla several smaller conical peaks or ridges are present. These are the *secondary papillae*.

FILIFORM PAPILLAE. These are the most abundantly present lingual papillae. They are spread over the entire surface of the body of the tongue. They are shaped like thick, conical hairs and are covered with a thick layer of keratinized epithelium. These papillae have a purely *mechanical* function, and they are the only lingual papillae *without* taste buds.

FUNGIFORM PAPILLAE. These papillae are far less numerous than the filiform papillae. They are distributed among the

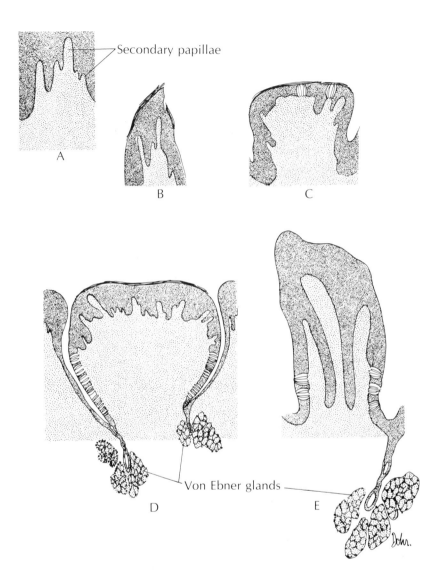

Fig. 3–15.   Diagrams of the various lingual papillae. *A,* All lingual papillae have a connective tissue core or primary connective tissue papilla, illustrated here. Several smaller,
conical secondary connective tissue papillae are present on top of the primary papilla.
B, Filiform papilla. Conical in shape. The only lingual papilla without taste buds. Heavily
keratinized epithelium. *C,* Fungiform papilla. Mushroom-shaped. Characterized by taste
buds on the top surface of the papilla. The epithelium is very thin, with some keratinization.
D, Vallate papilla. Mushroom-shaped. Characterized by a deep surrounding groove, into
which some small salivary (von Ebner) glands open. Several taste buds are present on the
sides of this papilla. *E,* Foliate papilla. Large, ridge-shaped. Deep grooves are present
between neighboring papillae. Von Ebner glands open into these grooves. Taste buds are
present on the side surfaces of these papillae.

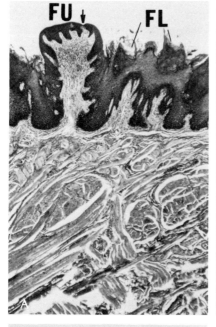

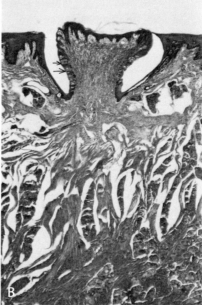

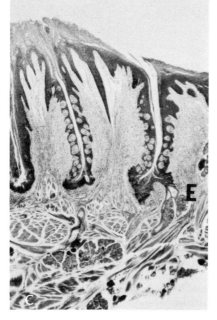

Fig. 3–16. *A,* Filiform papillae (FL), heavily keratinized, and one fungiform papilla (FU) in a histologic section of a monkey tongue. A taste bud *(arrow)* is present on the top of the fungiform papilla. Original magnification × 12.5. *B,* Vallate papilla in a histologic section of a monkey tongue. Notice the deep groove around the papilla and the several taste buds *(arrows)* on its side. No von Ebner gland is visible in this particular section. Original magnification × 12.5. *C,* Three foliate papillae, separated by deep grooves, in a histologic section of a rabbit tongue. A von Ebner gland (E) opens into one of the grooves. Many taste buds are present on the sides of the papillae. Original magnification × 12.5.

filiform papillae and show as reddish dots on the surface of the tongue. They are shaped like mushrooms. A thin, keratinized epithelium covers their surfaces. The thinness of the epithelium allows the red of the blood vessels in the connective tissue papilla to show through. This is responsible for the red color of these papillae. On its top surface a fungiform papilla may carry a variable number of taste buds.

VALLATE PAPILLAE. These large papillae are located in a V-shaped groove at the border between body and base of the tongue. There are only 8 to 12 of these papillae. Their shape resembles that of the fungiform papillae, but the vallate papillae are sunk below the surface of the tongue, so that they are surrounded by a groove and a low, circular wall of oral mucosa. These papillae are covered with keratinized epithelium. Numerous taste buds are present on the vertical (side) surfaces of the papilla, facing the surrounding groove.

FOLIATE PAPILLAE. Foliate papillae are 4 to 11 ridges, running parallel with each other on either side of the tongue, near the tongue base. These ridges may not easily be visible clinically. They are covered with keratinized epithelium and carry numerous taste buds on their sides.

The deepest parts both of the grooves surrounding the vallate papillae, and of the grooves separating adjacent foliate papillae contain the openings of ducts of special salivary glands, the *von Ebner* glands. Their serous saliva (Chap. 4) rinses the grooves continuously to enable the taste buds to perceive several different taste stimuli *in sequence.*

TASTE BUDS. Taste buds are barrel-shaped epithelial organs of special sense. While most of these organs are located on the lingual papillae, isolated taste buds may also be found on the soft palate and on the walls of the pharynx.

Taste buds extend from the basement membrane to the surface of the epithelium, across the entire epithelial thickness (Fig. 3–17). The epithelial cells of the taste buds are tall and spindle-shaped. Some of these cells are the actual *taste cells.* Each of these has a single cellular extension which protrudes into the *taste pore.* The taste pore is a superficial opening in the surface epithelium, which provides a direct connection between the taste bud cells and the contents of the oral cavity. Molecules of materials to be tasted come to this pore. The taste pore is filled with a *taste pore substance.* The chemical nature of this substance is unknown, but its role undoubtedly is to provide a selective filter and a barrier to protect the underlying taste bud cells from digestion by salivary enzymes.

Stimuli of the taste sensations, perceived by the taste cells, are transferred to nerve endings that are in contact with the bases of the

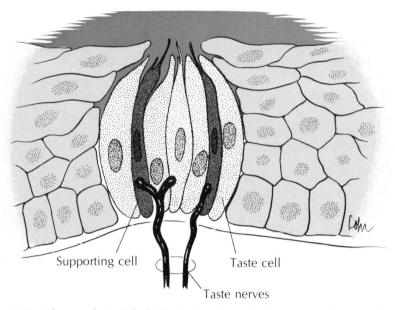

Supporting cell   Taste cell

Taste nerves

Fig. 3–17.   Diagram of a taste bud. The bud runs from the basement membrane to the top surface of the epithelium, where it is in contact with saliva via a taste pore. Taste cells (which are specialized epithelial cells) with taste hairs and supporting cells (also specialized epithelial cells) are present in the taste bud. Delicate endings of taste nerves pass through the basement membrane and are in contact with the taste cells.

taste cells. These nerves carry the stimuli to the central nervous system, where the taste is *perceived* and *identified.*

Additionally, the taste bud contains *supporting cells.* These cells support the actual taste cells and are responsible for the production of the taste pore substance, that fills the taste pore and surrounds the taste cell extensions.

A third population of taste bud cells is found in the basal region of the taste bud. Most likely they are involved in cell replacement, since there is a constant, rapid turnover especially of the taste cells.

SELECTED READING LIST

Abrahamson, D.R.: Recent studies on the structure and pathology of basement membranes. J. Pathol., *149*:257, 1986.

Arvidson, K., Cottler-Fox, M., and Friberg, U.: Fine structure of taste buds in the human fungiform papillae. Scand. J. Dent. Res., *89*:297, 1981.

Farbman, A.I.: Fine structure of the taste bud. J. Ultrastruct. Res., *12*:328, 1965.

Graziadei, P.P.C.: The ultrastructure of taste buds in mammals. In *Second Symposium on Oral Sensation and Perception.* Edited by J.F. Bosma, Springfield, IL, Charles C Thomas, 1970.

Halliday, G.M., and Muller, H.K.: The role of the Langerhans cell in local defence. IRCS J. Med. Sci., *12*:567, 1984.

Hashimoto, K.: Fine structure of Merkel cell in human oral mucosa. J. Invest. Dermatol., *58*:381, 1972.

Hume, W.J., and Potten, C.S.: Advances in epithelial kinetics—An oral view. J. Oral Pathol., *8*:3, 1979.

Kefalides, N.A. (ed.): *Biology and Chemistry of Basement Membranes.* New York, Academic Press, 1978.

Landmann, L.: The epidermal permeability barrier. Anat. Embryol., 178:1, 1988.

Laurie, GW., and Leblond, C.P.: What is known of the production of basement membrane components. J. Histochem. Cytochem., *31*:159, 1983.

Rowden, G.: The Langerhans cell. CRC Crit. Rev. Immunol., *3*:95, 1981.

Squier, C.A., and Meyer, J. (eds.): *Current Concepts of the Histology of Oral Mucosa. Part I: The Oral Epithelium.* Springfield, IL, Charles C Thomas, 1971.

Squier, C.A., Johnson, N.W., and Hopps, R.M.: *Human Oral Mucosa. Development, Structure and Function.* Oxford, Blackwell Scientific Publications, 1976.

Svejda, J., and Janota, M.: Scanning electron microscopy of the papillae foliatae of the human tongue. Oral Surg. Oral Med. Oral Pathol., *37*:208, 1974.

Svejda, J., and Skach, M.: The three-dimensional image of the lingual papillae. Folia Morphol., *22*:145, 1975.

Umeda, N., and Ikeda, A.: Scanning electron microscopic study of the capillary loops in the dermal papillae. Skin of the hand of the Japanese monkey *(Macaca fuscata).* Acta Anat., *132*:270, 1988.

Wyk, C.W. van, and Vyver, P.C. van der: Cytoplasmic granules in exfoliated buccal epithelial cells. J. Oral Pathol., *12*:177, 1983.

4

Oral Mucosa—Connective Tissue Proper

In the preceding chapter we learned that the lining of the oral cavity, the oral mucosa, consists of two tissue components—epithelium and connective tissue. The connective tissue component of the oral mucosa, called the *lamina propria,* itself consists of two layers: a *papillary layer,* comprising the connective tissue papillae and a thin common base, and a *dense fibrous layer,* comprising the bulk of the lamina propria. Between the oral mucosa and the underlying tissues (muscles for instance) there may be an intermediate layer of connective tissue, the *submucosa* (literally, *under* the mucosa) (Fig. 4–1).

Structurally, the submucosa is quite distinct from the lamina propria. It is a loose and delicate tissue. An oral surgeon uses this layer as a plane of dissection when placing the edge of the scalpel in the submucosa to lift the oral mucosa from the underlying tissues.

The submucosa is comparable, in structure and function, to the *hypodermis,* the connective tissue layer underneath the skin. Hypodermic needles owe their name to the fact that they are used to inject substances into the hypodermis. Similarly, for local anesthesia in the oral cavity, the submucosa is used for this purpose, *if it is*

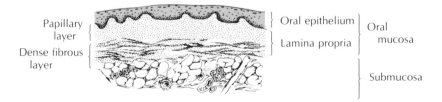

Fig. 4–1. The oral mucosa is composed of oral epithelium (dark) and a layer of connective tissue proper: the lamina propria, which is further subdivided into a papillary layer (lightly stippled), immediately underneath the epithelium, and a dense fibrous layer. Underneath the oral mucosa, another connective tissue layer, the submucosa, may be present.

present. Some areas of the oral mucosa have little or no submucosa. (This is especially true in the case of the masticatory mucosae: attached gingiva and mucosa of the hard palate.) If one attempts to give local anesthesia in such areas, the anesthetic will be able to infiltrate the dense tissue of the lamina propria only with difficulty, and this procedure is extremely painful. When possible, areas of the oral mucosa with a submucosa should be used instead (Fig. 4–2).

The tissues of the lamina propria and the submucosa are examples of *connective tissue proper.* This is only one tissue type within the larger group of *connective tissues.* Other connective tissues are bone and cartilage (Chap. 5), bone marrow, blood, lymphoid tissue (tonsils and lymph nodes) (Chap. 6), fat (this Chapter), as well as certain

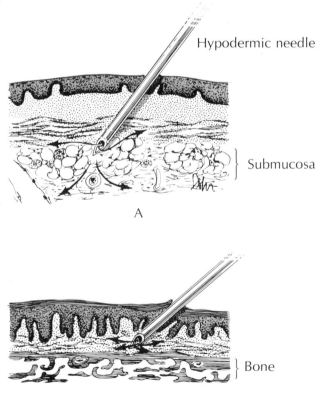

Fig. 4–2. When a thin hypodermic needle is used to inject substances underneath the oral mucosa, these substances will diffuse readily in the loose connective tissue of a submucosa, if present. This is the case in most areas of lining mucosae *(A)*. Underneath masticatory mucosae a submucosa is usually absent. The lamina propria, which consists of dense connective tissue, is tied firmly to the underlying (bone) tissue *(B)*. Injected substances do not diffuse readily, and the resulting localized pressure is uncomfortable.

tissues of the tooth: pulp, dentin (Chap. 10) and cementum (Chap. 12).

Collectively, connective tissues are a rather varied group. What these tissues have in *common* is that materials produced by connective tissue cells assume a prominent role in the overall organization of these tissues. The various types of connective tissues *differ* in the nature of their cell products and in the proportions in which these products are present in the tissues.

CONNECTIVE TISSUE COMPONENTS

All connective tissues develop from embryonic connective tissue or *mesenchyme.* Mesenchyme consists of relatively undifferentiated cells that produce intercellular material. As this intercellular material is deposited between them, the cells move apart, maintaining contact via small cell junctions, mostly tight junctions (Fig. 4–3).

The intercellular material generally consists of a fibrous matrix and a ground substance.

Fibrous Matrix

The fibrous matrix of a connective tissue may consist of one or more different types of collagen fibers and/or elastic fibers.

COLLAGEN FIBERS. Collagen is a protein. This means that collagen is produced in the rough endoplasmic reticulum of a col-

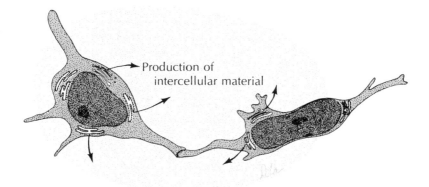

MESENCHYMAL CELLS

Fig. 4–3. Diagram of two mesenchymal cells. These cells have several long cell extensions, which are in junctional contact with similar extensions of neighboring mesenchymal cells. A few cisternae of rough endoplasmic reticulum, a medium Golgi complex, and some mitochondria are present in the cytoplasm. Mesenchymal cells produce a water-rich intercellular material.

lagen-producing cell. It is then moved through the Golgi complex (where some carbohydrates may be attached to it and other modifications occur) and the secretory granules to the outside of the cell. During its release from the cell collagen may be further modified.

The structure of collagen and the various steps in its synthesis are beyond the scope of this book. More than 10 different types of collagen (Types I through XI) are now known to exist. All these types have certain chemical and structural similarities, but they are sufficiently distinct from each other in other chemical and structural aspects to require different genetic instructions for their formation. For the purposes of this text we will limit our discussion here to collagen Types I through IV.

Types I through III are produced by connective tissue cells, while Type IV is the product of epithelial cells (basal lamina, described in Chap. 3). Types I through III are assembled in the form of fibers, while Type IV is intricately assembled into a sheet (the basic structure of a basal lamina).

All types of collagen initially are formed as coiled strands of amino acids. The strands of Types I through III are 300 nm long, while the strands of Type IV are 390 nm long. Outside the cells the individual strands are further assembled in a Type-specific fashion. In Types I through III three strands are wrapped around each other to form a *tropocollagen molecule.* Tropocollagen molecules are the basic units of collagen fibers. Some carbohydrates are attached to the surface of this molecule.

The tropocollagen molecules undergo an organized assembly into collagen fibers. Since the individual tropocollagen molecules are only 300 nm long and 1.4 nm wide, a large number of them is required to form the collagen fibers, which are visible with the light microscope (diameters: 1 to 15 μm), and the numbers needed to form a tendon (a structure consisting almost entirely of Type I collagen) are astronomical.

The tropocollagen molecules are securely attached to each other by chemical bonds, and they line up in an orderly manner according to the *quarter stagger* model (Fig. 4–4). Fully assembled collagen fibers are capable of resisting *tension,* and when they are assembled, the fibers tend to form in a direction optimally suited to resist the tensions to which the tissue is subjected (Fig. 4–4).

Type I collagen is most abundant in the human body. It forms the thick fibers traditionally identified as "collagen fibers." It is the dominant collagen in connective tissue proper and it is the principal collagen type found in calcified connective tissues: bone, dentin, and cementum.

Type II collagen forms more delicate collagen fibers, that are almost specifically found in cartilage tissue.

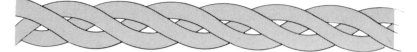

Tropocollagen molecule

Tropocollagen molecule schematically

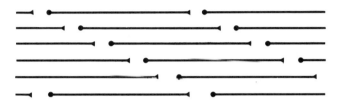

Tropocollagen molecules assembled in quarter stagger

Collagen fiber

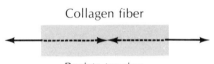

Resists tension

Fig. 4–4. The structural unit of collagen, tropocollagen, consists of three long protein strands, twisted around each other (top). For simplicity, the same tropocollagen molecule has been redrawn even more schematically. The tropocollagen molecules align themselves in an orderly "quarter stagger" model, forming a collagen fiber. The bottom diagram illustrates that a collagen fiber is capable of resisting tension imposed on it in the diagram of its long axis (arrows).

Type III collagen forms delicate fibers (usually not exceeding a diameter of 1 μm). These fibers were traditionally identified as "reticulin fibers." These fibers tend to be associated with a considerably larger amount of carbohydrates than are Type I collagen fibers. This accounts for the slightly different staining properties of the two fiber types. Type III collagen is found especially in immature connective tissues and in border areas between connective tissues and other tissues, for example, the reticular lamina of the basement membranes (Chap. 3).

Type III collagen is *not* found in calcified connective tissues.

ELASTIC FIBERS. Until recently, little was known about

this family of fibers. There are two principal types of fibers in this group: "elastic" and "oxytalan" fibers.

Elastic fibers consist of long fibrous proteins of a different composition from those in collagen. They are surrounded by a carbohydrate-rich mass. Certain components of this mass are only found in, and are specific for elastic fibers.

Oxytalan fibers are composed of the same long fibrous proteins, but are not surrounded by the carbohydrate rich mass. This chemical difference makes it possible to detect these fibers selectively.

Elastic fibers have diameters of 1 to 3 μm and they may be branched (collagen fibers are *not* branched). Elastic fibers are responsible for the return of a connective tissue to its original arrangement following deformation of this tissue. You may try this with the skin of your hand. Shift the skin over the underlying tissues as far as possible without hurting yourself. Then release. The resistance to this shifting movement came from the collagen fibers in the skin. The rapid recoil, following the release of this deformation, was due to the elastic fibers.

Oxytalan fibers appear to have a different, yet mechanical function. These fibers are found at several locations where they seem to "anchor" tissue components, such as blood vessels, smooth and striated muscle and epidermis.

Ground Substance

In addition to the fibrous matrix, connective tissue cells also produce a ground substance. This substance is frequently not visible in the light microscope, unless special stains are used, and is only barely visible in the electron microscope. The ground substance is characterized by the presence of relatively large molecules *(macromolecules)*. Some of these are proteins, others are complexes of proteins and carbohydrates. The principal macromolecules that have been identified are the following:

PROTEOGLYCANS. These are complexes of proteins to which long carbohydrate chains are attached. In some tissues, such as bone and dentin, the proteoglycans may be fairly simple, composed of a protein core with a few carbohydrate chains. In other tissues, such as cartilage, the proteoglycans form large and complicated aggregates.

GLYCOPROTEINS. These are proteins with only small amounts of carbohydrates attached.

PHOSPHOPROTEINS. These are proteins that are characterized by the presence of bound organic phosphate in the macromolecule.

The various groups of macromolecules of the ground substance appear to have different functions. The best understood of these is the mechanical function of the proteoglycans. The carbohydrate chains of the proteoglycans readily hold and bind water. They act somewhat as coils or springs as the result of their particular chemical characteristics. The carbohydrates are responsible for the gelatinous nature of the ground substance, which is highly resistant to *compression* (Fig. 4–5).

The preceding was a general introduction to the *intercellular* components of connective tissues. In the following section and in the next chapter we will discuss the specific details of certain types of connective tissues.

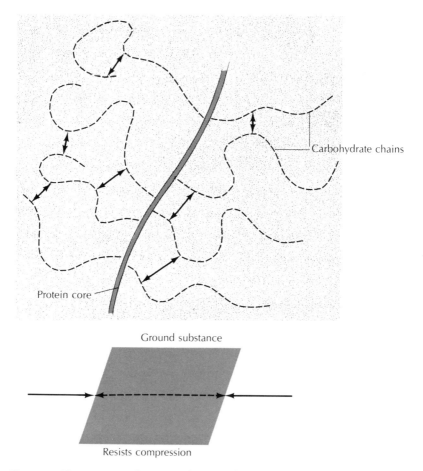

Fig. 4–5. The structure of a proteoglycan in the ground substance is shown in this simplified diagram. Long carbohydrate chains are attached to a central protein core. The particular chemical nature of the carbohydrates prevents them from approaching each other too closely. Thus they act as molecular springs and are responsible for the resistance of ground substance to compressive loadings imposed on it from any direction (arrows in diagram).

CONNECTIVE TISSUE PROPER

As does any other connective tissue, connective tissue proper consists of cells, fibrous matrix and ground substance.

CELLS. The cells of connective tissue proper are *fibroblasts,* the producers of the fibrous matrix and ground substance, and *other cell types* responsible for the maintenance and defense of the tissue.

FIBROUS MATRIX. The fibrous matrix consists of Types I and III collagen fibers, and variable amounts of elastic fibers. It has predominantly mechanical functions.

GROUND SUBSTANCE. The constituents of the ground substance are proteoglycans and glycoproteins, specific for connective tissue proper, with mechanical and physiologic support functions, e.g., as pathways for metabolic products.

Organization of the Fibrous Matrix in Connective Tissue Proper

We noted before that both the lamina propria and the submucosa are examples of connective tissue proper, but it appears that even within these tissues further differences are possible. In the papillary layer of the lamina propria, as well as in the submucosa, the fibrous matrix is relatively delicate. It consists of thin Type I collagen fibers, with relatively large, non-fibrous areas in between, and fair amounts of elastic and Type III collagen fibers. This type of connective tissue proper is called *loose connective tissue.* None of its three components (cells, fibrous matrix, and ground substance) is particularly prominent.

The dense fibrous layer of the lamina propria is an example of *dense connective tissue.* In this tissue type the fibrous matrix has become the dominant component. Dense connective tissue consists predominantly of heavy, tightly packed, Type I collagen fibers. You will remember that collagen is particularly well suited to resist *tension.* An understanding of the structure of this tissue leads to an understanding of its function. A dense connective tissue has a predominantly mechanical, tension-resisting function.

In the case of the dense fibrous layer of the lamina propria, the fibers are oriented in all directions, forming a three-dimensional meshwork. This means that this dense connective tissue is capable of optimally resisting tension in *any* direction.

There are other dense connective tissues, in which the collagen fibers are all oriented in a flat plane, forming a 2-dimensional meshwork. Such fibrous sheets: the fasciae surrounding the muscles and the periosteum surrounding the bones, resist tension, exerted largely in the plane in which the fibers are oriented.

In yet other dense connective tissues, the collagen fibers are all oriented in only one direction. In such cases, e.g., the tendons of muscles, most tension is exerted, and resisted only in the direction in which the collagen fibers are oriented.

In *loose connective tissue* Type I and Type III collagen fibers run in all directions, but because of their delicate nature, they have only a minor mechanical function. The major function of a loose connective tissue is one of physiologic support. It fills the spaces between tissues and organs and it carries blood vessels and nerves. In addition, it houses various types of cells engaged in the protection of the body. Thus, it should *not* be surprising that the loose connective tissue of the papillary layer carries the rich vascular network that supplies the overlying epithelium, as well as the sensory nerve terminals: *free nerve endings,* which cross the basal lamina and enter the epithelium, and *encapsulated nerve endings,* which remain in the connective tissue.

The submucosa similarly carries a rich vascular network as well as major nerves and blood vessels, fat and glandular structures. Relatively small amounts of elastic fibers are found in both types of connective tissue proper. These have mechanical functions.

Cells in Connective Tissue Proper

There are many types of cells, of varying and distinct functions, in connective tissue proper. A brief description of these cells will be given here. We distinguish two groups of cells: (1) cells that normally inhabit connective tissue (Fig. 4–6), and (2) wandering cells, normally circulating in blood, which enter the connective tissue by moving out of the blood vessels when needed (Fig. 4–7).

Cells that *normally inhabit* connective tissue are almost all highly specialized and differentiated cells of mesenchymal origin. Some *undifferentiated mesenchymal cells* may still remain in adult connective tissue. These cells are generally considered as a pool of reserve cells, which may differentiate at a later time, when needed.

FIBROBLASTS ("fiber-producers"). These cells have small cell bodies with several delicate cell extensions. Fibroblasts are responsible for the production of both fibrous matrix and ground substance. As might be expected, they all have the organelles necessary for the production of proteins and the attachment of carbohydrates to these proteins.

In addition, these cells are also capable of breaking down their own products. This enables them to continuously replace components of the intercellular materials, especially the rapidly "turned over" carbohydrate-rich substances.

MAST CELLS. These round-to-oval cells are important for the maintenance of health of a tissue. They are found throughout the

FIBROBLAST

MACROPHAGE

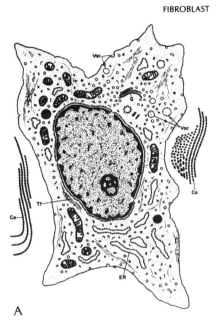

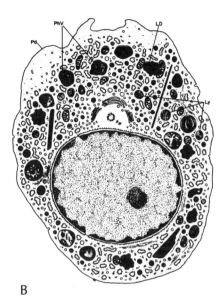

A

B

MAST CELL

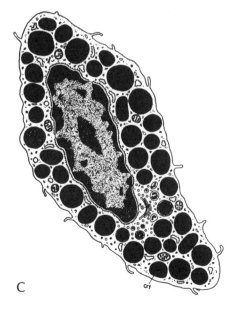

C

Fig. 4–6. *A,* Fibroblasts are spindle-shaped or star-shaped. They are responsible for the production of fibrous matrix and ground substance in connective tissue proper. ER = rough endoplasmic reticulum; G = Golgi complex; Vac = secretory vesicles; Tf = abundant tonofilaments (bundles of microfilaments in cytoplasm); Co = newly synthesized collagen fibers. *B,* Macrophage, or a histiocyte in which clear evidence of phagocytosis is present. PhV = phagocytic vacuoles, filled with various ingested materials; Ly = lysosomes; LD = lipid droplet; Pd = pseudopodium. An actively phagocytic cell may become mobile, and the small, transient pseudopodia are involved in the propagation of the cell. *C,* Mast cells are round to oval. The large granules in the cytoplasm have dense or crystalline (Cry) contents and are surrounded by a membrane. These granules contain the vasoactive substances heparin and histamine. Few organelles are present in these cells. (From Lentz, T.L.: Cell Fine Structure: An Atlas of Drawings of Whole-Cell Structure. Philadelphia, W.B. Saunders Co., 1971.)

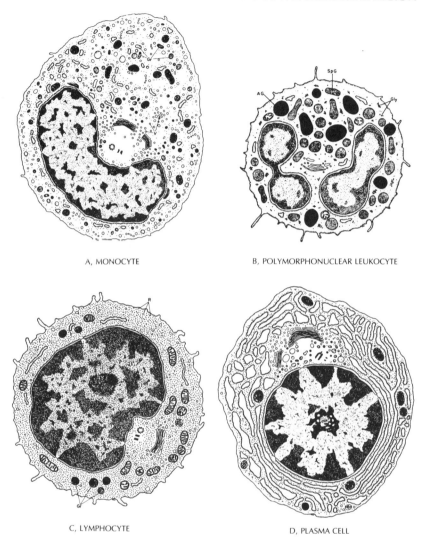

A, MONOCYTE

B, POLYMORPHONUCLEAR LEUKOCYTE

C, LYMPHOCYTE

D, PLASMA CELL

Fig. 4–7.   Wandering cells, which may be present in connective tissue proper. A, Monocytes have an abundant cytoplasm. An extensive Golgi complex and large numbers of lysosomes are indicative of the potential of this cell for digestive activities. When actively involved in phagocytosis, such cells become macrophages. B, A polymorphonuclear leukocyte is readily recognizable by its single, lobed nucleus, making it appear as if (in some sections) this cell had several nuclei. There are few organelles. Gly = several glycogen granules; SpG (specific granules) and AG (azurophilic granules) contain enzymes capable of digestion of phagocytosed materials. C, Lymphocytes have an almost spherical nucleus with a small indentation on one side. A narrow rim of cytoplasm surrounds the nucleus. Characteristically, large numbers of free ribosomes (R) are present in the cytoplasm. A few dense granules (Gr) are visible as well. D, A plasma cell has an ovoid, eccentrically placed nucleus, with a characteristic, cartwheel arrangement of chromatin. The cytoplasm contains an extensive rough endoplasmic reticulum and Golgi complex (active immunoglobulin synthesis). (From Lentz, T.L.: Cell Fine Structure: An Atlas of Drawings of Whole Cell Structure. Philadelphia, W.B. Saunders Co., 1971.)

connective tissue, but by preference close to the blood and lymphatic vessels. Under the light microscope, many "grains" are visible in their cytoplasm. These are vesicles filled with several substances, the most important of which are *heparin* and *histamine.* Heparin is an anticoagulant, a substance that prevents blood clotting. Histamine has a dilating (widening) effect on blood vessels. During an inflammation, mast cells discharge their contents in the ground substance. The resultant blood vessel reaction is one of the typical attributes of an inflammation, producing redness and later swelling of the tissues. In addition to these pre-formed, granule-contained substances, several other substances (such as prostaglandins, and leukotrienes, for example) are generated in the inflamed tissues under the influence of the mast cells.

HISTIOCYTES (MACROPHAGES). They belong to a widespread group of similar cells found in many tissues of the body. All these cells have in common that they are initially formed in the bone marrow, are transported as *monocytes* through the vascular system to the tissues in which they will be active, are capable of active movement through the tissue and are specialized in digestive activities. In connective tissue proper such cells become histiocytes. They are located predominantly alongside the blood vessels. They have several cell extensions and are rich in lysosomes.

Ingestion (uptake) and digestion (intracellular breakdown) of extracellular material is a process called *phagocytosis.* If a cell is involved in a great deal of phagocytosis, vacuoles filled with ingested materials become visible in its cytoplasm under the light microscope. When such clear evidence of phagocytosis is present, we no longer call such cells histiocytes, but *macrophages.* In addition to their phagocytic activities, these cells also assist in the immune responses of the tissue.

WANDERING CELLS. A number of cells normally carried in the blood stream may, when the need arises, move out of the blood vessels into the connective tissue proper (Fig. 4–7, Table 4–1).

Some of these cells are capable of *digesting* harmful agents, or breakdown products (thus assisting the resident population of histiocytes); others may be involved in the *immune responses* of the body, or in the *destruction* of other cells. These cells, which are normal components of blood, will be noted briefly here and more extensively in Chapter 6.

FAT

Fat is a special type of connective tissue. It is composed of *fat cells.* They have differentiated from mesenchymal cells and their

Table 4–1.   Wandering Cells of Connective Tissue Proper

Cell Type	Function	Where Found
Monocytes (Macrophages)	Phagocytosis. When large amounts of extracellular materials are ingested, monocytes, like histiocytes, are called macrophages	Areas of inflammation
Polymorphonuclear leukocytes (neutrophils)	Destruction and ingestion of cells, bacteria and other harmful agents	Areas of chronic and acute inflammation
Lymphocytes	Participation in immune response, both humoral and cell-mediated	Areas of chronic and acute inflammation
Plasma cells	Production of immuno-globulins	Areas of chronic inflammation

differentiation consists of an *intracellular* accumulation of fat (Fig. 4–8).

Frequently the cells are surrounded by delicate collagen fibers. While isolated fat cells may occur, they are more frequently assembled in groups, forming *fat tissue.* In the oral cavity some fat tissue is found in the submucosa of the hard palate, in the premolar region, making this a compressible area. Fat tissue may be present also in the submucosa, underneath the labial mucosa, and in the cheek, between cheek muscle and skin.

SALIVARY GLANDS

Small (or *minor)* salivary glands are commonly found in the submucosa. They are present in the submucosa of the lips, the cheeks, parts of the hard palate (especially near the soft palate), the soft palate itself, the top surface of the tongue and the sublingual areas.

In addition to these minor salivary glands, we have three pairs of *major* salivary glands: the parotid glands, the submandibular glands and the sublingual glands. The sublingual glands are located in the submucosa of the floor of the oral cavity. The two other pairs of major salivary glands are somewhat farther removed from the oral cavity. All salivary glands, however, carry their products via their duct systems into the oral cavity.

Organization of Salivary Glands

Salivary glands are organs consisting of an *epithelial* and a *connective tissue proper* component.

WHITE ADIPOSE CELL

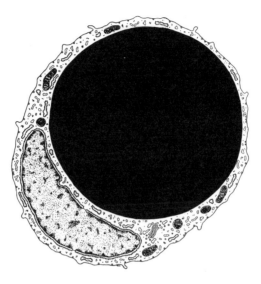

Fig. 4–8. A white fat (adipose) cell is large. A central lipid droplet (dark) occupies most of the cell volume, and is surrounded by a thin rim of cytoplasm. The nucleus is located in this peripheral cytoplasm and it is compressed into a crescent shape. A few organelles are scattered in the cytoplasm. (From Lentz, T.L.: Cell Fine Structure: An Atlas of Drawings of Whole Cell Structure. Philadelphia, W.B. Saunders Co., 1971.)

The *epithelium* resembles a tree, in which the "base" is the opening of the duct leading into the oral cavity and the "leaves" are the parts where the production of the saliva begins. The intervening "twigs" and "branches" are components of the duct system, through which the secretion product is moved and modified, until it reaches the oral cavity as saliva (Fig. 4–9).

Dense connective tissue surrounds the entire epithelial tree, forming a connective tissue *capsule* around the gland. Around the individual epithelial components of the gland, within the capsule, less dense connective tissue is present. The connective tissue gives mechanical support to the epithelium and it carries the physiologic support systems: the blood vessels and nerves.

Blood vessels and nerves have a branching pattern, similar to that of the epithelium, so that all epithelial components have rich blood and nerve supplies.

As a result of the branching pattern of the epithelial ductal tree, there is an uneven distribution of epithelial and connective tissue components in a salivary gland. The finer ducts and the "leaf" terminals form epithelium-rich *lobules,* in which most of the tissue

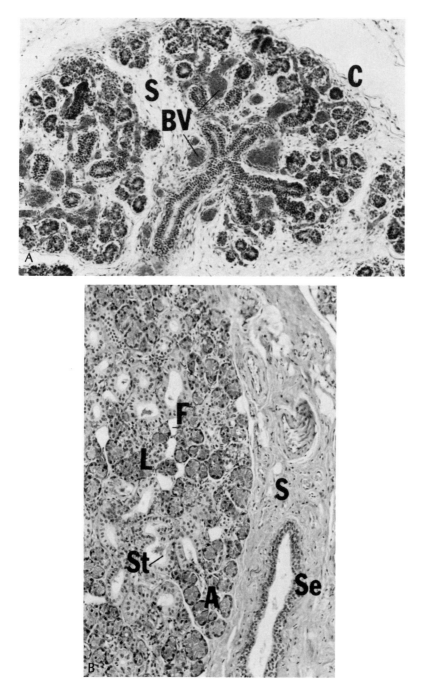

Fig. 4–9.

volume is occupied by epithelium (parenchyma) and a small part by delicate connective tissue (stroma), which surrounds the individual ducts and terminals.

Between the lobules are areas occupied by denser bands of connective tissue proper. These bands are called *septa.* They are like the walls that subdivide a house into smaller rooms. They run convergingly from the peripheral capsule in the glandular mass and carry the larger epithelial ducts and the blood vessels and nerves, which will further branch inside the lobules.

The different components of the epithelial ductal tree have different functions and the epithelial cells have specialized accordingly. Before we discuss the various epithelial components of a salivary gland, review the discussion of intracellular organelles (Chap. 2) and the classification of epithelia (Chap. 3).

Epithelial Ductal Tree

ACINUS. This is the "leaf" of the ductal tree of a salivary gland. Three-dimensionally an acinus is spherical. The epithelial cells forming the acinus are cuboidal and are arranged in a single layer. These are glycoprotein-producing cells and, therefore, have an abundant rough endoplasmic reticulum, Golgi complexes and secretory vesicles. Many secretory vesicles fill the slightly narrower top portion of the cell, where they will be released in the central space or *lumen* of the acinus.

An acinar cell may form one of two types of products. Depending on the product, one may have a *serous* cell (producing a somewhat watery product, in which proteins are prominent) or a *mucous* cell (producing a more viscous product, in which large carbohydrates are prominent). The distribution and proportions of the organelles in these different acinar cells vary with the nature of the product.

Fig. 4–9. *A,* Lobule of a developing salivary gland in a human fetus (second trimester of pregnancy). The tree-like arrangement of the darkly stained epithelium is clearly visible. Future saliva production will begin in the "leaves," and the saliva will be moved through the "twigs" and "branches" toward the oral cavity. Notice the rich blood supply (BV = blood vessels) in the lobule. C = developing connective tissue capsule; S = developing connective tissue septum. Original magnification × 40. *B,* Part of a connective tissue septum (S) and the parenchyma of an adjacent lobule (L) in a human parotid gland. A = acinus; St = striated duct; Se = excretory duct; F = fat cell. The tree-like structure of the epithelial component, while still existing, is no longer visible in a section of a mature salivary gland, owing to the increases in size and differentiation of the epithelial cells. Original magnification × 40.

Most *minor* salivary glands have mixed, largely mucous acini. The exception is formed by the purely serous, minor salivary glands that are associated with the vallate and foliate papillae of the tongue (von Ebner glands). Of the *major* salivary glands, the parotid has almost exclusively serous acini; the submandibular gland has both mucous and serous acini (mixed gland) and the sublingual gland has largely mucous and mucoserous acini.

DUCTAL SYSTEM. Once it is secreted, the product moves from the lumen of the acinus into the lumen of the *intercalated duct.* This duct is a hollow tube, lined by a single layer of small, cuboidal, epithelial cells. Some additional secretory activity occurs in these cells. This new secretory product is added to the initial acinar product, thereby beginning the process of modification of the final salivary product. This modification is continued as the product moves next into the *striated duct.* This duct is a hollow tube, lined by a single layer of tall, columnar, epithelial cells. These cells, which show light microscopically a series of stripes in their basal regions (hence the name: striated) are involved in a substantial modification of the salivary product. Sodium ions, chloride ions and water are removed from the product and moved back, across the cell, into the blood. Simultaneously, potassium ions are taken out of the blood and added to the salivary product in the lumen of the striated duct. Under the electron microscope, rows of mitochondria are found between deep folds of the basal membrane of these cells (under the light microscope these rows of mitochondria are visible as stripes). This arrangement supplies the energy to pump ions across the cells.

Acinar and ductal cells are firmly attached to each other, near their luminal surfaces, by tight junctions and complexes of junctions.

From the striated duct the salivary product moves into the *excretory duct.* This type of duct is the only component of the epithelial ductal tree, which is located entirely in a connective tissue septum (Fig. 4–10). All other components are located completely or partially inside the lobules. The excretory duct forms a hollow tube, and its epithelial lining shows all transitional forms between a single-layered columnar epithelium (near the striated duct) and a stratified squamous epithelium (nonkeratinized, near the oral epithelium). This duct carries the saliva to the oral cavity, while making final modifications in the composition of the saliva.

Clinically, the location of the *major* salivary glands frequently can be identified by spurts of saliva coming from the openings of the excretory ducts underneath the tongue and on the cheek, near the upper molars. Multiple openings of ducts of the *minor* salivary glands, especially at the border between hard and soft palate, may cause salivary discharge when you take an impression of the upper jaw.

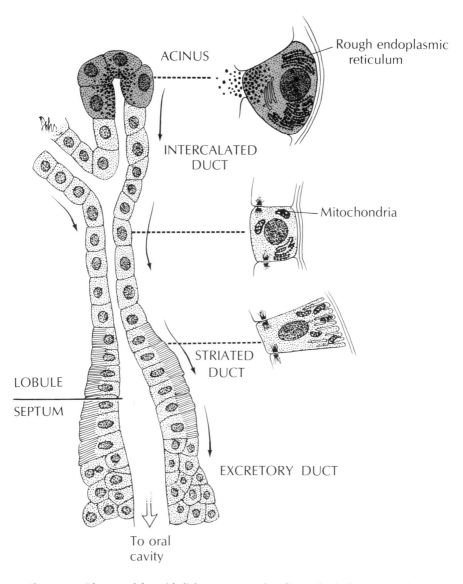

Fig. 4–10. Diagram of the epithelial components of a salivary gland. The arrows indicate the flow of the salivary product from acinus through intercalated, striated, and excretory ducts toward the oral cavity. The acinus consists of a spherical mass of cells with a central lumen. Illustrated separately is a serous acinar cell, producing a protein-rich product. An extensive rough endoplasmic reticulum is present. A basal lamina surrounds the epithelial cells, separating them from the connective tissue stroma. Secretion of the product, via secretory vesicles, takes place into the central lumen of the acinus. The intercalated duct cells (one is illustrated separately) are cuboidal cells, separated from the surrounding connective tissue stroma by a basal lamina. Tight junctions and desmosomes are present adjacent to the lumen. A similar arrangement of tight junctions, desmosomes, and basal lamina is found in the striated duct. Illustrated separately is a columnar striated duct cell, showing the rows of mitochondria between the basal membrane folds. The excretory duct is composed of transitional forms between a simple columnar epithelium, near the striated duct, and stratified squamous epithelium, near the oral mucosa. Part of the striated duct and the entire excretory duct are located in a connective tissue septum. The remainder of the ducts and the acini are located in a lobule.

VARIATIONS IN THE STRUCTURE OF THE ORAL MUCOSA

As we have seen, there are three types of oral mucosa: lining mucosa, masticatory mucosa and specialized mucosa. While all lining and masticatory mucosae have certain general characteristics (Chap. 3), there are some *regional differences.* A summary of the major differences is given in Tables 4–2, 4–3, and 4–4, pages 73–75.

SELECTED READING LIST

Böck, P.: Elastic fiber microfibrils: filaments that anchor the epithelium of the epiglottis. Arch. Histol. Jpn., *46*:307, 1983.

Buckwalter, J.A., and Rosenberg, L.: Structural changes during development in bovine fetal epiphyseal cartilage. Coll. Relat. Res., *3*:489, 1983.

Gordon, S., and Cohn, Z.A.: The macrophage. Int. Rev. Cytol., *36*:171, 1974.

Hascall, V.C.: Proteoglycans: the chondroitin sulfate/keratan sulfate proteoglycan of cartilage. I.S.I. Atlas of Science: Biochemistry, *1*:189, 1988.

Lentz, T.: *Cell Fine Structure. An Atlas of Drawings of Whole Cell Structure.* Philadelphia, W.B. Saunders Co., 1971.

Marom, Z., and Casale, T.B.: Mast cells and their mediators. Ann. Allergy, *50*:367, 1983.

Martin, G.R., et al.: The genetically distinct collagens. Trends Biochem. Sci., *10*:285, 1985.

Moss-Salentijn, L., and Moss, M.L.: Developmental and functional anatomy. In *Diseases of the Salivary Glands.* Edited by Rankow, R.M. and Polayes, I. Philadelphia, W.B. Saunders Co., 1976.

Narayanan, A.S., and Page, R.C.: Connective tissues of the periodontium: a summary of current work. Coll. Relat. Res., *3*:33, 1983.

Ross, R., and Bornstein, P.: Elastic fibers in the body. Sci. Am., *224*:44, 1971.

Smith, J.W.: Packing arrangement of tropocollagen molecules. Nature, *205*:356, 1965.

Sokol, R.J., et al.: Human macrophage development: a morphometric study. J. Anat., *151*:27, 1987.

Squier, C.A., and Meyer, J. (eds.): *Current Concepts of the Histology of Oral Mucosa. Part II: The Connective Tissue of the Oral Mucosa.* Springfield, IL, Charles C Thomas, 1971.

Squier, C.A., Johnson, N.W., and Hopps, R.M.: *Human Oral Mucosa. Development, Structure and Function.* Oxford, Blackwell Scientific Publications, 1976.

Testa-Riva, F., Puxeddu, P., Riva, A., and Diaz, G.: The epithelium of the excretory duct of the human submandibular gland: a transmission and scanning electron microscopic study. Am. J. Anat., *160*:381, 1981.

Uitto, J.: Biochemistry of the elastic fibers in normal connective tissues and its alterations in diseases. J. Invest. Dermatol., *72*:1, 1979.

Young, J.A., and van Lennep, E.W.: Gross anatomy. Microscopic anatomy. In *The Morphology of Salivary Glands.* New York, Academic Press, 1978.

Table 4–2. Lining Mucosa

	Epithelium	*Lamina propria*	*Submucosa*
General characteristics	Nonkeratinized, stratified squamous	Papillary layer has short papillae	Usually present
Differences Lip and cheek	Very thick (500 μm)	Irregular papillae Dense fibrous layer contains collagen and some elastic fibers Rich vascular supply	Contains fat and minor salivary glands, mostly mucous in nature Firm attachment between lamina propria and connective tissue covering of muscles
Alveolar mucosa	Thin (app. 150 μm)	Papillae sometimes absent Many elastic fibers Rich vascular supply, running close to surface (clinically: appears red)	Loose connective tissue with many elastic fibers Minor salivary glands of mixed, mostly mucous, nature
Floor of mouth	Very thin (app. 100 μm)	Broad papillae Extensive vascular supply	Loose connective tissue with fat and sublingual glands
Undersurface of the tongue	Thin (app. 150 μm)	Thin, with numerous papillae Some elastic fibers A few minor salivary glands, mostly mucous and mixed	*Absent* The lamina propria is bound directly to the connective tissue, covering the tongue muscles
Soft palate	Thin (app. 150 μm)	Thick, with numerous papillae *Elastic* fibers form a distinct elastic lamina	Loose connective tissue with numerous minor salivary glands, mucous in nature

An immediate *clinical* application of some of these characteristics is the administration of certain drugs, such as nitroglycerin, to a patient with heart disease. The tablet is placed on the mucosa of the floor of the mouth, underneath the tongue. The drug is readily absorbed through the thin epithelium, entering rapidly the extensive blood supply in the underlying lamina propria. In this way the drug becomes effective in a brief period of time.

Adapted from Squier et al. 1976.

Table 4–3. Masticatory Mucosa

	Epithelium	*Lamina propria*	*Submucosa*
General characteristics	Keratinized or parakeratinized, stratified squamous	Tall, narrow papillae Pronounced dense, connective tissue layer Moderate vascular supply	Only sporadically present
Differences			
Gingiva	Thick (app. 250 μm) Often stippled orange peel appearance	Extensive blood vessel loops in papillary layer	*Absent* Lamina propria is continuous with the fibrous covering of the underlying bone tissue
Hard palate	Thick. Surface thrown into transverse ridges (*rugae*)	Thick, especially in the rugae	Present *only* on the sides of the hard palate Contains fat in the premolar area Minor *salivary glands* in the molar area (mostly mucous) Elsewhere, the lamina propria is continuous with the fibrous covering of the underlying bone

An immediate *clinical* application of some of these characteristics is the *compressibility* of the mucosa of the hard palate in the areas containing fat or glandular tissue. These areas are used preferentially to support upper dentures or removable orthodontic appliances. When dentures or appliances rest on areas without submucosa (noncompressible), they cause pressure spots, extremely painful, on those surfaces of the mucosa.

Adapted from Squier et al. 1976.

Table 4-4. Specialized Mucosa

	Epithelium	Lamina propria	Submucosa
Top surface of the tongue only	Thick, keratinized, stratified squamous Some nonkeratinized areas Specialized surfaces of lingual papillae: taste buds	Distinct, specialized papillae Rich innervation, especially near taste buds Tonsillar tissue is present near the base or root of the tongue There are many minor salivary glands They are predominantly mucous or mixed, except near vallate and foliate papillae, where they are exclusively serous (Von Ebner glands)	Absent The lamina propria is continuous with the fibrous covering of the tongue muscles

Adapted from Squier et al. 1976.

5

Connective Tissues: Cartilage and Bone

Cartilage and bone are both skeletal tissues. In clinical practice these tissues usually are not visible, since they are always covered with skin, oral mucosa and other connective tissues, and occasionally with muscle tissue. But an awareness of the skeletal tissues must be an integral part of any dental treatment. More directly, you will encounter the images of one of these skeletal tissues: bone, on dental x-ray films *(radiographs)*.

X rays are used to study the structure of the so-called "hard tissues": bone and dental tissues. Such tissues owe their hardness to the presence of a mineral salt in their fibrous matrix and ground substance. This mineral salt forms a barrier for x rays. Soft tissues allow most x rays to pass through and hit an x-ray film, placed behind the tissues. Those parts of the film, which have been hit by x rays, become dark. Any light areas represent those areas of the film, which the x rays could not reach. Such areas (in the "shadows" of the hard tissues) show the shapes and the differential degrees of hardness of the structures which stopped the x rays, in general bone and teeth.

The radiographs shown in Figure 5–1 serve to illustrate this point. Notice the dense, solid (white) band, representing the bone at the periphery of the jaw: this is called *compact bone.* The compact bone layers enclose an area, which contains only delicate bone spangs, or *trabeculae.* This is called *spongy bone.* Between the bone trabeculae a soft, specialized connective tissue is present: bone marrow.

Any absence or disruption of the normal patterns of compact and spongy bone are indicative of bone loss or changes in the bone architecture, due to a disease process, such as an inflammation around the tip of a dental root, or advanced periodontal disease.

Bone and cartilage are both specialized types of connective tissue. While connective tissue proper has many different functions (see Chap. 4), which in part are illustrated by the variety of cell types in it, bone and cartilage are uniquely specialized for *support* functions.

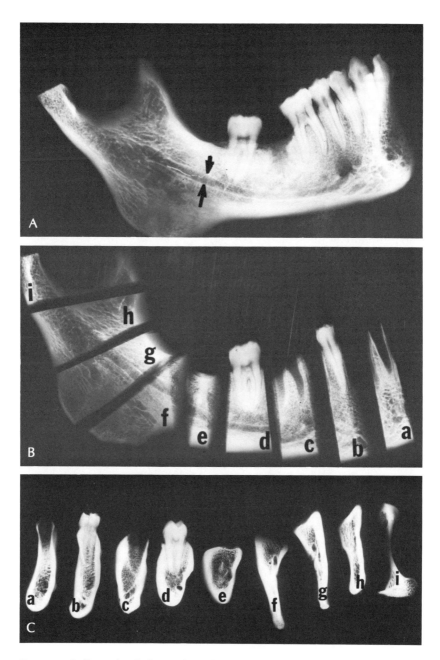

Fig. 5–1. Radiographs of a human lower jaw. *A,* Intact lower jaw. The second molar has been lost. Clearly visible within the jaw is the bony canal *(arrows),* which contains the nerves and the blood supply to the teeth and surrounding tissues. Notice that the peripheral parts of the jaw are lighter in the radiograph. This means that the bone in those parts is more compact than in the central regions. *B,* The same lower jaw as shown in *A.* The first molar and the first premolar have been removed, making the outlines of their bony sockets more clearly visible. The lower jaw has been cut into several sections (a through i). *C,* The cut sections of the lower jaw have been x-rayed individually, with their cut surfaces parallel to the x-ray film (turned 90 degrees from their orientation shown in *B).* The peripheral compact bone and the central spongy bone are clearly shown. In b through g, the dark openings of the cross-sectioned bony canal are visible.

77

This means that the intercellular substance of these tissues has assumed important properties.

Cartilage is a resilient "bouncy" tissue. It is uniquely suited to resist *compression* because 75% of its intercellular substance is composed of water and proteoglycan complexes.

Bone is a rigid tissue capable both of resisting *tension* and of giving *support.* It has these properties because almost 90% of the intercellular substance produced by the bone cells is composed of collagen fibers, and because the intercellular substance is impregnated with the mineral calcium salt: *hydroxyapatite.* This calcium salt does not allow x rays to pass through and thus is responsible for the images of bone on radiographs.

While bone is more important for the dental health professional, cartilage is found in several parts of the body that surround the oral cavity (Fig. 5–2). Furthermore, a knowledge of cartilage tissue is of use in understanding bone tissue. For this reason, we will start here with a description of cartilage.

CARTILAGE

Cartilage has the three components that are generally found in all connective tissues: *cells* (chondroblasts, chondrocytes), *fibrous matrix* (collagen and in special cases elastic fibers) and *ground substance* (mainly proteoglycans and glycoproteins in sizes and compositions that are specific for cartilage). Of these three components, the ground substance is the dominant one.

CELLS. Cartilage cells differentiate from the common forerunners of connective tissue cells: the mesenchymal cells. During their differentiation, these cells move closer together than the mesenchymal cells, which will form connective tissue proper. This *mesenchymal condensation* (Fig. 5–3) takes place before the cells start producing the fibrous matrix and ground substance characteristic of cartilage (review synthetic activities of a cell, Chap. 2).

With the production of these intercellular materials, the cells, now called *chondroblasts,* become eventually surrounded and enclosed by their own products. When this happens, they lose their contacts with the surrounding cells and come to lie in isolation in a small space or *lacuna* inside the intercellular substance. Once the cells are *enclosed* they are called *chondrocytes.* They slow down considerably in their synthetic activities, but they continue to be active in the turnover of the ground substance and some components of the fibrous matrix.

FIBROUS MATRIX. The fibrous matrix of cartilage contains several types of collagen that are unique to this tissue (Types II, IX,

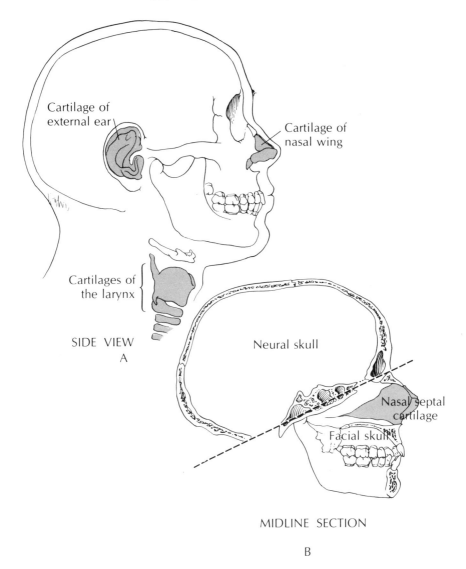

Fig. 5–2. Side View, *A,* and midline section, *B,* of a human skull, showing the bony components and the cartilaginous parts. In the adult, cartilage is found in the ear, the nose, and the larynx.

X, and XI). Among these, Type II collagen is dominant, forming a sparse meshwork of delicate collagen fibers.

GROUND SUBSTANCE. The ground substance of cartilage consists mainly of large proteoglycan complexes. The composition of those complexes and the chemical nature and relative sizes of their subunits are specific for cartilage. They largely determine the

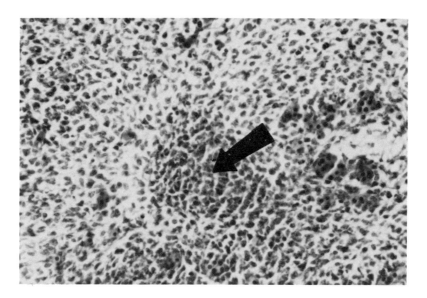

Fig. 5–3.   Histologic section through a mesenchymal condensation *(arrow)* in a 5½-week-old embryo. These condensed mesenchymal cells will soon start producing cartilage. Other mesenchymal condensations are present as well. Some of these will develop further into muscles, others into bone tissue. Original magnification × 100.

nature of this tissue. The ground substance is formed in such enormous amounts that it masks the fibrous matrix to the extent that it is no longer visible with conventional light microscopic techniques.

Cartilage Growth

Early cartilage resembles a gelatinous mass, in which chondrocytes are embedded. On the outside surface of this mass a layer of chondroblasts remains present. A cartilage mass may increase its size in two different ways (Figs. 5–4 and 5–5):

APPOSITIONAL GROWTH. This is the mechanism by which new cartilage is formed on the outside surface of the cartilage mass as the result of the synthetic activities of the layer of chondroblasts. These cells continue the production of new intercellular material, which is deposited at the circumference of the cartilage. Occasionally, one of the chondroblasts is enclosed in the matrix and becomes a new chondrocyte (Fig. 5–4).

INTERSTITIAL GROWTH. This is the mechanism by which a cartilage mass increases in size as the result of mitoses and the production of new intercellular substance by chondrocytes that are already surrounded by intercellular substance.

Once a chondrocyte is enclosed in a lacuna, it is still able to

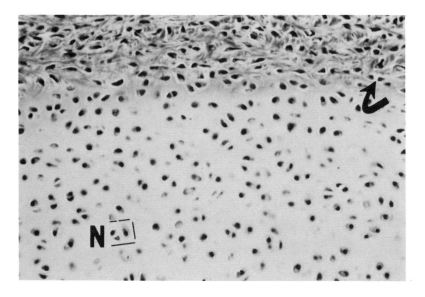

Fig. 5–4.   Histologic section through a cartilage structure in a newborn. The cartilage ground substance is the dominant component of this tissue, masking the fibrous matrix completely. Chondrocytes, fully enclosed within lacunae, are present throughout the tissue. Some are grouped in nest-like arrangements (N). At the periphery of the cartilage, the cell-rich zone of the perichondrium is visible. This zone contains chondroblasts, some of which are partially enclosed in lacunae (arrow), in the process of becoming chondrocytes. Original magnification × 100.

undergo some cell division or mitosis. The two resulting daughter cells utilize the somewhat fluid nature of the intercellular substance to "float apart," while producing a little more matrix in the process. As a result of the mitosis and of the synthetic activity, the daughter cells are found in *"cell nests,"* groups of two, three, or four chondrocytes, close enough to show their common descent, but enclosed in separate, individual lacunae.

The Perichondrium

With further development, the cartilage mass becomes more and more organized. The cartilage, with its peripheral layer of chondroblasts, becomes completely surrounded by a dense fibrous connective tissue layer. This layer, together with the layer of chondroblasts, is called *perichondrium* (literally, around the cartilage).

The perichondrium, in addition to its mechanical functions as a site of attachment for muscles and as an outer membrane, defining the shape of the cartilage mass, also contains most of the blood vessels, supplying the nutriments for the cartilage cells. The liquid nature of the intercellular substance of cartilage allows easy move-

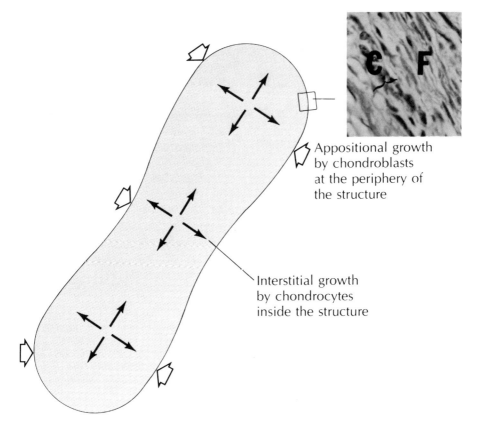

Appositional growth
by chondroblasts
at the periphery of
the structure

Interstitial growth
by chondrocytes
inside the structure

GROWTH OF A CARTILAGINOUS STRUCTURE

Fig. 5–5. Diagram of a cartilage structure. The small arrows within the structure indicate that it can increase its size "from within" by mitoses of the chondrocytes and production of new intercellular substance (interstitial growth). The larger, open, arrows indicate the second mechanism of growth of a cartilage structure by production of new cartilage "on the outside" (appositional growth). The chondroblasts in the inner layer of the perichondrium are responsible for the appositional growth. *Insert*, Histologic section showing the two-layered structure of perichondrium in a human fetus. An inner layer, adjacent to the cartilage, is cell-rich (C) and contains the chondroblasts. The outer layer of the perichondrium consists of densely arranged collagen fibers (F). There are some collagen fibers in the inner layer and some cells in the outer layer, but the layers of the perichondrium are named after their dominant components. Original magnification × 125.

ment *(diffusion)* of gases and nutriments to the chondrocytes and of metabolic waste products away from the chondrocytes. Thus, there is relatively little need for blood vessels to be present *inside* the cartilage tissue. Cartilage is sometimes called an *avascular* tissue (no blood vessels at all), but this is only true for small cartilage masses. Some blood vessels may run for some distance into *larger* masses of cartilage. We therefore prefer to call cartilage a *relatively avascular* tissue.

Different Types of Cartilage

The cartilage tissue we have described up to this point is *hyaline cartilage*, one of three types of cartilage found in the human body. We distinguish hyaline cartilage, fibrous cartilage and elastic cartilage.

HYALINE CARTILAGE. This is predominantly a compression-resistant tissue. Its intercellular substance is dominated by the ground substance, which masks the collagenous fibrous matrix. This "reinforced gelatin" type tissue is found in many areas of the body. In the head and neck region, hyaline cartilage is found in the skeleton of the nose, in the growing skull base, in the condylar head of the lower jaw and in the larynx.

All cartilages in the human body start out as hyaline cartilages, but depending on their specific locations and loading patterns, some cartilages may specialize further and become either fibrous or elastic cartilage.

FIBROUS CARTILAGE. In this type of cartilage, such large amounts of collagen fibers are added to the intercellular substance that the ground substance loses its relative prominence and the fibers are no longer masked, becoming visible with the light microscope. Microscopically, this tissue somewhat resembles tendon tissue, with the exception that the cells (chondrocytes) are enclosed in lacunae. There are no lacunae in tendon tissue. Fibrous cartilage is found in areas that are subjected to combinations of compression and tension, such as the discs in the vertebral column. In the head, only the temporomandibular joint of an older individual may contain some fibrous cartilage.

ELASTIC CARTILAGE. Normally, few or no elastic fibers are found in cartilage, but sometimes such fibers are *added* to the intercellular substance in cartilages that are in need of elastic rebound, such as the external ear and the epiglottis. The elastic fibers form a delicate fibrous matrix. They are not seen with conventional light microscopy, unless they are made visible with a specific elastic stain.

BONE

Bone has the three components commonly found in connective tissues: *cells* (osteoblasts, osteocytes, osteoclasts), *fibrous matrix* (Type I collagen fibers) and *ground substance* (mainly proteoglycans and glycoproteins in sizes and compositions that are specific for bone tissue). Of these three, the fibrous matrix is the dominant component. *In addition,* the nature of the bone tissue is determined, to a large extent, by the presence of calcium salts *(hydroxyapatite)* in its intercellular substance.

Biomechanically, bone is particularly well suited to resist tension and brief periods of compression. If placed under any prolonged compression, bone tissue will yield readily by disappearing (see discussion of bone resorption in this chapter).

Bone tissue has two principal functions: (1) it gives biomechanical support and protection to the associated tissues and organs; and (2) it serves as a large reservoir for calcium and phosphorus ions (hydroxyapatite is a calcium phosphate salt). Calcium and phosphorus ions are critical for the maintenance of life. To this end, these ions must be constantly present in the circulating blood, where their concentration levels have to be maintained within narrow limits— 10 mg Ca/100 ml blood and 6 mg P/100 ml blood. If these concentrations drop, immediate endocrine action stimulates increased breakdown of bone to liberate more ions. If the concentrations become too high, a different kind of endocrine action slows down the breakdown of bone.

For an understanding of bone tissue, it is necessary to understand not only its mode of formation, but also its constant *remodeling* throughout life: breakdown of bone tissue *(resorption)* and new formation of bone *(deposition).* In healthy adults, about 4% of all bone tissue is broken down at any given time.

Bone tissue is formed by *osteoblasts,* differentiated mesenchymal cells, but despite this common denominator, bone may develop in one of two different ways:

1. *Intramembranous ossification.* Mesenchymal cells move closer together (mesenchymal condensation), differentiate into osteoblasts and begin to produce the intercellular substance of bone directly.

2. *Endochondral ossification.* This is a process of bone formation with an intermediate stage. The future bone is preformed as a cartilage model. This is subsequently destroyed, and on its remains newly differentiated osteoblasts deposit bone tissue.

Figure 5–6 illustrates which parts of the bony skull are formed by intramembranous ossification and which by endochondral ossification. Without discussing each individual bone, it should be clear from this figure that the bones of the *cranial base,* between the neural skull and the facial skull, form by endochondral ossification, whereas the bones of the facial and neural skulls form largely by intramembranous ossification. Minor exceptions are a few bones in the nasal skeleton and the articulating condylar head of the lower jaw, all of which form endochondrally.

Intramembranous Ossification and Appositional Bone Growth

The initial stages of intramembranous ossification are similar to those of cartilage development. Mesenchymal cells move closer to-

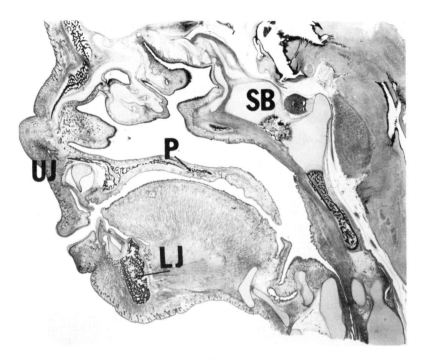

Fig. 5–6.   Histologic section, near the midline, through the facial region of a human fetus in the second trimester of pregnancy. Intramembranous ossification [direct bone formation] is taking place in the lower jaw (LJ), upper jaw (UJ), and palate (P). Endochondral ossification (bone formation, with an intermediate cartilage stage) occurs in the skull base (SB). Original magnification × 2. (Courtesy the late Dr. E. Applebaum.)

gether into mesenchymal condensations, differentiate into *osteoblasts* and begin to produce the intercellular substance that is characteristic for bone. As in the case of cartilage, the earliest osteoblasts soon become surrounded by their own products and they are enclosed in small spaces *(lacunae)* inside the bone tissue. The enclosed cells are *osteocytes.*

Bone formation involves one *additional* step, however: after some intercellular substance has been laid down by the osteoblasts, these cells now deposit calcium salts in it. The process of deposition of calcium salts in a previously formed intercellular substance is called *calcification.* In this case we speak of the calcification of bone. Many aspects of this very complicated process are understood; others are as yet to be elucidated. A calcifiable intercellular substance has specific chemical characteristics, which enable it to undergo calcification. Enzymes and a host of other compounds can act on this substance and modify it, thereby either stimulating calcification or inhibiting it.

The intercellular substance has a role in calcification, in that it permits calcium salts to be deposited in it. Whether it has also a more active role in promoting nucleation of calcium salts is unclear at this time. It is generally accepted that the cells (osteoblasts in this case) of a calcifying tissue play a role in the calcification process. In most cases calcium and phosphorus pass through the cells and are stored in the mitochondria, before being released in the intercellular substance as precursors of hydroxyapatite.

There is always a lag period between the time of intercellular substance synthesis and the full calcification of the bone tissue. Because of this, there is usually a thin, uncalcified layer of inter-cellular substance (the *osteoid seam)* immediately underneath the osteoblasts. This seam represents the most recently formed fibrous matrix and ground substance (Fig. 5–7).

OSTEOCYTES. Osteocytes differ from chondrocytes in two important aspects:

1. They do not become isolated in their *lacunae* like the chondrocytes, but retain gap junction contacts with neighboring osteocytes and osteoblasts. The cell processes, which make these contacts, are thin and are located inside narrow bony channels *(canaliculi),* which run from lacuna to lacuna and from lacuna to outside surface of the

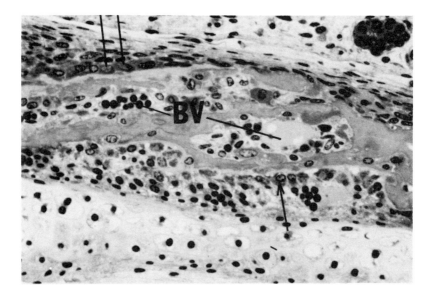

Fig. 5–7.   Histologic section, illustrating early intramembranous ossification in the upper jaw region. A delicate network of bone trabeculae alternates with a network of thin-walled blood vessels (BV). Osteoblasts *(arrows)* line the surfaces of the bone trabeculae. A thin band of uncalcified bone (osteoid) intervenes between osteoblasts and calcified bone. A few cells have become trapped in lacunae inside the bone substance. These cells (osteocytes) have slowed down their synthetic activities considerably. Original magnification × 125.

bone mass. The osteocytic lacunae, therefore, do not have a smooth, rounded outline, but are rather spider-shaped instead.

2. They are surrounded by a *calcified* intercellular substance. This means that there is no room for further cell divisions and therefore the bone *cannot* grow by interstitial growth.

Furthermore, the calcified bone is an effective barrier, preventing diffusion of nutrients, gases and waste products. Instead, all this transport must take place through canaliculi between the outside of the bone and the individual lacunae. This type of transport can only take place over a limited distance (about 200 μm), which is the farthest distance an osteocyte may be removed from a blood vessel. Thus, while cartilage is relatively avascular, bone tissue is vascular.

Because of the high metabolic activities of osteoblasts and osteocytes, *and* because blood vessels are needed in the proximity of all bone cells, the entire appearance of a developing bone is from the start different from that of a developing cartilage structure (Fig. 5–8).

A cartilage structure develops as one solid, homogeneous mass. A bone structure develops as a loose network of bone trabeculae, associated with a network of blood vessels in the spaces between the trabeculae. Each bone trabecula consists of a mass of calcified bone substance with osteocytes in their lacunae. Along the periphery of the trabecula is an osteoid seam, covered by a layer of osteoblasts. Each individual bone trabecula grows by *appositional growth* only. Interstitial growth is not possible in bone tissue.

PERIOSTEUM. Individual trabeculae are surrounded only

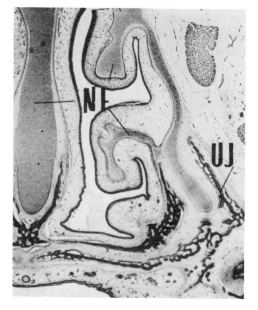

Fig. 5–8. Histologic section through one half of the upper jaw region of a human fetus in the second trimester of pregnancy. This section shows a fundamental difference in appearance between developing cartilage and bone tissues. The cartilage of the nasal frame (NF) is one solid, homogeneous mass, somewhat thickened at the edges. The bone of the developing upper jaw (UJ) and palate consists of a delicate network of bone trabeculae, which alternates with a network of blood vessels (the latter are not visible at this magnification). Original magnification × 2. (Courtesy the late Dr. E. Applebaum.)

by cells (mainly osteoblasts). The activities of the osteoblasts that surround the individual bone trabeculae, produce an increase in the size of the trabeculae. This does *not* make the bone as a whole larger, just more compact.

Around the developing bone as a whole (the entire complex of bone trabeculae and blood vessels), a *periosteum* develops in time. It consists, as does a perichondrium, of a dense fibrous layer on the outside and an inner cellular (osteoblasts) layer, next to the surfaces of the outermost bone trabeculae.

The activities of the osteoblasts of the inner layer of the periosteum are responsible for an increase in the external dimensions of the bone (Fig. 5–9).

Compact and Spongy Bone; Woven and Lamellar Bone

When a bone is studied on a radiograph or cut open and inspected with the unaided eye, *compact* and *spongy bone* may be distinguished in it. This is a gross distinction, based on how much of the volume of the bone actually is occupied by bone tissue.

At the microscopic level another kind of distinction is possible, between two types of bone tissue: *woven* and *lamellar* bone. This distinction is based on the organization of the fibrous matrix within the tissue.

WOVEN, *Spongy* BONE. The earliest formed bone has a fibrous matrix, which consists of a three-dimensional collagenous meshwork. These collagen fibers have no distinct preferential orientation. Such bone tissue is called woven bone. Woven bone is usually composed of trabeculae and is therefore classified as *spongy* (see Fig. 5–8).

LAMELLAR BONE. When bone tissue becomes functionally

Fig. 5–9.   *A,* The trabecular network of spongy woven bone in a histologic section through the lower jaw of a human fetus. Each trabecula is lined with osteoblasts. Continued bone deposition by these cells makes the individual trabeculae thicker and thus the bone as a whole more compact. A fibrous layer of periosteum (P) is forming at the periphery of the entire complex of bone trabeculae. This periosteum outlines the shape of the future bone. Original magnification × 40. *B,* Compact lamellar bone at the periphery of the lower jaw of an adult. The only interruptions in this bone mass are the channels *(large arrows)* carrying the blood supply of the bone cells in the osteocytic lacunae. This compact bone was formed, in part, as the result of bone deposition around the individual trabeculae, making the bone more compact, and, in part, as the result of deposition of lamellar bone by the osteoblasts in the periosteum. The dark lines in the bone are arrest lines (A) and reversal lines (R), evidence of the constant remodeling of bone tissue. Original magnification × 40.

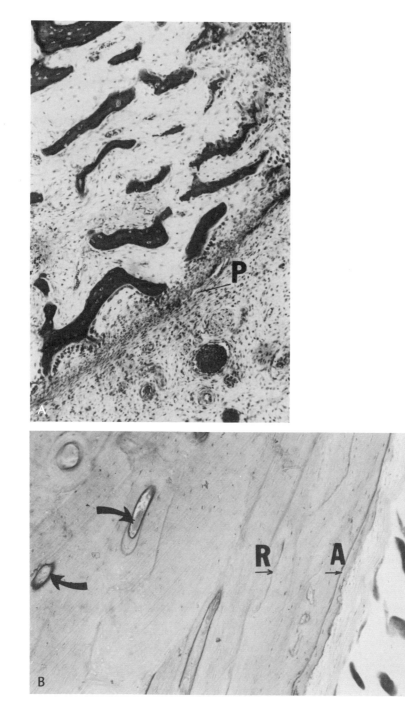

loaded, it is in need of a better engineering design, and the woven bone is gradually replaced by *lamellar bone.* Lamellar bone is somewhat comparable to plywood. It consists of a series of thin sheets, or *lamellae,* 4 to 7 μm wide. Within each sheet the collagen fibers run parallel to each other, but in a different direction from that of the collagen fibers in the adjacent sheets. This arrangement gives the mature bone tissue an optimal ability to withstand the varieties of loading patterns imposed on it. Generally, all bone tissue that is formed after birth is lamellar. Lamellar bone may be either *compact* or *spongy.*

Lamellar Compact Bone. At the periphery of a bone, such as the lower jaw, the osteoblasts of the periosteum produce a series of lamellae, parallel to each other and to the bone surface. These lamellae form a dense, *compact* layer of bone. However, the thickness of this layer is limited by the nutritional needs of the osteocytes. This need may be solved in different ways (Fig. 5–10): (1) inclusion of a blood vessel from the surrounding periosteum; and (2) breakdown of some older lamellar bone and outgrowth of a branch of a neighboring blood vessel in this newly created space. This blood vessel is subsequently surrounded by new bone.

A special type of lamellar compact bone is the bone that is deposited around existing blood vessels. As the result of its particular location, this bone forms a hollow cylinder of *concentric lamellae,* an *osteon.* Owing to its arrangement, an osteon has particular biomechanical properties that make it well suited to resist a large variety of loading patterns, such as those applied to the long bones of the limbs, where osteons are found in large numbers.

In the flat bones of the skull, osteons are not as numerous. The predominant pattern of compact bone in these bones is one of flat, parallel lamellae.

Lamellar Spongy Bone. The trabeculae in the spongy bone areas of the jaws consist of lamellar bone as well. Just as with compact bone, the spongy bone undergoes constant remodeling. The orientation of the trabeculae is a good indication of the loading patterns imposed on the bone. In general, the trabeculae are oriented in two main directions: one is parallel with the principal loading direction; the other is at right angles with the first. If the loading pattern changes, bone remodeling follows, adjusting the size and/or orientations of the bone trabeculae to the new condition.

Between the bone trabeculae *bone marrow* may be found. This specialized connective tissue consists of fat and/or blood forming cells. A characteristic of spongy bone is that the overall volume of the marrow is greater than that of the bone mass.

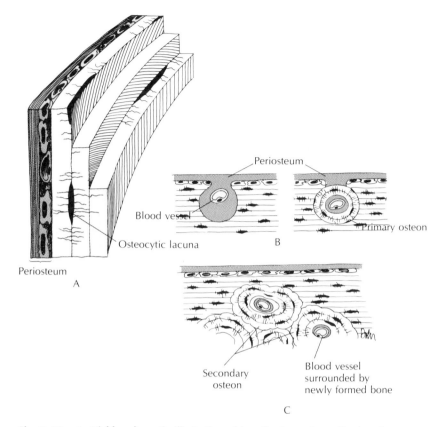

Periosteum

Blood vessel

Osteocytic lacuna

B

Primary osteon

Periosteum

A

Secondary
osteon

Blood vessel
surrounded by
newly formed bone

C

Fig. 5–10. *A,* Highly schematic illustration of lamellar bone, immediately adjacent to periosteum. Osteoblasts comprise the inner layer of the periosteum, between the dense fibrous outer layer and the bone lamellae. Three lamellae are illustrated, with some (dark) osteocytic lacunae. The collagen fiber direction in the bone of the individual lamellae is indicated by parallel lines. Note that, within each lamella, all collagen fibers run parallel to each other, but in a different direction than the collagen fibers in adjacent lamellae. *B,* Enclosure of a periosteal blood vessel and formation of a primary osteon around it. The periosteal osteoblasts produce layer upon layer of bone lamellae, parallel to the outer bone surface. Occasionally, a blood vessel of the periosteum is left behind in the developing bone. Osteoblasts line the surface of the hollow space around the blood vessel and these cells produce concentric bone lamellae, forming a primary osteon around the blood vessel. *C,* Formation of secondary osteons. If continued bone lamella production by periosteal osteoblasts is not accompanied by occasional blood vessel inclusion, some of the older lamellar bone will be broken down. This older bone is located more centrally (deeper). After the breakdown, branches of neighboring blood vessels grow out into this newly established space. Around each of these blood vessel branches, new, concentric bone lamellae are deposited and a secondary osteon is formed. A secondary osteon differs from a primary osteon in that a secondary osteon has a scalloped, not smooth, outer surface. The surface is scalloped because bone breakdown precedes the formation of a secondary osteon. The scalloped edge reflects the final resorption surface, with resorption lacunae— the "last bites," as it were, into the bone tissue, during the process of breakdown.

Bone Resorption

Several times in the foregoing discussion the concept of *bone breakdown* or *resorption* has been mentioned. Bone resorption may take place for two different reasons:

1. Adaptation of the internal and/or external structure of the bone to altered loading conditions. In this case, resorption is usually a *localized* process.,

2. Liberation of calcium and phosphorus ions in response to endocrine activity. In this case, resorption is a *general* process throughout the body.

Bone resorption involves two activities, dissolution of bone salts (by acid from the lysosomes, released outside the cell) and breakdown of intercellular bone substance (a digestive activity, also involving lysosomes). While osteoblasts and osteocytes are moderately capable of some bone resorption (of intercellular substance), the resorption of calcified bone tissue is done by a special cell type, which differentiates when the need arises and disappears again when the job is done.

This cell is the *osteoclast.* It forms by fusions of several cells of bone marrow origin. These cells are related to the cells of the monocyte line (macrophages, see Chap. 4) and are carried to the bone resorption site via the blood vessels. The osteoclast is *large* and it contains several nuclei (usually 4 to 10). It has a large number of lysosomes for its digestive activities (Fig. 5–11).

The resorption process is inititated by the *osteoblasts.* These cells prepare the bone surface that will be broken down and then move away to allow the osteoclasts to move next to the bone surface (see the two possible configurations in Fig. 5–12). An osteoclast seals off the area with a seal reminiscent of a suction cup. In this way the cell can discharge acid and lysosomal enzymes without harming other parts of the surrounding tissues, which should be preserved.

If an osteoclast is located on a flat bone surface, the localized bone resorption results in a concavity or *resorption lacuna* (Howship's lacuna). At the end of the resorption period a bone may have many of these concavities. Before disappearing from the scene the osteoclast prepares the bone surface for osteoblasts to start depositing new bone again.

Arrest Lines and Reversal Lines

A histologic section of bone can reveal much of the history of this tissue because of the presence of *arrest lines* and *reversal lines.* A layer of osteoblasts involved in bone deposition occasionally takes a rest stop before continuing with further bone deposition. In the

OSTEOCLAST

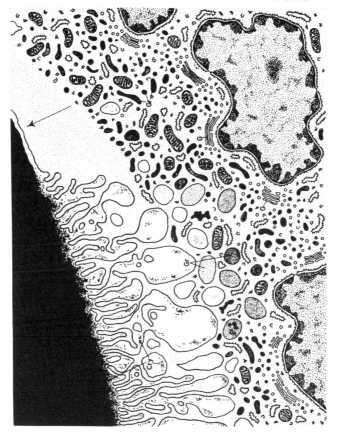

Fig. 5–11.   Diagram illustrating the ultrastructure of part of an osteoclast. The dark mass in the lower left hand corner is the bone, which is about to be resorbed. In the osteoclast, parts of three nuclei are visible. The cell contains an extensive Golgi complex (G), numerous mitochondria and lysosomes. A small section of the cell membrane lies flat against the surface of the bone *(arrow)*, and the adjacent cytoplasm is very clear. This is the region of the seal, which completely surrounds the digesting surface of the osteoclast. That part of the osteoclast's membrane which is engaged in bone resorption (digestive activity) is thrown into large folds (ruffled border). This substantially increases the surface area of the cell. Gr = granules (lysosomal). (From Lentz, T.L.: *Cell Fine Structure. An Atlas of Drawings of Whole Cell Structure.* Philadelphia, W.B. Saunders Co., 1971.)

bone tissue such a rest stop shows up as a clearly marked *arrest line.* Arrest lines are relatively smooth. They consist of intercellular substance with less collagen and relatively more ground substance than is present in the rest of the tissue. Because of this, arrest lines stain differently (they are more acid) and remain visible in the bone tissue formed before and after the rest stop (Fig. 5–13, A).

Reversal lines are lines that stain much the same as arrest lines,

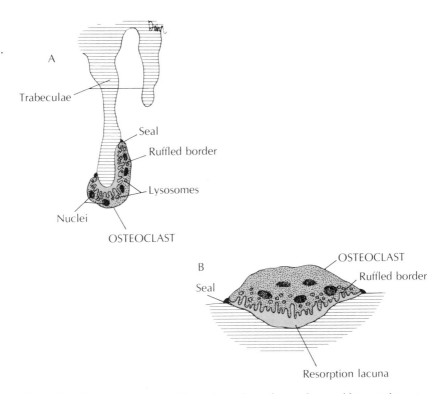

Fig. 5–12. Diagrams of two possible configurations of osteoclasts and bone surface. *A,* **An osteoclast is perched on the tip of a bone trabecula, partially surrounding it. The resorption will result in a reduction in length of the trabecula.** *B,* **An osteoclast is located on a flat surface of bone. In this case, resorption will result in the illustrated depression (or resorption lacuna) in the bone surface. Notice, in both cells, the seal, which surrounds the ruffled border area and localizes the resorption process. Multiple nuclei and lysosomes are illustrated.**

but reversal lines are scalloped, not smooth. They represent the terminal location of a series of resorption lacunae. Following the termination of the resorption process, new osteoblasts differentiated and deposited bone tissue. Thus, the resorption cavities were filled with new bone, and the bone surface was gradually smoothed in the process (Fig. 5–13, B).

Endochondral Ossification

In areas where there is an early need for skeletal support, during prenatal development, some bones are preformed as cartilaginous models. The advantage of such cartilage models is that they provide early, resilient support for the developing body and, at the same

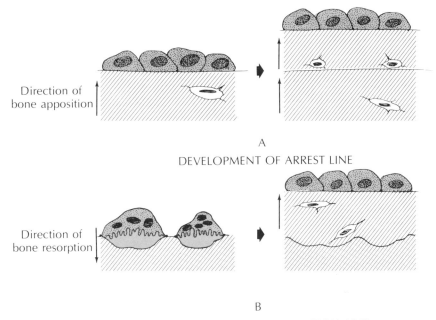

A

DEVELOPMENT OF ARREST LINE

B

DEVELOPMENT OF REVERSAL LINE

Direction of
bone apposition

Direction of
bone resorption

Fig. 5–13. *A,* An arrest line is formed in bone when the process of bone deposition, by a layer of osteoblasts, is temporarily halted and subsequently resumed. The small arrows indicate the direction in which the bone surface moves. *B,* A reversal line is formed in bone when the process of bone resorption, by a layer of osteoclasts, is halted and followed by the deposition of a new layer of bone by osteoblasts. The small arrows indicate the opposite directions in which the bone surface moves during the resorption and the apposition of bone. Since a bone surface, which undergoes bone deposition, is smooth, an arrest line is smooth. Since resorption creates resorption lacunae on a bone surface, a reversal line, reflecting the final resorption surface, is scalloped.

time, serve as important sites of growth because of the ability of cartilage to grow interstitially.

Bone tissue gradually *replaces* the cartilage models. This is done by breakdown of the cartilage tissue, in localized areas, and deposition of bone tissue on the cartilage remnants. The cartilage must undergo two important changes before it can be broken down and replaced by bone: chondrocytic hypertrophy and calcification of the intercellular substance of cartilage (cartilage matrix).

In *chondrocytic hypertrophy* the individual chondrocytes become much larger and vacuolated.

In *cartilage matrix calcification* the hypertrophic chondrocytes change the composition of the cartilage matrix and then deposit hydroxyapatite salts in it.

The process of endochondral ossification in the skull is rather complex, and so we will demonstrate its principles on one of the long limb bones, which also form by endochondral ossification (Fig. 5–14).

Chondrocytic hypertrophy and cartilage calcification occur first in the middle and then slowly spread toward the two ends of the long bone model. Simultaneously, a collar of bone is deposited by osteoblasts on the outside surface of the cartilage, at the level of the earliest cartilage changes. This bone collar expands toward the two ends of the model at approximately the same rate at which the cartilage changes spread inside the model. The bone collar serves as an external scaffold, taking over the support function of the changed cartilage tissue, which will be removed.

A blood vessel, accompanied by differentiating osteoblasts and osteoclasts, invades the cartilage model and begins its destruction and replacement. The calcified cartilage with the hypertrophic chondrocytes is invaded by numerous branches of this blood vessel. The osteoclasts remove much of the calcified intercellular substance. On some of the cartilage remnants the osteoblasts begin to deposit bone tissue. While the already changed cartilage is thus broken down and replaced by the first bone trabeculae, the processes of chondrocytic hypertrophy and cartilage calcification spread farther in opposite directions toward the two ends of the cartilage model.

If no further growth activity would take place in the remainder of the cartilage model, the process of its replacement would be finished rapidly. However, before the chondrocytes hypertrophy and participate in the calcification of the intercellular substance, they usually undergo several mitoses, thus further enlarging the cartilage model interstitially.

In the long bones, all growth in length is due to the interstitial enlargement, resulting from mitoses and hypertrophy, of the cartilage, before it is replaced by bone. Once bone tissue has replaced the cartilage, only appositional growth is possible, leading largely to an increase in the width of these bones. No significant amounts of bone form on the joint surfaces at the ends of the bones. These remain covered with hyaline cartilage, which is able to resist the compressive loading placed on the joint surfaces in function. Once all the cartilage of the original model is removed (with the exception of the cartilage on the joint surfaces), the growth in length of a long bone stops. Any further bone formation can only produce a wider bone with greater density, but not a longer bone.

Frequently, more than one site of bone formation is found in the cartilage model of a long bone. Such *ossification centers* spread individually, so that soon only narrow strips of cartilage, *growth plates,* remain. Usually, two growth plates are found in the long bones of growing individuals. When skeletal maturity is reached, generally in the teenage years, the chondrocytes in the growth plates stop

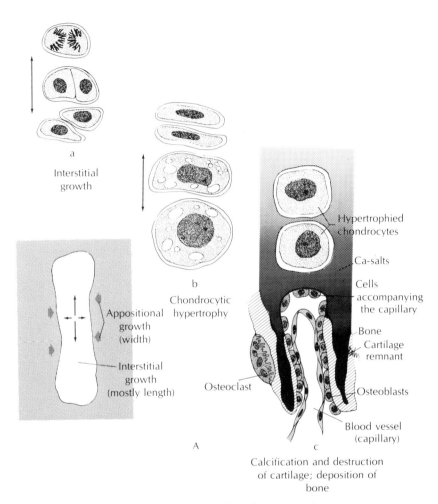

Interstitial growth

a

Interstitial
growth

Appositional
growth
(width)

Interstitial
growth
(mostly length)

A

b

Chondrocytic hypertrophy

Osteoclast

Hypertrophied
chondrocytes

Ca-salts

Cells
accompanying
the capillary

Bone

Cartilage
remnant

Osteoblasts

Blood vessel
(capillary)

c

Calcification and destruction
of cartilage; deposition of
bone

Fig. 5–14. *A,* In a cartilaginously preformed model of a long bone, most appositional growth results in an increase in width of the model, while interstitial growth is largely responsible for the increase in length. In *a* we show diagrammatically how, during this interstitial growth, the cells stack vertically into a column after mitosis. The next event, illustrated in *b*, hypertrophy of the chondrocytes, also leads to an increase in the vertical dimensions of the cartilage mass. In the final stages of chondrocytic hypertrophy, the cartilage matrix, between the columns of hypertrophied chondrocytes, is calcified. Once the matrix is calcified, the cartilage can be resorbed and replaced by bone. As illustrated in *c*, small blood vessels grow toward this calcified cartilage. Some mesenchymal cells, which accompany them, break down most of the cartilage. Other cells come along with blood vessels, differentiate into osteoblasts and begin to deposit bone on the cartilage remnants. This new bone is not long lived. Remodeling (by osteoclasts) soon follows, removing most of the young bone and leaving behind a marrow cavity. As is stated in the text, *b* and *c* must occur before endochondral ossification can take place. Although *a* usually precedes *b* and *c*, it is not a necessary condition for endochondral ossification.

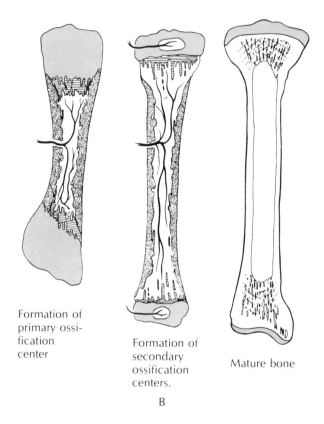

Formation of primary ossi-fication center

Formation of secondary ossification centers.

Mature bone

B

Fig. 5–14 *(Continued)*.   *B,* Three stages in the ossification of a long bone in the limb are illustrated. *Formation of a primary ossification center:* The earliest destruction of cartilage and replacement by bone occur in the middle of the shaft of a long bone model. The processes then continue, in two opposite directions, toward the ends of the model. Notice that most of the cartilage is not replaced by bone and that a large central marrow cavity remains. *Formation of secondary ossification centers:* In the cartilage masses at the ends of the long bone model, smaller, separate ossification centers are established. Endochondral ossification spreads in these areas from the center toward the periphery. Note that two narrow plates of cartilage remain between the primary and secondary ossification centers. These are the growth plates of the long bone. They are responsible for the further (interstitial) growth in length of the bone and will remain in existence until skeletal maturity is reached and growth ceases. In these growth plates, endochondral ossification, as illustrated in Figure 5–14 *A,* continues. At puberty, the growth plates disappear. The long bone now consists entirely of bone, with a central marrow cavity. Some spongy bone is found near the ends, but most of the shaft consists of compact lamellar bone, with many osteons. The two joint surfaces at the ends remain covered with hyaline cartilage throughout the individual's life.

undergoing mitoses. The remaining cells hypertrophy, the cartilage is calcified, and then the whole growth plate is broken down and replaced with bone.

Once endochondral ossification is completed and the growing cartilages are resorbed, the individual bone has attained its final length. However, if a growth cartilage is destroyed *before* it has stopped growing, for instance, as the result of an accident or a bad infection, further growth in length of the bone is halted, and it will be abnormally shorter for the rest of the individual's life. A well-known example of what can happen to the growth of long bones, when cartilage stops growing before sexual maturity is reached, is the growth retardation in poliomyelitis.

JOINTS

Joints are the structures between two adjacent bones. The following joints are found in the skull (Fig. 5–15): sutures, synchondroses, and the temporomandibular joint.

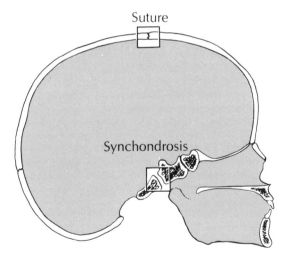

Fig. 5–15.   Diagram, showing locations of a suture and a synchondrosis in a child's skull. A third type of joint, the temporomandibular joint, is found between the lower jaw and the rest of the skull, just in front of the ear. There are several sutures in the skull, many of which remain visible throughout life. During fetal life, there are also several synchondroses in the endochondrally ossifying skull base. Only one of these, however, persists after birth until skeletal maturity is reached. This synchondrosis, the spheno-occipital synchondrosis, is illustrated in this figure.

Sutures

Sutures are dense, fibrous connections between adjacent *intra-membranously* formed bones. Some minor movements between these bones are made possible by the sutures. Sutures have several functions:

1. They allow passage of a baby's head through the narrow birth canal, by letting adjacent bones of the skull overlap, thus temporarily reducing the size of the skull.

2. They serve as shock breakers. If sutures were not present, the skull would more easily fracture on impact.

3. They serve as sites of appositional bone growth, at the free edges of the bones, during the period of growth. This results in an increase in the size of the individual bones and thus in an increase in overall skull size.

Histologically, a suture is composed of the meeting edges of the adjacent bones, their periosteal coverings and an intermediate connective tissue layer.

The bone edges may be smooth or irregular, straight or beveled. Each bone is covered with a layer of periosteum, composed of an inner layer of osteoblasts and occasionally osteoclasts, next to the bone surface, and an outer fibrous layer. The osteoblasts are capable of increasing the dimensions of the bones by appositional growth. If the dimensions of the individual bones increase, the skull as a whole increases in size. Between the two opposing fibrous layers of periosteum, a middle layer is present. This layer consists of dense fibrous connective tissue, with many collagen fibers running from one fibrous layer to the other. The middle layer also contains the blood supply for the periosteal osteoblasts (Fig. 5–16).

SYNCHONDROSES. A synchondrosis is a cartilaginous joint between two adjacent endochondrally formed bones of the skull. This joint allows a little movement between the bones, but its major role is to serve as a site of growth, by endochondral ossification, of the two adjacent bones.

Synchondroses are found in the skull base of a *growing* individual only. One synchondrosis, the spheno-occipital synchondrosis (located between sphenoid and occipital bones), continues to undergo endochondral ossification until skeletal maturity at about 16 years of age. At that time, it generally disappears. The structure of a synchondrosis resembles two growth plates mounted "back to back." We call this structure bipolar, which means that endochondral ossification takes place at both ends of a synchondrosis, leading to an increase in the length of the bones of the cranial base and of the cranial base itself (Fig. 5–17).

TEMPOROMANDIBULAR JOINT. The joint between the

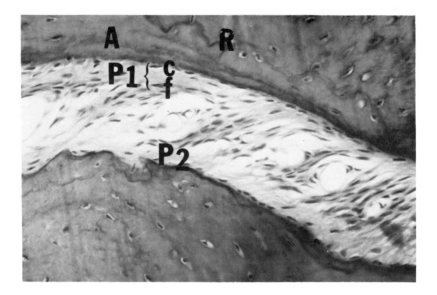

Fig. 5–16. Suture in a histologic section through the midline of the hard palate in a young primate. The two bone edges are visible with several distinct layers of intervening soft tissues: cellular layer, mostly osteoblasts (c), and fibrous layer (f) of the periosteum of one bone edge (P1) and cellular and fibrous layers of the periosteum (P2) covering the second bone edge form a sandwich arrangement with a richly vascularized middle layer. In this last layer, collagen fibers run obliquely between the two periostea (P1 and P2). A reversal line (R) and several arrest lines (A) are visible in the bones themselves, attesting to a certain amount of bone remodeling in the suture. Original magnification × 100.

lower jaw (mandible) and the rest of the skull, the temporomandibular joint, is the only joint in the skull with joint cavities, making this a freely moveable joint. The joint is between the endochondrally formed part of the mandible, the *condylar head* (the rest of the mandible is formed by intramembranous ossification), and the intramembranously formed *articular tubercle* on the zygomatic process of the temporal bone. The structure of the joint is shown in Figure 5–18. Since both the mandibular condyle and the articular tubercle have convex surfaces, a bi-concave disc of dense collagenous tissue intervenes between the two surfaces, to make them compatible for joint motion.

The articular surfaces of the temporomandibular joint are somewhat unlike the joint surfaces of most other joints in the body in that they are covered with a dense fibrous connective tissue (later in life they may become covered with fibrocartilage), rather than with hyaline cartilage.

In growing individuals the condyle consists of a mass of hyaline cartilage, in which the chondrocytes are undergoing hypertrophy and the cartilage matrix becomes calcified. This endochondral os-

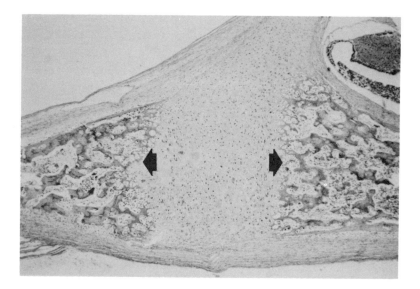

Fig. 5–17.   Midline section through the spheno-occipital synchondrosis in the skull base of a newborn primate. The surface facing the brain is at the top, while the surface facing the pharynx is at the bottom. The cartilaginous synchondrosis undergoes the process of endochondral ossification at both ends (arrows) somewhat resembling a bipolar growth plate. Original magnification × 12.5.

Fig. 5–18.   *A*, Histologic section through the temporomandibular joint of a young primate. AT = articular tubercle; D = articular disc; C = mandibular condylar head. The articular disc and the covering layers of the articular tubercle and mandibular condylar head consist of dense collagenous, fibrous connective tissue (1). Between the bone and the fibrous layer of the articular tubercle, a darkly staining layer of calcified cartilage is present (3). In the mandibular condylar head, endochondral ossification of the hyaline cartilage layer (2) is taking place, allowing for vertical growth of that part of the lower jaw. There is little interstitial growth in this cartilage. Most growth is the result of the appositional activities of the chondroblasts, located underneath the fibrous layer *(arrow)*. When skeletal maturity is reached, most cartilage will be replaced by bone in the condylar head, which will resemble histologically the articular tubercle. Original magnification × 10. *B,* The temporomandibular joint of a young adult man, seen in histologic section. AT = articular tubercle; D = articular disc; C = mandibular condylar head. Some fibers of the lateral pterygoid muscle are visible, inserting into the periosteum of the neck of the condyle *(arrow).* The upper and the lower joint cavities appear as light spaces. In the back, part of a section through the joint capsule is seen (at the right side). Original magnification × 2. (Courtesy the late Dr. E. Applebaum.)

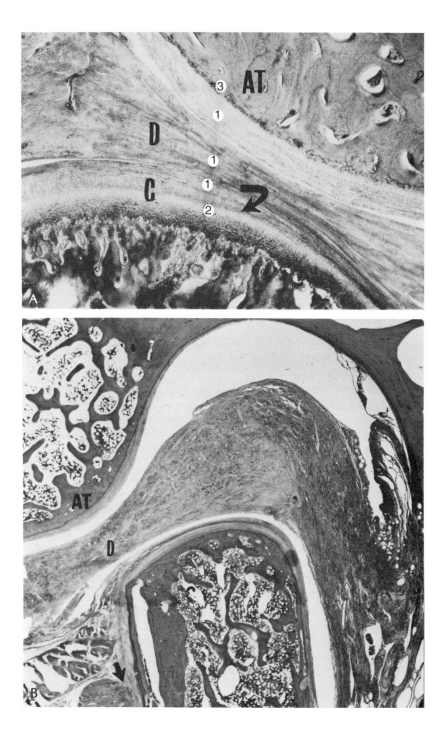

sification process occurs at a slow pace and is responsible for the increase in height of the ramus of the mandible.

An unusual feature is that no interstitial mitotic activity takes place in this cartilage. We see mostly *appositional* growth here, with a layer of chondroblasts located underneath the fibrous articular surface layer. This process of endochondral ossification is completed between the ages of 18 and 30 years. At that time all hyaline cartilage underneath the fibrous layer is calcified and/or replaced by bone tissue.

The *articular tubercle* is also covered with a fibrous layer. This may become fibrocartilage in the deeper areas of this layer, which covers the bone of the tubercle directly.

Surrounding the temporomandibular joint components is an *articular capsule,* consisting of an outer layer of dense fibrous connective tissue and an inner layer of loose connective tissue with a rich network of blood vessels. The innermost lining or *synovial lining* of this capsule faces directly the joint cavities (upper and lower, separated from each other by the *articular disc)* and consists of a layer of fibroblasts. These cells produce macromolecular (protein-carbohydrate) substances, which are added to the fluid that has filtered out of the blood vessels. This filtered fluid with the macromolecular substances is the *synovia,* the lubricant of the joint cavities.

On the outer surface of the joint capsule, at the level of the disc, and on the neck of the mandibular condyle, two parts of the lateral pterygoid muscle attach. This muscle moves both disc and condyle forward during mouth opening and is one of the four major *masticatory* muscles.

SELECTED READING LIST

Betts, F., Blumenthal, N.C., and Posner, A.S.: Bone mineralization. J. Crystal Growth, *53*:63, 1981.

Bloom, W., and Bloom, M.A.: Calcification and ossification. Calcification of developing bones in embryonic and newborn rats. Anat. Rec., *78*:497, 1940.

Boyde, A., and Jones, S.J.: Early scanning electron microscopic studies of hard tissue resorption: their relation to current concepts reviewed. Scanning Microsc., *1*:369, 1987.

Durkin, J., Heeley, J., and Irving, J.T.: The cartilage of the mandibular condyle. Oral Sci. Rev., *2*:29, 1973.

Enlow, D.H.: *The Human Face. An Account of the Postnatal Growth and Development of the Craniofacial Skeleton.* New York, Harper & Row, 1968.

Enlow, D.H.: *Handbook of Facial Growth.* 2nd Ed. Philadelphia, W.B. Saunders Co., 1982.

Hall, B.K.: Earliest evidence of cartilage and bone development in embryonic life. Clin. Orthop., *225*:255, 1987.

Hall, B.K.: The embryonic development of bone. Am. Sci., *76*:174, 1988.

Hancox, N.M.: *Biology of Bone.* London, Cambridge University Press, 1972.

Lacroix, P.: The internal remodeling of bones. In *The Biochemistry and Physiology of Bone. Vol. III. Development and Growth.* 2nd Ed. Edited by G.H. Bourne. New York, Academic Press, 1971.

Lentz, T.: *Cell Fine Structure. An Atlas of Drawings of Whole Cell Structure.* Philadelphia, W.B. Saunders Co., 1971.

Moss-Salentijn, L., Moss, M.L., Shinozuka, M., and Skalak, R.: Morphological analysis and computer-aided, three dimensional reconstruction of chondrocytic columns in rabbit growth plates. J. Anat., *151*:157, 1987.

Roughley, P.J., and Mort, J.S.: Ageing and the aggregating proteoglycans of human articular cartilage. Clin. Sci., *71*:337, 1986.

Sperber, G.H.: *Craniofacial Embryology.* 4th Ed. Dental Practitioners Handbook #15. London, Wright, 1989.

Uhthoff, H.T., and Wiley, J.J. (eds.): *Behavior of the Growth Plate.* New York, Raven Press, 1988.

Vaes, G.: Cellular biology and biomechanical mechanism of bone resorption. A review of recent developments on the formation, activation, and mode of action of osteoclasts. Clin. Orthop., *231*:239, 1988.

Vaughan, J.: *The Physiology of Bone.* 3rd Ed. Oxford, Oxford University Press, 1981.

Wagemans, P.A.H., Velde, J.P. van de, and Kuijpers-Jagtman, A.M.: Sutures and forces: a review. Am. J. Orthod. Dentofac. Orthop., *94*:129, 1988.

Wijngaert, F.P. van de, Schipper, C.A., Tas, M.C., and Burger, E.H.: Role of mineralizing cartilage in osteoclast and osteoblast recruitment. Bone, *9*:81, 1988.

6

Muscle and Nerve Tissue;
Blood Vessels and Blood;
Lymphatics

During inspection of the oral cavity, you may observe that some parts, such as the lips and cheeks, tongue and soft palate, can be moved at will. These parts contain a central core of *muscle tissue,* a tissue specialized in contractions, which is responsible for the observed movements.

In this chapter we will have a closer look at the constituents of muscle tissue and their relationship to the other structures of the oral cavity. In addition, we will describe components of two other systems essential to the function and maintenance of tissues around the oral cavity: the *vascular* system and the *nervous* system. This chapter will end with a brief description of lymph vessels and lymphatic tissue, as they relate to the orofacial region.

MUSCLE TISSUE

Muscle tissue consists predominantly of *cells* that have differentiated from embryonic mesenchymal cells to become highly specialized in *contracting* or shortening. This specialization, compared with specialization in other cell types, involves the production of considerable amounts of *intracellular,* contractile protein filaments. These protein filaments largely determine the appearance of the muscle cells, because of their abundance and their organization inside the muscle cells and also because of their staining properties.

The contraction of the individual muscle cells would have little effect on the tissues to be moved as the result of the muscle contraction if these cells were not organized, packed together, and tied to each other and the surrounding tissues in a specific manner. Muscle tissue proper consists of *specialized muscle cells* that are bound together functionally by a *connective tissue framework.* This same connective tissue also carries the rich blood vessel and nerve supplies needed for the function of the muscle.

There are *three types* of muscle tissue: skeletal (striated) muscle tissue, smooth muscle tissue, and heart muscle tissue.

SKELETAL (STRIATED) MUSCLE TISSUE. In skeletal muscles, contractions are generally under our own control and are therefore called *voluntary.* By and large, these contractions are rapid, short in duration and powerful (although these characteristics may show some variation, depending on the function of the particular muscle).

Skeletal muscle contractions are initiated by stimuli of motor nerves (this chapter). These muscles are found wherever skeletal elements are to be moved relative to each other (example: masticatory

Table 6–1.   Nomenclature of Striated Muscle Tissue

	Intracellular structures
Myofibrils	Bundles of contractile protein filaments found in the muscle fibers.
Myofilaments	Contractile protein filaments composed of either actin or myosin.
Sarcomere	The contractile unit of a myofibril.
Sarcolemma	The outer membrane of a muscle fiber, consisting of the lipoprotein membrane of the cell, plus a basal lamina.
Sarcoplasm	The cytoplasm of the muscle cell.
Sarcoplasmic reticulum	A modified type of agranular endoplasmic reticulum, composed of tubules and cisternae; it is found in the sarcoplasm and forms a canalicular arrangement around each myofibril.
Transverse tubules (T-tubules)	A narrow transverse tubule that extends inward from the sarcolemma. Two cisternae of the sarcoplasmic reticulum are found on either side of the T-tubule. This arrangement is referred to as the *triad* of the reticulum. In human skeletal muscle there are two triads per sarcomere. The T-tubules play a vital role in facilitating skeletal muscle contraction. When a nerve impulse is propagated along a nerve fiber in the area where the motor-endplate meets the muscle, the sarcolemma lining the synaptic trough becomes permeable to ions. The increase in flow of the ions generates an action potential, and a wave of depolarization spreads over the entire muscle fiber and into its interior via the T-tubule system. This causes the muscle to contract.
	Connective tissue frame structures
Epimysium	The thick, highly organized connective tissue layer that encloses the muscle as a whole. Gross anatomically known as *fascia.*
Perimysium	The connective tissue layer that envelops a *bundle* of muscle fibers.
Endomysium	The connective tissue that extends from the perimysium into the muscle bundle. This connective tissue branches into progressively finer branches, until each individual muscle fiber or cell is surrounded by a delicate sheath ("body stocking").

muscles between lower jaw and the rest of the skull); where the skin has to be moved relative to the underlying skeletal elements (example: muscles of facial expression between facial bones and facial skin); and where a muscular organ (the tongue) has to be moved relative to the lower jaw (muscles running from several points of the skull into the tongue) or has to change its own shape (muscles running inside the tongue only).

SMOOTH MUSCLE TISSUE. In smooth muscle tissue, the contractions generally do not require our conscious control, although they may be brought under our control with a good deal of practice. These *involuntary* muscle contractions are under the control of our autonomic nervous system. They are slow, but may be maintained over long periods of time without the use of much energy. This is quite in contrast with contractions of skeletal muscles, which require a great deal of energy and rapidly exhaust the muscles.

Structures in which smooth muscle tissue is found include the walls of the stomach, intestines, urinary bladder, uterus and *arteries.*

HEART MUSCLE TISSUE. This type of muscle tissue has characteristics of both skeletal and smooth muscle tissue. It is an *involuntary* muscle, capable of fast, powerful contractions. This type of muscle will not be discussed further here, since it is beyond the immediate scope of this text.

Organization of Skeletal Muscle Tissue

The organization of a skeletal muscle is best illustrated by the structure of a cut of meat (most meat we eat consists of skeletal muscle). Meat, or skeletal muscle tissue, is usually not homogeneous, but may be separated into distinct parts or *bundles.* The separation takes place along connective tissue sheaths, which cover and surround the muscle bundles (as well as the individual muscle fibers). Connective tissue also ties the muscle bundles to each other and to the dense, highly organized connective tissue sheath, which surrounds the entire muscle (Fig. 6–1).

If you take part of a muscle bundle and gently tease it with a fine needle, you will be able to separate it into fine strands, which are called *muscle fibers* (*Note:* These muscle *fibers* are in fact the *muscle cells* and are *not* comparable to the intercellular fibers of connective tissues).

The reason skeletal muscle cells are visible with the unaided eye is their large size. Striated muscle cells may be 30 to 100 μm thick and up to 300 mm long. These unusual cell dimensions are produced during the prenatal development of striated muscle. The large cells actually are produced as the result of *fusion* of many differentiating

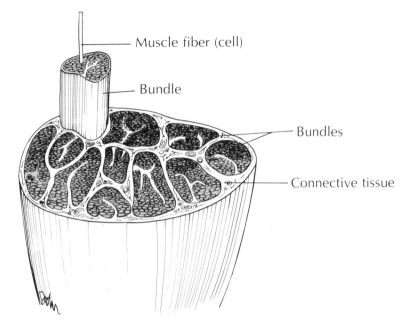

Muscle fiber (cell)

Bundle

Bundles

Connective tissue

Fig. 6–1. Diagram of the structure of a small skeletal muscle. The entire muscle is surrounded by a thick connective tissue sheath (epimysium). Within the muscle several smaller bundles of muscle fibers are present, each of which is surrounded by a thin connective tissue sheath (perimysium). The individual muscle fibers of which a fiber bundle is composed each have their own delicate connective tissue sheaths (endomysium).

mesenchymal cells. This fusion produces one giant cell, with many oval-shaped nuclei (Fig. 6–2).

Skeletal, or striated, muscle cells are shaped like elongated cylinders, with rounded ends. Their cytoplasm contains large amounts of tightly packed bundles of contractile protein filaments, seemingly pushing the nuclei and other organelles, such as the mitochondria, to the sides of the cell.

The bundles of contractile protein filaments, located inside the cell, are about 1 μm thick and are therefore visible with the light microscope. They have cross striations along their length. Many of these bundles neatly line up inside the muscle cell, making it appear as if the cell itself is striated. These cross striations are responsible for the name *striated muscle,* which is frequently used for skeletal muscle. In the section on muscle contractions, we will briefly discuss the structural basis for these striations.

The following is a *summary* of the organization of a skeletal muscle from the cellular level to the anatomically identifiable muscle (see Fig. 6–1).

1. Individual *muscle cells* (fibers) are surrounded by a delicate

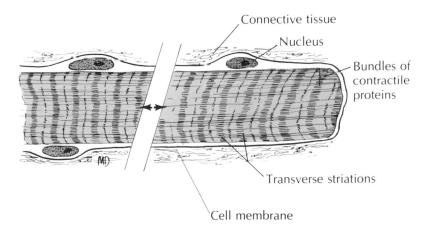

Fig. 6–2. Simplified diagram of a striated muscle fiber (cell). This big cell has blunt, rounded ends and many oval nuclei, all peripherally located within a thin band of cytoplasm. Most of the cell's volume is occupied by bundles of contractile protein filaments with cross-striations. A delicate connective tissue sheath, predominantly consisting of Type III collagen fibers, surrounds the cell. The double-headed arrow indicates that this cell type is far too long to be shown in its entirety in this diagram.

connective tissue sheath, consisting predominantly of fine Type I and Type III collagen fibers. This sheath fits around an individual muscle cell like a "body stocking."

2. A group of cells, with their connective tissue sheaths, is packed together in a *bundle,* surrounded by a layer of connective tissue consisting predominantly of Type I collagen fibers.

3. Several bundles together form a *muscle,* which is surrounded by a layer of dense connective tissue.

The *connective tissue frame* around cells, bundles and whole skeletal muscle performs important functions: biomechanical and physiologic support functions.

Biomechanical Support Functions

1. The connective tissue frame supports the individual muscle cells and holds them together in a particular orientation and shape.

2. Because of their intimate contacts with all individual muscle cells, the connective tissue elements *transmit* the *contractions* of these cells to the connective tissue at the points of attachment of the muscle.

3. The connective tissue frame of the muscle *binds* the muscle to its points of attachment, either *directly,* by forming numerous short fibers, which run into periosteum, perichondrium, lamina propria of the oral mucosa, or dermis of the skin; or *indirectly,* by attaching the muscle mass to a highly oriented rope (tendon) or sheet (apo-

neurosis) of collagenous connective tissue, which in turn inserts into a skeletal element (see: skeletal muscle attachments, below).

Physiologic Functions

The connective tissue elements between muscle bundles contain blood vessels and nerves, both of which branch inside this connective tissue into progressively finer branches. A rich network is formed of fine blood vessels inside the connective tissue elements around the individual muscle cells, and each cell is individually innervated.

The rich vascularization is responsible in part for the red color of muscle tissue. The contents of the muscle cells themselves further contribute to this color.

Skeletal Muscle Attachments

Skeletal muscle attachments are formed by elements of its connective tissue frame. The precise nature of an attachment depends on the site and the function of the muscle. For example, the muscle, which by its contraction changes the *shape* of the *tongue,* is attached on both sides to the lamina propria of the oral mucosa of the tongue. In contrast to this, the muscles which, by their contraction, *move* the *tongue* relative to the skeletal elements are attached on one end only to the oral mucosa of the tongue and on the other end to the skeletal element in question. The muscles of *facial expression* either attach with both ends into the dermis of the skin or, more frequently, attach with one end to the skin and with the other end to the skeleton. Certain muscles in the *lips* attach with one end into the skin and with the other into the oral mucosa. Their contractions change the thickness and shape of the lips. *Masticatory* muscles, which move the lower jaw complex relative to the rest of the skull, attach with both ends to skeletal elements.

In many instances, the connective tissue elements, which surround and support the muscle components, run directly into the *periosteum,* when the attachment is to bone, into the *perichondrium* when the attachment is to cartilage, into the *dermis* when the attachment is to skin, or into the *lamina propria* when the attachment is to oral mucosa. The collagen fibers of the connective tissue frame mesh with the meshwork of collagen fibers in any of these structures, thus fastening the muscle securely to them.

Occasionally, an intermediate structure, a *tendon,* may be involved in the muscle attachment. This may be a heavy, rope-like structure, or a sheet-like tendon, sometimes called *aponeurosis.* If a tendon is present, the connective tissue elements of the muscle mesh with the collagen fibers of the tendon. The tendon itself consists of dense connective tissue, with highly oriented and compact Type I collagen fibers. This structure may insert into periosteum or perichondrium, but in some locations it runs directly into the bone tissue. In such cases, the tendon fibers, which are embedded in the bone, become calcified (hydroxyapatite is deposited in them) to a large extent.

Because of the dense organization of a tendon, its fibroblasts are compressed between the thick cords of collagen fibers. These are *not* actively synthesizing cells, and the turnover time of tendon components is long.

The vascular supply of a tendon is minimal, reflecting the tissue's low metabolic activity. Blood vessels tend to run inside narrow strands of loose connective tissue, interposed between the thick collagen fibers. We will see later a similar arrangement in the principal fiber bundles of the periodontal ligament. Because of its minimal blood supply and its low metabolic activity, a ruptured tendon does not heal readily.

Organization of Smooth Muscle Tissue

In the orofacial area, smooth muscle cells are found in the wall of the trachea and in the walls of blood vessels, mostly arteries and arterioles. Smooth muscle cells are somewhat longer than most other cells in the body, but they are by no means as long as the striated muscle cells. Their lengths are between 15 and 500 μm and their diameters between 5 and 10 μm. Whereas striated muscle cells are large conglomerates, formed prenatally by fusion of many differentiating mesenchymal cells, the smooth muscle cells are formed prenatally by *single*, differentiating mesenchymal cells.

Smooth muscle cells are elongated and spindle-shaped, with one long, sausage-shaped nucleus. This nucleus is located centrally in the cell. While contractile protein filaments, somewhat similar in nature to those in striated muscle cells, are present in substantial amounts in the smooth muscle cytoplasm, they are not as rigidly organized in thick bundles and thus are not visible in the light microscope (Fig. 6–3).

Each striated muscle cell is individually innervated, but only a few smooth muscle cells are innervated. Nevertheless, smooth muscle cells can contract in an organized and coordinated fashion. This is because once the impulse for contraction is received by the few cells that are innervated, this impulse is immediately communicated to the non-innervated cells via the low-resistance *gap junctions,* by which the smooth muscle cells are functionally coupled.

Each individual smooth muscle cell is surrounded by its connective tissue "body stocking," consisting of fine Type I and Type III

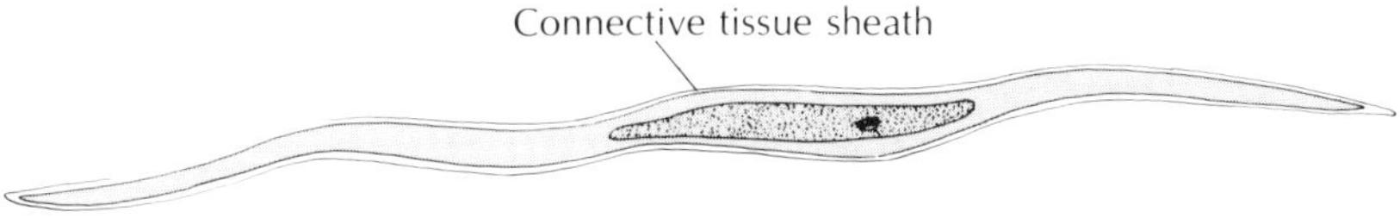

Connective tissue sheath

Fig. 6–3. A simplified diagram of a smooth muscle cell. This long, spindle-shaped cell has a single, sausage-shaped nucleus, which is located centrally. The protein filaments in the cytoplasm of these cells are not as strictly organized as the filaments in striated muscle cells, and they are not visible by light microscopy. A delicate "stocking" of Type III collagen fibers surrounds the cell.

collagen fibers, except in the areas of the gap junctions, where no connective tissue is present.

As in striated muscle, a connective tissue frame with both bio-mechanical and physiologic support functions is associated with an organized group of smooth muscle cells. Since smooth muscle cells tend to be located in the walls of hollow structures, such as blood vessels, the mechanical functions of the connective tissue consist largely of the *transmission* of muscle contraction, which decreases the size or diameter of the hollow structure, and the provision of *mechanical support* for the muscle cells and the wall of the hollow structure itself.

Mechanism of Muscle Contraction

Although the principles of muscle contraction appear to be comparable in both smooth and striated muscle cells, most investigations on muscle contraction have been performed on striated muscle cells. Their high degree of organization enables us to give a simple account of muscle contraction, without going into the intricate physiology of the contraction process, for which the interested reader is referred to more extensive texts on this particular subject.

As may be seen in Figure 6–4, the cytoplasm of a striated muscle contains many *bundles* of contractile protein filaments. The organization of these protein filaments within the bundles is shown.

The bundles of contractile protein filaments in a striated muscle cell are usually called *myofibrils.* Each myofibril, in turn, consists of two types of regularly arranged protein filaments, *actin* and *myosin* filaments. In regularly stained histologic sections, the darker striations are produced by the presence of myosin filaments, while the lighter areas contain only actin filaments. The actin filaments are attached "back-to-back" to a "backbone" or *Z-line.* That section of a myofibril that is located between two Z-lines is the contractile unit or *sarcomere* of the myofibril. Each sarcomere is composed of one dark striation and two half light striations.

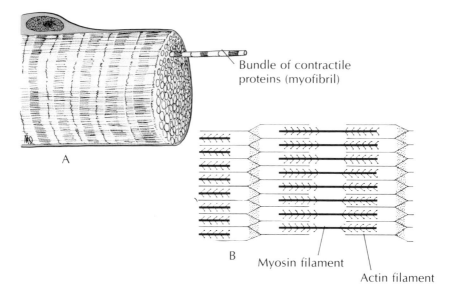

Bundle of contractile
proteins (myofibril)

A

B   Myosin filament

Actin filament

Fig. 6–4. From the cut end of a striated muscle cell, shown in this diagram, one bundle of contractile proteins (a myofibril) protrudes, A. A small segment of this myofibril is enlarged, B, to show the arrangement of the protein filaments (actin and myosin filaments) that are responsible for the striations and for the contraction mechanism. The stippled, vertical bands are the Z-lines. Actin filaments are attached back to back to the Z-lines. The heavier myosin filaments alternate with the actin filaments. The segment between two Z-lines is a sarcomere, the unit of contraction of a striated muscle cell.

During muscle contraction, the actin and myosin filaments form a series of links with each other, which allow the myosin filaments to pull themselves closer to the Z-lines. The lengths of the individual sarcomeres are thereby shortened in a fashion known as the *sliding mechanism.* The shortening of the individual sarcomeres leads to the shortening of the total length of the muscle cell, which is somewhat more than the sum of all sarcomeres (Fig. 6–5).

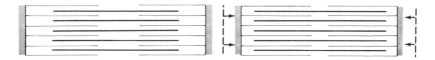

Fig. 6–5. Two diagrams of a sarcomere, the unit of contraction of a striated muscle cell, located between two Z-lines (grey vertical bands). During contraction, the actin filaments slide past the myosin filaments toward each other, bringing the two Z-lines closer together and thus decreasing the length of the sarcomere *(arrows).* If this occurs simultaneously in all sarcomeres along the length of a muscle fiber, this fiber shortens considerably.

NERVE TISSUE

The nervous system, composed of nerve tissue, might be compared with a large central computer (*central nervous system:* brain and spinal cord) with numerous input and output channels (*peripheral nervous system:* nerves and small aggregates of nerve cells [ganglia]).

In Figure 6–6 some pathways of the nervous system are shown. There are nerves that transmit impulses from the periphery to the central nervous system (example: *sensory input* from the skin is transmitted this way, via *afferent* nerves). Other nerves transmit impulses or commands from the central nervous system to the periphery (example: the *somatic motor output,* which provides the impulse for muscle contraction is transmitted this way, via *efferent* nerves. Another example: the *autonomic, secretomotor output,* which provides the impulse for secretion in a salivary gland is also transmitted via *efferent* nerves). In the central nervous system, the input is sorted out and processed. When necessary, the information is converted into appropriate output signals.

Within the nervous system we distinguish 2 principal types of *cells:*

1. Nerve cells or *neurons:* involved in impulse transmission. The cell bodies of these cells are located in the central nervous system or in the ganglia of the peripheral nervous system. The long processes of these cells are located in the peripheral nerves.

2. Supporting cells: *glia cells* in the central nervous system; *Schwann cells* in the peripheral nerves and *satellite cells* in the ganglia. These cells are involved in support and service functions of the nervous system.

NEURONS. Neurons are cells that are specialized in the conduction of impulses (an electric current flow) along their cell membranes. The differentiated neuron is no longer capable of mitosis. A neuron generally consists of a relatively large cell body (4 to 135 μm) and one, two or more cell processes, which may be of variable lengths. The number and the lengths of these processes depend on the location of the neuron within the communication system.

1. The neurons of the *central nervous system* and in the *autonomic ganglia* have several cell processes *(multipolar neurons).* Usually one of these, the *axon,* is considerably longer than the others *(dendrites).* Dendrites generally receive and conduct impulses toward the neuronal cell body. The axon conducts impulses *away* from the cell body (Fig. 6–7). Numerous cell contacts *(synapses)* exist between the neurons in the central nervous system, resulting in a very complex circuitry.

Within the central nervous system, groups of neurons, *centers,*

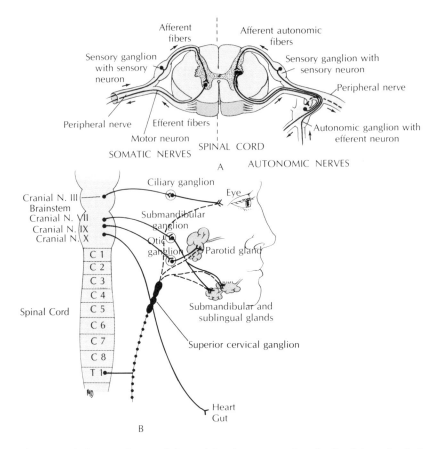

Afferent fibers

Afferent autonomic fibers

Sensory ganglion with sensory neuron

Sensory ganglion with sensory neuron

Peripheral nerve

Peripheral nerve

Efferent fibers

Motor neuron

Autonomic ganglion with efferent neuron

SPINAL CORD

SOMATIC NERVES

A

AUTONOMIC NERVES

Ciliary ganglion

Eye

Cranial N. III

Brainstem

Cranial N. VII

Cranial N. IX

Cranial N. X

Submandibular ganglion

Otic ganglion

Parotid gland

C 1

C 2

C 3

C 4

Spinal Cord

C 5

C 6

C 7

C 8

T 1

MO

Submandibular and sublingual glands

Superior cervical ganglion

Heart

Gut

B

Fig. 6–6. *A,* Some pathways of the peripheral nervous system, leading into and out of a section of spinal cord, are shown in this diagram. The spinal cord is seen from the front. For clarity, pathways of autonomic nerves are illustrated on the right side, while pathways of somatic nerves are shown on the left side. It should be understood that both types of nerves are found on both sides. Input signals (afferent) reach the sensory neurons in the peripherally located sensory ganglia. These signals may then be transmitted further centrally, where the motor neurons and autonomic neurons are located. From these neurons, output signals (efferent) may leave the central nervous system for an appropriate peripheral response. Notice that the autonomic output signals use two autonomic neurons (one whose cell body is located in the spinal cord and one whose cell body is located in a peripheral autonomic ganglion). The somatic output signals use only one neuron, the cell body of which is located in the spinal cord, while the input signals similarly use only one neuron, the cell body of which is located in a peripheral sensory ganglion. *B,* The autonomic pathways for the head and neck region are shown in this diagram. The sympathetic outflow from the thoracic level of the spinal cord (dotted line from T1). The second group of neuronal cell bodies is located on the superior cervical ganglion (black). From there, all sympathetic output signals travel further along nerve fibers associated with blood vessels (broken lines). The parasympathetic neurons are located in the brain. Parasympathetic output signals travel in nerve fibers associated with four cranial nerves emerging from the brainstem. The second group of neuronal cell bodies is located in four parasympathetic ganglia. From those, the parasympathetic output signals travel further toward the viscera (especially salivary glands) that are innervated by them (solid lines). For clarity, the fourth parasympathetic ganglion in this area, the pterygopalatine ganglion, has been omitted from this diagram. Parasympathetic signals from this ganglion travel to all parts of the face and pharynx.

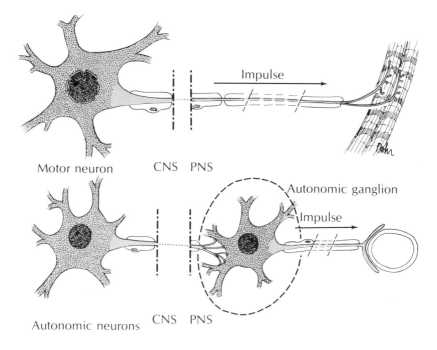

Motor neuron   CNS   PNS

Autonomic neurons   CNS   PNS

PSEUDO-UNIPOLAR NEURON

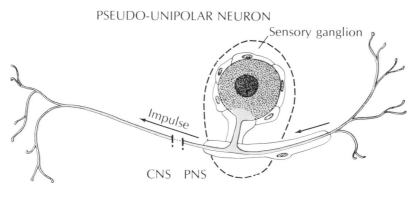

Sensory neuron

Fig. 6–7. Diagrammatic representation of three multipolar neurons and one pseudo-unipolar neuron. The vertical broken line in all diagrams represents the border between central nervous system (CNS) and peripheral nervous system (PNS). The arrows indicate the direction in which the signal impulses move. One of the cell processes of a multipolar motor neuron, whose cell body is located in the CNS, is a long axon, innervating a skeletal muscle. Some light, supporting cells (Schwann cells) are illustrated along the length of the axon. Of the two autonomic multipolar neurons, one is located in the CNS. Its axon communicates with a second multipolar neuron in an autonomic ganglion. From this cell, a second axon runs toward the structure to be innervated (a blood vessel in this case). Supporting cells are illustrated around the axons. A neuron in a sensory ganglion is pseudo-unipolar. One cell process leaves the cell body, but it divides almost immediately into two long branches: one running toward the CNS and one running toward the periphery of the body (skin, oral mucosa). The impulse travels in the direction of the arrows from periphery to CNS.

subserve specific functions in processing sensory information and control of motor output. Most of these cells do not have cell processes beyond the central nervous system.

2. Neurons in *sensory ganglia* have one single process that later bifurcates (T-shape). These are called *pseudo-unipolar neurons* (Fig. 6–7).

The maintenance of the long cell processes of a neuron (especially a motor neuron, whose cell body lies in the central nervous system, while its cell process, the axon, ends in a skeletal muscle) is demanding and therefore the cell body is actively involved in protein synthesis. A constant flow of proteins takes place in the axon from the cell body toward the periphery. An extensive cytoskeleton is present in the cell processes.

SYNAPSES. A synapse is a specialized, localized region of cell contact between 2 neurons or between a neuron and its effector tissue (muscle or gland). The cell membranes of the 2 cells that are involved in a synapse usually do not come together completely; a 20-nm wide *synaptic gap* remains between them (Fig. 6–8).

An impulse is transmitted from one cell to the next across the synaptic gap by *neurotransmitter substances.* These substances are released into the synaptic gap from small vesicles present in the cytoplasm of the first (presynaptic) cell.

SUPPORTING CELLS. Supporting cells are not involved in

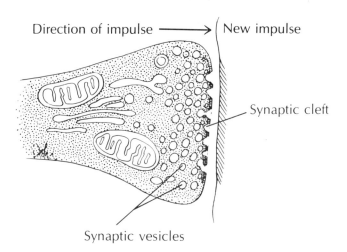

Fig. 6–8.   Synapse between a neural cell process and either another neuron or an effector tissue (a muscle cell, for example). In this diagram, the impulse travels from left to right. In the left (presynaptic) cell, numerous synaptic vesicles are present. The vesicles contain the neurotransmitter substances, which are to be released in the synaptic neuron or effector cell.

impulse conduction. These cells support and nourish the neurons. Unlike the neurons, the supporting cells are capable of mitosis.

In the central nervous system the supporting cells are *glia* cells. There are several types of glia cells, each with different functions. Some produce a sheath of fatty material, *myelin,* around the axons. Others cover the nonsynaptic surfaces of the neuronal cell bodies as well as the blood vessel walls, thereby controlling the environment of the neurons by regulating the flow of nourishment, ions and gasses to the neurons.

In the peripheral nervous system *satellite* cells cover the nonsynaptic surfaces of the neuronal cell bodies in the ganglia. *Schwann* cells support the individual axons in the peripheral nerves. The Schwann cells in the afferent (sensory) nerves and in the efferent (somatic motor) nerves surround the axons with a sheath of myelin.

Autonomic nerves and the terminal parts of peripheral afferent and efferent nerves are unmyelinated. In these nerves Schwann cells support the axons in depressions of their cell surfaces (Figs. 6–9 and 6–10).

Organization of a Peripheral Nerve

A *nerve,* which may be identified in a gross anatomic dissection or in a histologic slide, consists of a group of axons with their supporting Schwann cells and an encapsulating frame of connective tissue with blood vessels. One axon with its associated sheath of Schwann cells, lined up along the lengths of the axon, is called a *nerve fiber* (Fig. 6–11).

Let us review the differences in the use of the term *fiber* in the various tissues. In *connective tissue,* a fiber is an *inter*cellular matrix component, produced by connective tissue cells and consisting largely of proteins and some carbohydrate chains. We distinguish different types of collagen and elastic fibers. In *striated muscle,* a fiber is a large, multinucleated muscle *cell.* In a *nerve,* a fiber is a long *cell process* (axon) of a neuron, with a sheath of several *supporting cells.*

Nerve Terminals

There is a variety of nerve terminals at both output and input ends of the peripheral nervous system. We will discuss here the nerve terminals of importance in the orofacial region (Fig. 6–12).

In *striated muscle,* an efferent (motor) nerve terminates on the surface of individual muscle cells in *motor endplates,* resembling synapses. The impulse, propagated along the nerve, is transmitted

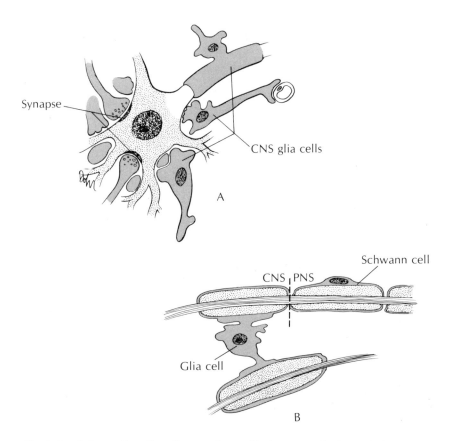

Fig. 6–9. *A*, Supporting glia cells around a multipolar neuron in the central nervous system (CNS). All nonsynaptic neuronal surfaces are covered by glia cells. In the upper right hand corner, a glia cell has produced a myelin sheath around the axon. Just below it, a glia cell has cell processes, covering both a blood vessel wall (right) and part of the neuronal surface. *B*, Axons running from central nervous system (CNS) to peripheral nervous system (PNS). In the CNS, the axons are given anatomic and physiologic support by the glia cell, whose cell processes form myelin sheaths around them. One glia cell may support several adjacent axons. In the PNS, Schwann cells support the axons, surrounding them with a myelin sheath. A Schwann cell cannot participate in the formation of more than one myelin sheath. Several Schwann cells are found along the length of an axon.

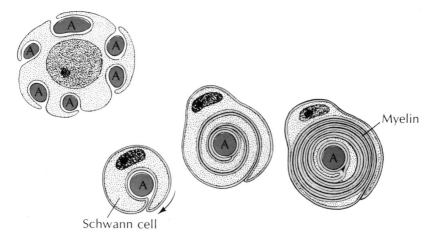

Myelin

Schwann cell

Fig. 6–10. The relationships between axons (A) and Schwann cells is illustrated in these diagrammatic cross sections through an unmyelinated and a myelinated nerve. At left, a Schwann cell (with stippled cytoplasm) is shown, supporting several axons in depressions on its cell surface. The number of axons thus supported is variable. In some cases, only one axon may be found in this type of relationship. No myelin sheath is formed by these Schwann cells. The three diagrams below show the steps in the formation of a myelin sheath around a single axon. The Schwann cell wraps itself progressively further around the axon. The concentric layers of the Schwann cell membrane, fused together, constitute the myelin sheath.

across the synaptic trough, increasing the permeability of the muscle cell membrane and stimulating muscle contraction.

Within both muscles and tendons, specialized *sensory receptors* are present, feeding back information to the central nervous system about the state of contraction of the muscle and the positions of the moving parts of the body.

Within the *oral mucosa* and *periodontal ligament,* two main types of sensory receptors should be recognized: free nerve endings and encapsulated nerve endings.

FREE NERVE ENDINGS. These are the terminal portions of afferent (sensory) axons, no longer covered by supporting Schwann cells. In the oral mucosa, such nerve endings penetrate, across the basal lamina, into the oral epithelium, where they are associated with Merkel cells. In the dental pulp, free nerve endings are the principal nerve terminals, associated with *pain* perception. Toothaches are transmitted via nerves that terminate as free nerve endings either in the pulp or in the periodontal ligament.

ENCAPSULATED NERVE ENDINGS. These consist of several terminal portions of afferent axons, surrounded by a bulbous capsule of several Schwann cells, without myelin, and some connective tissue elements. Encapsulated nerve endings are probably associated with *touch* perception. In the oral mucosa, they are highly

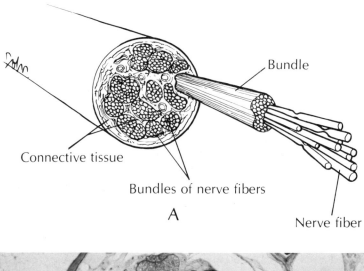

Bundle

Connective tissue

Bundles of nerve fibers

A

Nerve fiber

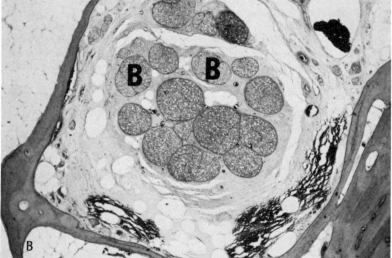

Fig. 6–11. *A,* The organization of a peripheral nerve is shown diagrammatically. The nerve is surrounded by a predominantly collagenous connective tissue sheath. It is composed of several bundles of nerve fibers. Both bundles and individual nerve fibers are further encapsulated in connective tissue sheaths. An individual nerve fiber consists of an axon surrounded by its sheath of Schwann cells. *B,* Histologic cross section through the mandibular nerve, located in the bony canal of a lower jaw. The several bundles (B) of nerve fibers, each surrounded by its connective tissue sheath, are clearly visible. The individual nerve fibers appear in cross section as tiny, open rings, some with a dot (axon) inside. The myelin is lost during histologic processing, which accounts for the seeming emptiness of the nerve fibers in histologic section. Original magnification ×10.

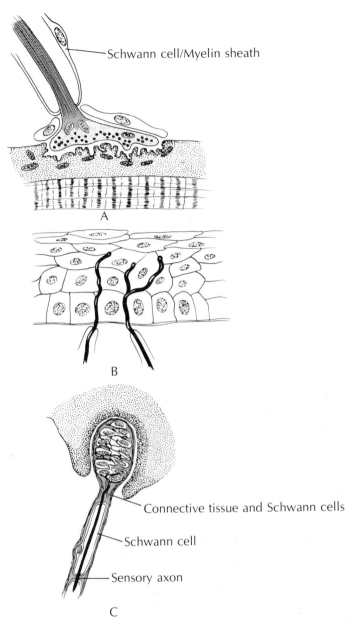

Schwann cell/Myelin sheath

A

B

Connective tissue and Schwann cells

Schwann cell

Sensory axon

C

Fig. 6–12. Various nerve terminals are shown diagrammatically in this figure. *A,* Motor endplate. The axon of a motor neuron forms a flat extension, which is located in a depression on the surface of a striated muscle fiber (stippled cytoplasm; a few myofibrils are visible). A synaptic cleft, into which the synaptic vesicles may release their neurotransmitter substances, is present between muscle membrane and presynaptic axon membrane. *B,* Free nerve endings. Single sensory axons, no longer covered with Schwann cells, cross the basal lamina and terminate inside stratified squamous epithelium. *C,* Encapsulated nerve endings. A specific example of an encapsulated sensory terminal is illustrated: Meissner's corpuscle. It is located characteristically in a connective tissue papilla, occupying nearly all of its volume, immediately beneath the epithelium. A bulbous capsule of nonmyelinated Schwann cells and connective tissue elements surrounds the sensory axon terminals.

organized *Meissner's corpuscles,* generally found in connective tissue papillae of the lamina propria. In the periodontal ligament, the encapsulated nerve endings are small and poorly organized.

BLOOD AND BLOOD VESSELS

In order to function and stay alive, the cells of an organism have to be supplied constantly with all requirements for their metabolism and must be relieved of their metabolic waste products. This is the principal function of the *vascular system.* Other functions of this system include the transport of inflammatory cells and antibodies, and, in warmblooded individuals, the maintenance of a constant body temperature.

The vascular system consists of a pumping organ, the *heart,* and a closed system of blood vessels, running from the heart to the organs and back to the heart. Between the heart and the organs, the blood vessels *(arteries)* branch progressively into finer vessels, until, in the organs, a network of extremely delicate vessels *(capillaries)* is formed. Between the organs and the heart, many smaller vessels combine to form progressively larger vessels *(veins),* which carry the blood back to the heart.

For tissues and organs, the essential part of the vascular system is the capillary bed, where the exchange of gases and metabolic substances occurs. The heart and the larger vessels have the role of moving blood to and from the capillary beds.

The vascular system develops embryologically from mesenchymal cells, which form a network of delicate tubular structures, composed of differentiated cells. These cells, *endothelial cells,* are flat (squamous), and they are arranged in an epithelium-like fashion. With further development and function, the several distinct types of blood vessels are formed, each with its characteristic wall structure. But all of the blood vessels, as well as the heart, retain an innermost lining of endothelial cells.

ARTERIES. Around the simple endothelial lining a thick layer of smooth muscle cells and elastic membranes is present. In the largest arteries, closest to the heart, there are relatively more elastic membranes (composed of elastic fibers), while in the smaller arteries, further away from the heart, there are mostly smooth muscle cells in the arterial wall (Fig. 6–13, A).

The heart contracts rhythmically. If the walls of the arteries were rigid, the blood would reach the organs in squirts. In fact, when the heart contracts, the walls of the larger arteries distend and then slowly return to their original position (this is elastic rebound, a result of the action of the elastic membranes), thereby ensuring a steady flow of blood in the smaller vessels.

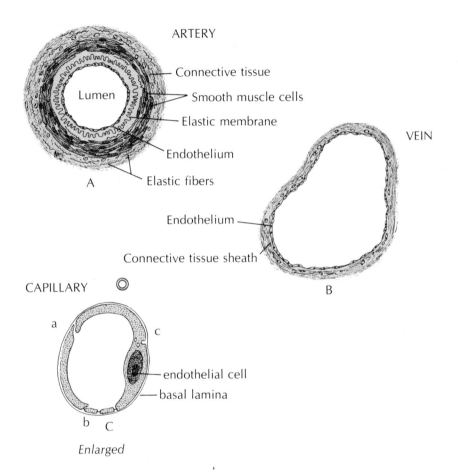

Enlarged

Fig. 6–13. **Diagrammatic representations of cross sections through a small artery, *A*, a small vein, *B*, and a capillary, *C*. The artery has a relatively cylindrical lumen, round in cross section, surrounded by a single layer of endothelial cells and a thick wall of elastic membranes, concentrically arranged smooth muscle cells and a small amount of connective tissue proper. The vein has an irregular, wide lumen, surrounded by a single layer of endothelial cells and a thin wall, consisting predominantly of connective tissue elements. A capillary, if shown proportionally, would be no larger than the small circular outline, drawn here. To show more detail, the capillary cross section is further enlarged. The capillary wall, in cross section, consists of a single endothelial cell, wrapped around a narrow lumen. A basal lamina is present between this cell and the surrounding tissues. a, openings at the cell junctions; b, pores; c, pinocytotic vesicles (see text for explanations).**

The contractions of smooth muscle cells in the arterial walls further aid the distribution of blood. This is particularly important in the microvascular system.

VEINS. Veins generally accompany arteries, but carry blood in the opposite direction. These vessels consist of an endothelial lining with a connective tissue reinforcement around it. Occasionally, a few smooth muscle cells are present in the walls of the largest veins. Veins contain about 70% of the total blood volume of the body at any time (Fig. 6–13, B).

CAPILLARIES. Capillaries are simple endothelial tubes approximately 5 to 7 μm in diameter. The endothelial cells and a peripheral basal lamina are the only components of a capillary wall, forming a selective barrier between the blood and the tissues. Transport across the capillary wall may take place via (1) openings in the line of contact between adjacent endothelial cells, (2) openings across the endothelial cells, which are filled with some selective filtering material and are called *pores,* and (3) *pinocytotic vesicles,* small vesicles engulfing some material on one side of the cell, shuttling it across the cytoplasm, and releasing it at the other side of the endothelial cell (Fig. 6–13, C).

MICROVASCULATURE. Arteries and veins branch progressively into smaller blood vessels as they approach the capillary bed. The smallest arteries *(arterioles)* and the smallest veins *(venules)* form, together with the capillary bed, the microvasculature.

The terminal branch of an arteriole is called a *preferential channel,* a blood vessel leading directly into a venule. This channel has several side branches, which are entrances into the capillary bed. At any given time, most of these entrances are closed and the blood passes "by preference" through the preferential channel from the arterial side to the venous side of the microvasculature.

As may be seen in Figure 6–14, at each entrance to the capillary bed a *precapillary sphincter* is present. This sphincter consists of a smooth muscle cell, wrapped around the entrance, which by contracting closes off this entrance.

Selective, temporary closure of parts of the capillary bed is important. If all capillaries of the body would be open at the same time, we would not have enough blood to fill the entire vascular system and would go into *shock.* The selective opening and closing of parts of the capillary bed is presumably regulated by the specific metabolic needs of the tissue supplied by the capillary bed.

Soon after the blood enters a capillary bed, a number of substances, including fluid from the blood plasma, passes through the capillary wall into the surrounding tissues. This movement out of the capillaries is due largely to the hydrostatic pressure that is present in the arterioles of the microvasculature. Since larger molecules, particu-

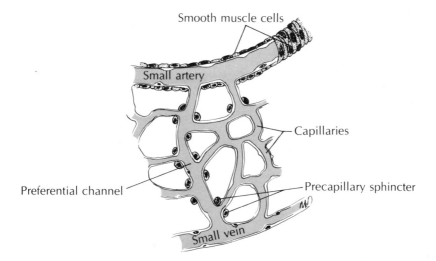

Fig. 6–14. Simplified diagram of a microvascular bed. A small arteriole, with an inner layer of endothelial cells and a single peripheral layer of smooth muscle cells, has terminal branches, one of which is shown here, which form preferential channels to small venules (endothelial cells surrounded by a thin connective tissue sheath). From a preferential channel, several branches lead into the capillary network. At the entrance of each of these branches, a precapillary sphincter (a smooth muscle cell) is present. These sphincters control how much blood is admitted into which capillaries.

larly albumin, cannot pass through the capillary walls, the concentration of these molecules increases in the blood that remains in the capillaries, which is now also reduced in fluid volume.

Because of the distribution of the remaining blood over many small capillaries, the hydrostatic pressure is decreased in those vessels and the movement of fluid and substances out of the capillaries stops. However, because of the high concentration of the larger molecules in the blood, some of the fluid that did move out of the capillaries is now attracted back into the blood stream (by a process of osmosis).

Usually, not all fluid returns to the capillaries in this manner, and so the tissues need another mechanism to remove the fluid that is left behind. The needed mechanism is provided by the *lymphatic vessels* (this chapter).

BLOOD AND BLOOD CELLS

Blood consists of two component parts, a liquid phase *(plasma)* and a cellular phase *(blood cells)*.

Plasma transports all nutritive substances. It contains also several important proteins: *albumin,* a protein that serves to maintain the osmotic pressure of blood; circulating *antibodies;* and *fibrinogen,* a protein involved in the initiation of the blood clotting process. Blood *serum* is blood plasma from which certain clotting factors, especially fibrinogen, have been removed.

Blood cells comprise about 45% of the total blood volume. A listing of the characteristics of the cells found in the circulating blood is presented here. The cellular phase of blood can be subdivided into 3 main groups (Fig. 6–15):

  I. *Red cells* (erythrocytes)

 II. *White cells* (leukocytes)

    A. Granular leukocytes

      1. Neutrophils

      2. Eosinophils

      3. Basophils

    B. Nongranular leukocytes

      1. Monocytes

      2. Lymphocytes

III. *Platelets*

Red Cells (Erythrocytes)

The cytoplasm of these cells is filled with hemoglobin (which binds oxygen). The hemoglobin gives the cells their red color, which in turn is responsible for the red color of the blood. The red cells have no nucleus; it is lost during cell development.

Function: transport of O_2 and facilitation of transport of CO_2

Size: 7 μm

Prevalence: 4 to 6 million/mm³ of blood

  in men the average is 5.7 million/mm³

  in women the average is 4.5 million/mm³

Where formed: red bone marrow

Where destroyed: red bone marrow and spleen

Survival time in circulating blood: about 120 days

White Cells (Leukocytes)

Prevalence: 5000 to 10,000/mm³ of blood

Granular Leukocytes

The cytoplasm of all granular leukocytes is filled with distinctive granules, that may be seen in the light microscope. These granules are lysosomes, filled with specific enzymes. The primary function of these cells lies not in the blood, but in the connective tissues. They all are capable of ameboid movement, which allows them to leave the capillaries and enter the tissues where they are needed.

Where formed: red bone marrow

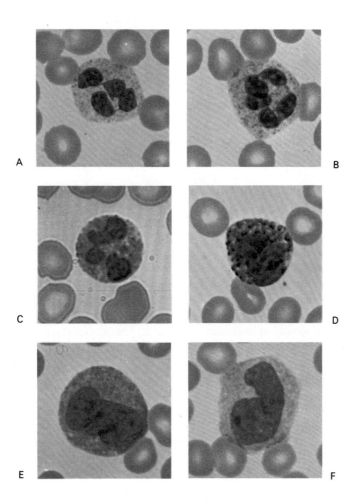

Fig. 6–15.   Normal white blood cells (leukocytes), photographed in a surrounding of red blood cells (erythrocytes). *A,* Neutrophil (polymorphonuclear leukocyte). *B,* Neutrophil. *C,* Eosinophil. *D,* Basophil. *E,* Monocyte. *F,* Monocyte. (From Wintrobe, M.M., et al.: *Clinical Hematology.* 7th Ed. Philadelphia, Lea & Febiger, 1974.)

Where destroyed: connective tissue, alimentary tract; lungs
Survival time: unknown; estimated between 1 day and 2 weeks

NEUTROPHIL (polymorphonuclear leukocyte). This is an actively ameboid cell. The nucleus has several lobes. The granules contain mostly lysosomal, proteolytic enzymes. The granules are neither acid nor alkaline, reacting in a neutral fashion with the histologic stains.
Function: first defense against bacterial invasion, *phagocytosis.*
Size: 11 μm
Prevalence: 60% of all leukocytes

EOSINOPHIL. This is a somewhat ameboid cell. The nucleus has 2 lobes. The cytoplasm contains large alkaline granules, staining preferentially with eosin. These granules contain specific lysosomal enzymes.
Function: defense against strange proteins; involvement in allergy reaction
Size: 12 μm
Prevalence: 2% of all leukocytes

BASOPHIL. This is a somewhat ameboid cell. The nucleus is bent in a U-shape or S-shape. This nucleus is barely visible due to the presence of large acid granules in the cytoplasm. These granules stain preferentially with the base hematoxylin. They contain histamine, heparin (vaso-active substances) and serotonin.
Function: Release of granular material in the presence of an antigen (?)
Size: 10 μm
Prevalence: 0.5% of all leukocytes

Nongranular Leukocytes

MONOCYTE. This cell has small granules (lysosomes) in its cytoplasm. In the mature cell, the nucleus is placed in a somewhat eccentric position and is kidney-shaped.
Function: precursor of several types of phagocytic cells in different tissues (macrophages in various tissues, osteoclasts in bone tissue).
Size: 17 μm
Prevalence: 3 to 8% of all leukocytes
Survival time: circulates in blood 1 to 2 days; *months* in tissues
Where formed: red bone marrow
Where destroyed: tissue

LYMPHOCYTE. No specific granules are present in the cytoplasm of this cell type. In small lymphocytes the nucleus fills most of the cell. Several types of lymphocytes exist, with different functions, although all are involved in immune defense. An exhaustive description is beyond the scope of this book.

Function: promotion of phagocytosis (cellular defense, T cells), and production of antibodies (humoral defense, B cells). Once activated, B cells differentiate into *plasma cells.*
Size: 6 to 8 μm (small); 12 to 15 μm (large)
Prevalence: 25 to 33% of all leukocytes
Where formed: bone marrow (B cells), bone marrow and thymus (T cells) and lymphoid tissues.
Where destroyed: spleen
Survival time: unknown, variable

Platelets

Platelets are cell fragments of a specific cell type in red bone marrow (megakaryocyte). They have no nuclei.
Function: promote blood clotting
Size: 2 to 3 μm
Prevalence: 300,000/mm³
Where formed: red bone marrow
Where destroyed: spleen and liver; blood clot
Survival time: 4 to 6 days

LYMPHATICS

Lymph is the fluid that is collected from the tissues and is returned to the blood stream by a system of lymphatic vessels. Lymph differs from blood in that it does *not* contain red blood cells, platelets, fibrinogen or albumin. It does, however, contain lymphocytes, some granular leukocytes and antibodies. Antibodies are added to the lymph as it passes through the lymph nodes.

Lymphatic Vessels

Lymphatic vessels do *not* carry anything to the tissues. They only carry lymph away from the tissues.
Lymphatic capillaries run parallel with the blood capillaries. Lymphatic capillaries consist, as do blood capillaries, of endothelial cells, but there is no clear basal lamina around the vessels and large openings are present between the endothelial cells. Thus, there is easy access for fluid and substances from the tissues into the lymphatic capillaries.

A system of increasingly larger lymphatic vessels collects the contents of the smaller lymphatic capillaries, and finally the lymph is returned to the blood stream, just before it returns to the heart.

In addition to the normal components of lymph, lymphatic vessels occasionally carry other matter away from the tissues: breakdown products resulting from inflammation in the tissues, or metastatic cells from malignant tumors may be carried from their original locations to other parts of the body via the lymphatic vessels.

Some safeguards against such components reaching the blood stream and producing systemic illness throughout the body, are provided by the presence of small organs, *lymph nodes,* which are found along the lymphatic pathways. These nodes consist of an encapsulated mass of lymphoid tissue and serve, not always perfectly, as filters of the lymph. Several lymphatic vessels, arriving at the outside surface of a lymph node, break up into a capillary network inside the node. During the passage through this capillary net, "foreign" matter may be removed from the lymph and digested by the cells of the lymphoid tissue. Following passage through the lymph node, the capillaries come together again into one large lymphatic vessel. This carries the lymph away from the lymph node.

In healthy individuals, lymph nodes are inconspicuous, but in disease, when the nodes are actively performing filtering functions, they become swollen and sometimes painful. Diagnostically, such nodes are important. They may indicate the presence of an inflammation or the spread of a malignant tumor. A gross anatomy atlas should be used to help you locate the lymph nodes that are critical for the "drainage" of the orofacial area.

Lymph Nodes

Lymph nodes are lymphoid organs. They consist of an encapsulated mass of lymphoid tissue. Lymphoid tissue is a specialized, loose connective tissue, consisting of reticular cells in intimate relation with a delicate network of Type III collagen fibers, in which accumulations of lymphocytes are present. These accumulations are called lymphatic nodules, and they are areas where lymphocytes are actively proliferating. The lymphocytes, both B and T cells, interact with each other in developing specific immune defenses against any foreign material that might pass through the lymph nodes. In addition, macrophages are present in the lymph nodes capable of phagocytosis of any undesired foreign matter.

Tonsils

Tonsils are special lymphoid organs, located around the passageway between oral cavity and pharynx. These organs consist of lymphoid tissue, which is arranged underneath and around deep grooves and pits, formed by the oral and pharyngeal epithelium in this tissue (Fig. 6–16).

Many lymphocytes are located in all layers of the epithelium. The

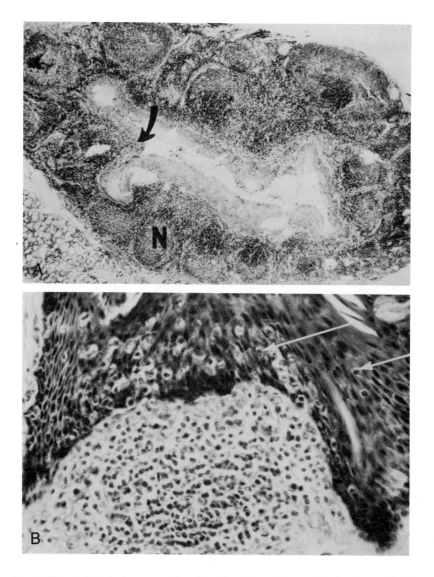

Fig. 6–16.   A, Histologic cross section through a deep pit (crypt) in a human tonsil. The crypt is lined with stratified squamous epithelium *(arrow)*. Lymphoid tissue is arranged underneath the epithelium. Some accumulations of the darkly staining lymphocytes, lymphatic nodules (N), are visible in the lymphoid tissue. No clear connective tissue capsule surrounds the tonsillar tissue. Original magnification × 10. B, Stratified squamous epithelial lining of a human tonsillar crypt. Several lymphocytes *(arrows)* have invaded the epithelium and are located among the epithelial cells. Original magnification × 100.

tonsil may be thought of as an early warning system, which serves to detect the nature of the substances, entering the body via the digestive tract, and to prepare an early immune defense against any dangerous substances.

In contrast with the lymph nodes, tonsils have lymphatic vessels at their periphery *only*. These carry lymph away from the tonsil. Frequently, tonsils are not well separated from the underlying connective tissue by a dense fibrous capsule. As a result, surgical removal of these organs is difficult.

SELECTED READING LIST

Bülbring, E., and Bolton, T.B. (eds.): Smooth muscle. Br. Med. Bull., *55*:27, 1979.

Cooper, S.: Muscle spindles and other muscle receptors. In *Structure and Function of Muscle. Vol. I.* Edited by G.H. Bourne. New York, Academic Press, 1960.

Davison, A.N., and Peters, A.: *Myelination.* Springfield, IL, Charles C Thomas, 1970.

Drinker, C.K., and Yoffey, J.M.: *Lymphatics, Lymph and Lymphoid Tissue.* Cambridge, MA, Harvard University Press, 1941.

Eccles, J.C.: *The Physiology of Nerve Cells.* Baltimore, Johns Hopkins Press, 1957.

Florey, H.: Exchange of substances between the blood and tissues. Nature, *192*:908, 1961.

Gauthier, G.E.: The motor endplate. In *The Peripheral Nerve.* Edited by D.N. Landon. London, Chapman and Hall, 1976.

Glees, P.: *Neuroglia: Morphology and Function.* Springfield, IL, Charles C Thomas, 1955.

Grossman, R.C., and Hattis, B.F.: Oral mucosal sensory innervation and sensory experience: a review. In *Symposium on Oral Sensation and Perception.* Edited by J.F. Bosma. Springfield, IL, Charles C Thomas, 1967.

Huxley, H.E.: The mechanism of muscular contraction. Science, *164*:1356, 1969.

Huxley, A.F., and Simmons, R.M.: Mechanical properties of the cross-bridge of frog striated muscle. J. Physiol., *218*:59, 1971.

Kuntz, A.: *The Autonomic Nervous System.* 4th Ed. Philadelphia, Lea & Febiger, 1953.

Lavelle, C.L.B.: The blood supply of the oral tissues. In *Applied Physiology of the Mouth.* Edited by C.L.B. Lavelle. Bristol, John Wright and Sons, 1975.

McMahon, T.A.: *Muscles, Reflexes, and Locomotion.* Princeton, NJ, Princeton University Press, 1984.

Munger, B.L., and Ide, C.: The structure and function of cutaneous sensory receptors. Arch. Histol. Cytol., *51*:1, 1988.

Noback, C.R., and Demarest, R.J.: *The Nervous System: An Introduction and Review.* New York, McGraw-Hill Book Co., 1972.

Ogata, T.: Structure of motor endplates in the different fiber types of vertebrate skeletal muscles. Arch. Histol. Cytol., *51*:385, 1988.

Palade, G.E., Simionescu, M., and Simionescu, N.: Structural aspects of the permeability of the microvascular endothelium. Acta Physiol. Scand. (Suppl.), *463*:11, 1979.

Rhodin, J.A.G.: Fine structure of the vascular walls in mammals with special reference to smooth muscle component. Physiol. Rev., *42*:49, 1962.

Rhodin, J.A.G.: Fine structure of the vascular wall in mammals. Physiol. Rev., *42* (Suppl. 5):48, 1962.

Rhodin, J.A.G.: The ultrastructure of mammalian arterioles and precapillary sphincters. J. Ultastruct. Res., *18*:181, 1967.

Rhodin, J.A.G.: Ultrastructure of mammalian venous capillaries, venules and small collecting venules. J. Ultrastruct. Res., *25*:452, 1968.

Schwartz, J.H.: Axonal transport. Components, mechanisms, and specificity. Ann. Rev. Neurosci., *2*:467, 1979.

Sims, D.E.: The pericyte—a review. Tissue Cell, *18*:153, 1986.

Small, J.V., and Sobiezek, A.: The contractile apparatus of smooth muscle. Int. Rev. Cytol., *64*:241, 1980.

van Furth, R., et al.: The mononuclear phagocyte system: a new classification of macrophages, monocytes, and their precursor cells. Bull. WHO, *46*:845, 1972.

Weiss, L.: *The Cells and Tissues of the Immune System: Structure, Functions and Interactions*. Englewood Cliffs, NJ, Prentice-Hall, 1972.

Wintrobe, M.M., et al.: *Clinical Hematology*. 7th Ed. Philadelphia, Lea & Febiger, 1974.

Zweifach, B.W.: *Functional Behavior of the Microcirculation*. Springfield, IL, Charles C Thomas, 1961.

Zweifach, B.W.: *Microcirculation*. Ann. Rev. Physiol., *35*:117, 1973.

7

Embryologic Development of the Face and Oral Cavity

The human body consists of many groups of specialized cells forming tissues, organs and organ systems. In this chapter we will give a brief description of some of the developmental events that transform one single cell (the *fertilized ovum*) into a human body. Special emphasis will be placed on the development of the facial region.

Embryologic development requires complex interactions and differentiations of cells. If there is any disturbance in the normal sequence of events, especially during the first 3 months of pregnancy, a *malformation* is likely to result. Such malformations, which are evident at birth, are called *congenital* malformations.

As a dental health professional, you must be concerned about congenital malformations in at least two situations:

1. Congenital malformations of the head and neck region occur in 1 out of every 700 live births. The chances that you will treat patients, who were born with such malformations are real. These malformations may range from serious facial deformities to small deficiencies of the soft palate or cysts underneath an otherwise intact oral mucosa. It is hoped that such patients will have undergone surgical treatment for these defects by the time they seek your professional service. However, in the more serious cases, special consideration and adaptation of your treatment still may be necessary.

2. The development of certain congenital malformations, such as facial or palatal clefts, may be related to "environmental" conditions, for example, the use of certain drugs by pregnant women during susceptible stages of their pregnancy. Women in the first 3 months of pregnancy are particularly vulnerable in this respect. Treatment of such patients must be directed toward prevention of congenital malformations.

In human prenatal development, three distinct periods may be distinguished (Fig. 7–1):

THE FIRST WEEK (the period of the *unattached conceptus*).

136

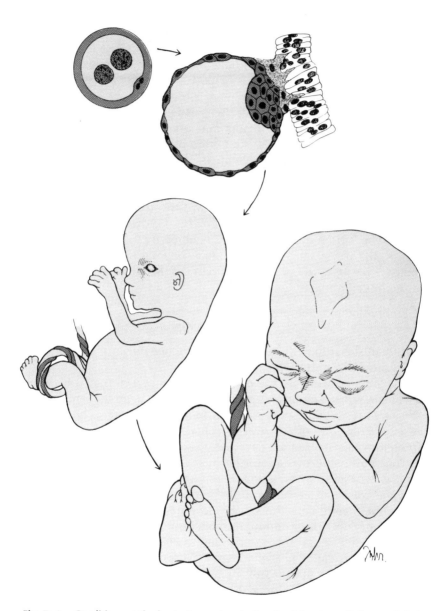

Fig. 7–1. Conditions at the beginning and end of each of the three distinct periods in human prenatal development. The first period begins with the newly fertilized ovum and ends with the attachment of the conceptus to the wall of the uterus. The second or embryonic period begins with the small vesicle of the conceptus attaching to the wall of the uterus and ends with an individual of recognizably human appearance. The third, or fetal, period begins with the small, but recognizably human, fetus and ends with the newborn baby.

In this week the fertilized ovum travels from the site where it was fertilized to the womb (uterus) and becomes attached to the wall of this organ by the end of the first week. At that time, a number of changes have occurred, which have transformed the single cell into a vesicle, consisting of a layer of peripheral cells and a small accumulation of embryonic cells.

THE EMBRYONIC PERIOD (the second through eighth week). In this time most organs and organ systems of the future individual are formed. This is a period of *differentiation*, and most congenital malformations develop in this time. At the end of the embryonic period, the developing individual has a recognizably human appearance.

THE FETAL PERIOD (the third through the ninth month). This is predominantly a time of *growth* of existing structures and will not be further described in this chapter. By the end of the fourth month, the physician is able to detect the fetal heartbeat; and only some weeks later, the pregnant woman is able to feel the movements of the fetus (quickening).

FERTILIZATION

Human development begins when one female germ cell and one male germ cell unite. This is fertilization.

The female germ cell, the *ovum*, develops in 1 of the 2 ovaries of a woman. Once a month, during the period between menarche (usually in early puberty) and menopause (45 to 50 years), the ovum is released from one of the ovaries. This process is called ovulation. Ovulation takes place 14 days before the next expected menstrual period. Following ovulation, the ovum is normally swept into the *uterine tube* and moved along the tube toward the uterus. An ovum survives for about 24 hours in the female genital tract.

The male germ cell, the *sperm,* develops in 1 of the 2 testes of a man. Generally sperm production is continuous from puberty until death. During sexual intercourse 300 to 500 million sperms are deposited in the vagina near the uterus. The sperms begin to move into the uterus and the uterine tubes at a considerable speed. The survival time of these germ cells, once they have been deposited in the female genital tract, is 3 to 4 days.

About 10 hours after intercourse, a relatively small number of the fastest moving sperms (300 to 500) have traveled two-thirds the length of the uterine tube. *If a living ovum is present at that time* in the tube, one of these germ cells will unite with the ovum (fertilization) and prenatal development begins (Fig. 7–2).

Each germ cell contains only one-half the normal number of chromosomes in its nucleus (23 chromosomes instead of 46). During

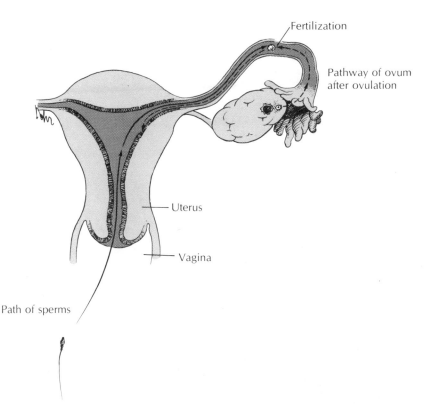

Fig. 7–2. Pathways of ovum and sperms before and immediately after fertilization. The ovum, released from one of the ovaries, is swept into the uterine tube and moves through the tube in the direction of the uterus (*broken line*). The sperms, deposited in the vagina, move through the uterus and up into the uterine tube *(solid line).* One sperm cell is illustrated, disproportionately large. The size of the projectile-shaped cell body of this cell is about $\frac{1}{20}$ that of an ovum. The length of the long tail, used to propel the sperm cell into the uterine tube, is about $\frac{1}{2}$ the diameter of an ovum. In the uterine tube, one sperm cell fertilizes the ovum. The fertilized ovum is moved slowly (*broken line*) from the site of fertilization toward the uterus, where it becomes attached to the uterine wall.

fertilization the nuclei of both germ cells are combined, restoring the number of chromosomes to 46, 23 from the male and 23 from the female parent.

THE FIRST WEEK

While the ovum is traveling to the uterus, following fertilization, it undergoes a series of mitotic divisions (Fig. 7–3).

On the *fourth day* after fertilization, the structure, consisting of 16 to 32 cells, enters the uterus. On the *fifth day* a central cavity develops inside this previously solid mass of cells. The structure

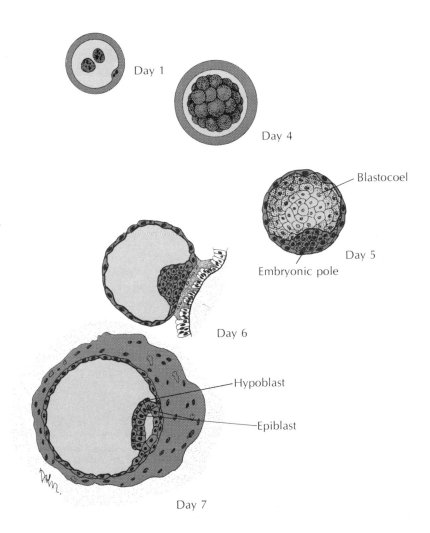

Fig. 7–3.   The appearance of the human conceptus during the first week of prenatal development. On day 1, the day of fertilization, the nucleus of the sperm cell is about to fuse with the nucleus of the ovum, thus restoring the chromosome number to 46. On day 4, the conceptus still moves about freely. The number of cells has increased from 1 to 16 by a few mitoses. The size of the conceptus, however, has barely increased. On day 5, the membrane, which surrounded initially the ovum and later the conceptus, has been lost. A central cavity (blastocoel) has developed. There is a distinct, single layer of peripheral cells and an accumulation of cells at the embryonic pole. The conceptus is called a blastocyst and is shown diagrammatically (cut open) to reveal its 3-dimensional structure. On day 6, the conceptus becomes attached to the wall of the uterus. The first attachment site is the embryonic pole. On day 7, the conceptus becomes further attached and embedded (implanted) in the uterine wall. In the cell accumulation at the embryonic pole, 2 distinct layers of cells are becoming visible: an epiblast layer and a hypoblast layer. Between epiblast and peripheral cell layers, a second cavity is forming. Epiblast and hypoblast now constitute a clearly delineated embryonic disc.

now develops into a *blastocyst,* which consists of a single layer of peripheral cells surrounding a fluid-filled cavity (blastocoel). At one site the cellular layer is thicker, because of the presence of about 8 slightly larger cells. This site is called the *embryonic pole,* and the larger cells will give rise to the actual embryo, which later becomes the fetus. The smaller peripheral cells give rise to most of the fetal membranes that will surround the developing individual (Fig. 7–3).

On the *sixth day* the developing structure, or conceptus, becomes attached to the wall of the uterus and *implantation* begins. This is essential for the success of the pregnancy, since implantation ensures the development of the placenta, which is necessary for the interaction between fetal and maternal circulation. An adequate placenta is needed to meet the metabolic and respiratory requirements of the developing human. The conceptus slowly invades the uterine tissues to some depth and, by the end of the second week, it is completely surrounded by these tissues.

On the *seventh day* the actual embryonic cells begin to form 2 distinct cell layers.

THE EMBRYONIC PERIOD

During this period, the second, third and fourth weeks of development have distinct characteristics.

THE SECOND WEEK. During the second week, the process of implantation continues. By further mitoses and differentiation, the actual embryonic cells have formed two distinct cell layers (Fig. 7–4, A): *epiblast,* facing the peripheral cell layer, and *hypoblast,* facing the fluid-filled blastocoel cavity. Between epiblast and peripheral cells a second cavity, the *amniotic cavity*, forms. Epiblast and hypoblast now constitute a clearly separate *disc* two cell-layers thick, suspended between two fluid-filled cavities. The disc will give rise to the embryo and is therefore called the *embryonic disc.*

For the sake of simplicity, we will not discuss here the further development of the fetal membranes, placenta, yolk sac and umbilical cord. The interested reader is referred to the standard texts of human embryology. The descriptions in this chapter will be limited to the fate of the head end of the embryonic disc.

THE THIRD WEEK. This week is characterized by the establishment of a rod-shaped thickening on the epiblast surface of the embryonic disc. This thickening is called the *primitive streak,* and it is the first external manifestation of the long axis of the future human body. We can now visualize a *bilateral symmetry* in the disc, as well as a head (cephalic) end and a tail (caudal) end (Fig. 7–4).

The continually proliferating epiblast cells now move in a wavelike fashion *toward* the primitive streak. At the primitive streak many

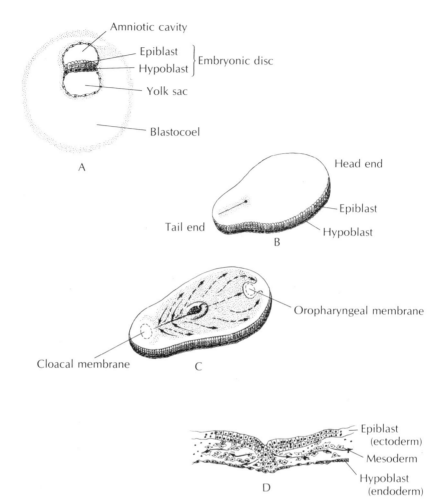

Fig. 7–4. Development in the second week, *A,* and third week, *B–D,* of human prenatal development are shown diagrammatically. *A,* During the second week, the epiblast and hypoblast are clearly defined within the embryonic disc. The second cavity, formed between epiblast and peripheral cells, becomes clearly established as the amniotic cavity. An outgrowth of hypoblast cells lines a yolk sac, thus subdividing the blastocoel cavity. In the following diagrams, only the structures of the embryonic disc have been depicted in three dimensions. *B,* The embryonic disc seen from "above" (epiblast side) at the beginning of the third week. A central thickening, the primitive streak, has formed at the tail end of the epiblast layer. *C,* Several epiblast cells, while undergoing further mitosis, move to the primitive streak (*solid arrows*), where they descend to a position between epiblast and hypoblast layers and establish a middle layer (*broken arrows*). This third (middle) layer is formed everywhere in the embryonic disc, except in the areas of oropharyngeal and cloacal membranes, which continue to consist of only two cell layers. *D,* A diagrammatic section through the embryonic disc, at the level of primitive streak, shows the movement of the epiblast cells. Most of these cells form the mesoderm. Some cells become inserted in the hypoblast layer, which now becomes the endoderm. The remainder of the epiblast layer becomes the ectoderm.

epiblast cells move "downward" to a position between the epiblast and hypoblast layers. Here they distribute themselves, establishing a *middle layer* sandwiched between epiblast and hypoblast. This middle layer is present in all parts of the embryo, except in two small, circular regions, the *oropharyngeal membrane* and the *cloacal membrane.* These membranes continue to consist of two cell layers only, and they represent the beginning and end points of the future digestive tract.

By the end of the third week, the embryonic disc consists of three distinct layers *(germ layers)* (Fig. 7–5): *ectoderm*, from the original epiblast, *mesoderm* (the *new* layer, between ectoderm and endoderm), derived from epiblast cells that have moved down through the primitive streak, and *endoderm,* derived in part from the original hypoblast and in part from epiblast cells, which moved down through the primitive streak and pushed into the original hypoblast layer. The cells in each of these three germ layers have already undergone certain differentiations, which make them different from the cells in the other two germ layers.

THE FOURTH WEEK. During the fourth week of development, the formation of the central nervous system is initiated. The central nervous system is derived from cells that are located in a thickened central band of ectoderm *(neurectoderm)*, running from the cephalic to the caudal end of the embryonic disc.

This thickened band, or *neural plate,* is first folded into a *neural groove*, which subsequently closes to become a *neural tube.* During the closure of the neural tube, the adjacent ectoderm grows over it and covers it. The closed neural tube lies, therefore, between endoderm and ectoderm, in mesoderm territory (Fig. 7–6). Closure of the neural tube occurs first in the neck region of the embryo and then continues, in a zipper-like fashion, in the direction of both the head and the tail.

During closure of the neural tube, two peripheral strips of neurectodermal cells, the *neural crest,* become separated from the neural

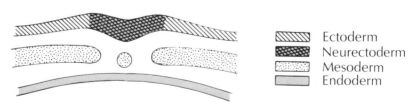

Ectoderm
Neurectoderm
Mesoderm
Endoderm

Fig. 7–5. Simplified diagrammatic transverse section through the embryonic disc, which consists of three germ layers by the end of the third week. The key to the right indicates the ectoderm, mesoderm, and endoderm. A small, central strip of ectoderm will differentiate further into neurectoderm, which will form the central nervous system.

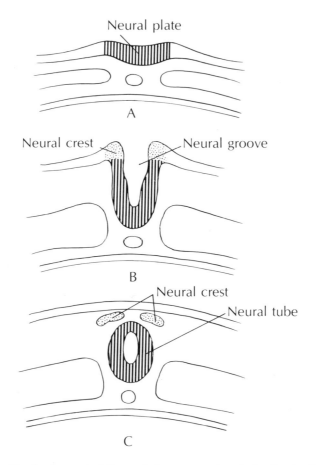

Fig. 7–6. The development of the central nervous system during the fourth week of prenatal development. *A, B,* **and** *C,* **represent chronologically sequential cross sections through the embryonic disc.** *A,* **A central strip of ectoderm, neurectoderm, has thickened into a neural plate.** *B,* **The neural plate has become folded into a neural groove. The two strips of neural crest (stippled) are clearly visible.** *C,* **The neural groove has closed into a neural tube. The neural tube and the two strips of neural crest are covered over by ectoderm.**

tube, but are covered over by ectoderm as well. The cells of those two strips, which come to lie on either side of the neural tube, will eventually migrate to many regions of the body, where they will differentiate into several different types of cells. Important to this discussion is the fact that these cells will become ganglion cells (both sensory and autonomic) and melanocytes.

In the *facial region* the *neural crest cells* play a rather exceptional role. Here, they migrate *among* the already present mesoderm cells, where they further differentiate and give rise to several tissues: (1) bone and cartilage, (2) connective tissue proper, and (3) some dental tissues (dental pulp and dentin, cementum and periodontal ligament). The *mesoderm* in the facial region gives rise to (1) blood vessels, and (2) muscle tissue.

Please *note* that the facial region is an *exceptional* region. In the rest of the body, neural crest cells do *not* differentiate into bone, cartilage or connective tissue cells and *certainly not* into cells that form dental tissues.

It is now possible to give, in general outline, a list of tissues and organs in the human body and to indicate from which of the three germ layers each is derived. Table 7–1 provides a *general* outline of the derivatives of the three germ layers.

Folding and Curving of the Embryo

In the foregoing discussion, we have considered the embryo as a flat disc, consisting of three distinct cell layers (except in the areas of the oropharyngeal and cloacal membranes, which consist of two cell layers). Actually, the flat embryonic disc is transformed during the third and fourth weeks of development into a curved, tubular structure, as the result of folding and curving (Fig. 7–7).

As a result of these events, the ectoderm comes to lie on the outside of the tubular structure and the endoderm on the inside. The foldings are produced by the extensive growth of both ectoderm and neural tube (especially the developing brain), compared with the much

Table 7–1.   Derivatives of 3 Germ Layers

Germ Layer	Derivatives
Ectoderm	Nerve tissue (from neurectoderm)
	Neural crest (from neurectoderm)
	Facial connective tissues, bone, cartilage, dental connective tissues
	Other derivatives: ganglion cells, melanocytes, etc.
	Epithelium
	Oral epithelium
	Epidermis
Mesoderm	Connective tissues
	Connective tissue proper
	Skeletal tissue (bone, cartilage)
	Circulatory system (heart, blood, blood vessels)
	Lymphatics
	Muscle tissue
	Heart
	Striated muscle
	Smooth muscle
	Urinary system
	Epithelium and connective tissue
Endoderm	Epithelial lining of digestive tract (except oral cavity)
	Epithelial lining of respiratory tract

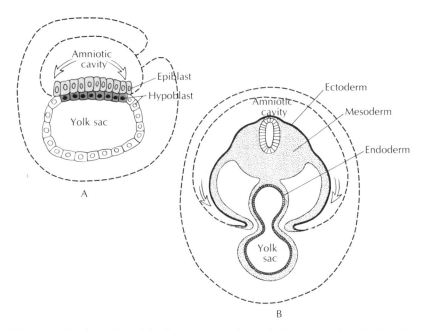

Fig. 7–7. Transformation of the flat embryonic disc at the beginning of the third week, *A*, to a tubular structure at the end of the fourth week, *B*, of development, seen in cross sections. During this period of folding, the ectoderm comes to lie on the outside of the embryo, while the endoderm is gradually enclosed at the inside, becoming the lining of the digestive and respiratory tracts. The arrows indicate the direction in which the amniotic cavity is enlarged, until it finally almost completely surrounds the embryo (later the fetus). Concurrently with the enlargement of the amniotic cavity, the blastocoel cavity becomes reduced in size and finally disappears.

slower growth of the endoderm. The faster growing regions, there-fore, have to "bulge" out of the way (Fig. 7–8).

The Facial Region

Development of the facial region begins in the fourth week of prenatal life and is completed during the twelfth week. However, the most critical events in the development of the face take place *before* the fetal period begins, at 8 weeks.

In the fourth week of development, the rapidly growing brain bulges over the oropharyngeal membrane. The latter is disintegrating, establishing access into the digestive tract from the amniotic cavity (Fig. 7–9). The area of the future face is squeezed between the fore-brain and the heart. A bulging strand of tissue runs between the forebrain region and the developing heart, on either side of the dis-integrating oropharyngeal membrane. This is called the *mandibular arch.*

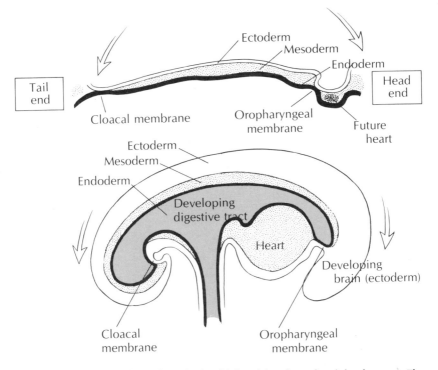

Fig. 7–8. Curving of the embryo in the third and fourth weeks of development. The embryonic disc is shown in a section along its entire length (top figure). The three germ layers are illustrated. Cloacal and oropharyngeal membranes consist of two germ layers. The amniotic cavity (on the ectoderm side) enlarges in the direction of the arrows. Since the ectoderm (which includes the central nervous system in this diagram) grows much more extensively than the endoderm, the embryo becomes curved, with ectoderm at the larger, bulging side (bottom figure).

The mandibular arch is the first of 5 pairs of swellings (the four others are indicated in Fig. 7–9 as the second through the fifth arches). The four other pairs of swellings are involved predominantly in the formation of the neck region. The organization of the skeletal elements in the adult neck is a reflection of this original, *segmental* organization in arches.

However, for the development of the face proper, only the first or mandibular arch will be considered, in addition to the swelling of the tissues over the forebrain: the so-called *frontonasal process.*

In the adult face, the parts formed by the tissues of the frontonasal process are (1) the forehead and (2) the nose. The parts formed by the tissues of the mandibular arch are (1) the midface, except for the nose, and (2) the lower face (Fig. 7–10).

The development of the face is best considered as the forward growth, around nasal and oral cavities, of a number of swellings or

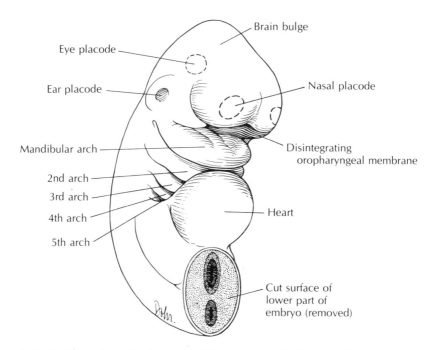

Fig. 7–9.   **Three-dimensional diagram of the upper part of a human embryo at about 4 weeks of prenatal development. The cut surface, where the lower part of the embryo has been removed, is shown. The facial region is located between the bulge of the developing forebrain and the large developing heart. Five pairs of swellings (mandibular or first arch and second through fifth arches) are illustrated in the neck region of the embryo. Between mandibular arch and bulging forebrain is the primitive oral cavity. At this location, the oropharyngeal membrane is disintegrating, establishing an open connection between amniotic cavity and primitive gut. The organs of special sense are represented at this stage by rounded placodes of thickened ectoderm. There are 3 pairs of these placodes: nasal, eye, and ear placodes.**

processes arising from the frontonasal process and the mandibular arch. These swellings have a core of embryonic connective tissue (mesenchyme), derived from neural crest cells and mesoderm cells, and an outer covering of ectoderm.

DEVELOPMENT OF THE NOSE. The nasal epithelium which will be responsible for the sensation of smell, develops on the surface of the frontonasal process of the embryo in the form of 2 *nasal placodes.* Placodes are rounded areas of specialized thickened ectoderm, which is comparable to the neurectoderm of the neural plate. Placodes are found at the locations of developing *organs of special sense*—eyes, ears and nose. The nasal placodes will develop into the olfactory epithelium.

Parts of the frontonasal process begin to swell around these nasal placodes. The placodes themselves do not grow forward very much,

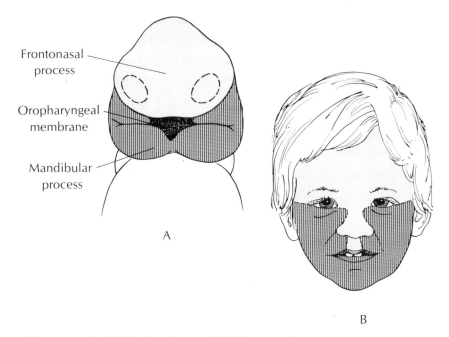

Frontonasal process

Oropharyngeal membrane

Mandibular process

A

B

Fig. 7–10. The facial region of a 4-week-old human embryo. A, and of a young child, B, are shown, seen from front. The lightly stippled frontonasal process in A, will give rise to forehead, nose, and midsection of upper lip, similarly stippled in B. The mandibular arch darkly shaded in A, will give rise to a large part of the midface and all of the lower face, similarly shaded in B.

while the surrounding swellings do. As the result of this unequal growth, the nasal placodes stay behind and come to lie in deep pits: the future nasal cavities.

The swellings around these pits, all derived from the frontonasal process, are identified as *two lateral nasal processes* and *two medial nasal processes* (Fig. 7–11). The lateral nasal processes will form the sides of the nose, while the medial nasal processes will form the bridge of the nose and the central band (philtrum) of the upper lip.

DEVELOPMENT OF THE MIDDLE AND LOWER FACE. The lower face is formed directly by the bilateral swellings *(mandibular processes)* of the mandibular arch. The middle face is formed by a pair of separate swellings *(maxillary processes)*, which develop from the mandibular arch, just above the mandibular processes.

Each maxillary process rapidly grows forward between lateral nasal process and mandibular process, and then makes contact with the lower edge of the medial nasal process (Fig. 7–12).

Initially, grooves of various depths separate the facial processes from each other. Required for the *normal* development of the face are (1) correlated speeds and amounts of forward growth of the var-

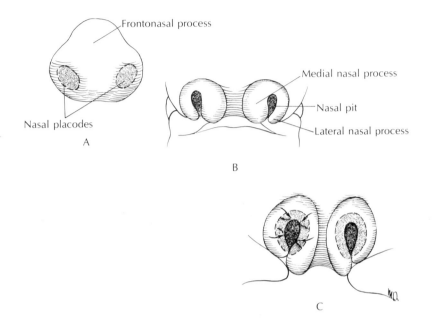

Fig. 7–11. *A*, At 4 weeks of development, the nasal placodes are still located on the ectodermal surface of the frontonasal process. The nasal placodes do not grow forward as much as the surrounding tissues. As a result, at a slightly later stage, *B*, the nasal placodes have stayed behind and are now located in nasal pits, surrounded by several swellings (lateral nasal and medial nasal processes), which have developed from the frontonasal process. In *C*, the situation in the sixth week of development, the placodes are lying deeper in the nasal pits, which are in contact with the primitive oral cavity below. The lateral nasal processes will form the sides of the nose. The medial nasal processes will form the bridge of the nose and the central strip of the upper lip.

ious facial processes, and (2) elimination of the grooves between the processes.

On the external surface of the face, grooves between adjacent facial processes are eliminated by the proliferation of the mesenchyme underneath the ectoderm that lines the deepest part of the groove. Because of this proliferation, the groove area "catches up" with the forward growth of the facial processes and the groove is eliminated (Fig. 7–13, A, B). If a groove is not eliminated, or is partially eliminated, a *facial cleft* may result. Facial clefts may be complete or incomplete; bilateral or unilateral (Figs. 7–14 and 7–15).

TIMETABLE. The groove in the future chin area, between the 2 mandibular processes, is the first to be eliminated at about 4 weeks. The grooves between maxillary and medial nasal processes are the last to be eliminated, at about 6 weeks.

DEVELOPMENT OF THE PALATE. By the age of 6 weeks,

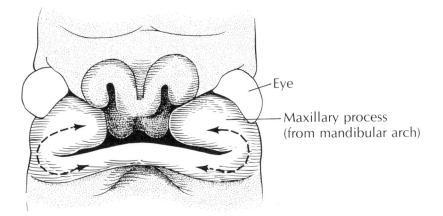

Fig. 7–12. Contributions to the development of the face by components of the mandibular arch during the fifth and sixth weeks of development. The mandibular arch will form the lower face directly, by further increase in size. In addition, two maxillary processes will form as additional swellings on the upper surfaces of the mandibular arch and will give rise to a large part of the midface. The maxillary processes grow forward (*two top arrows*), first establishing contact with the lateral nasal processes and subsequently with the medial nasal processes.

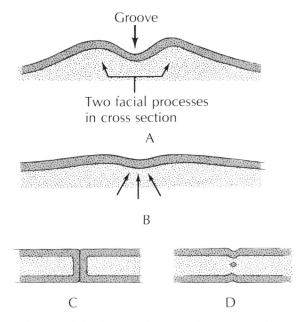

Fig. 7–13. During normal development, the groove between two adjacent facial processes (swellings) is eliminated by increased tissue growth in the groove region, *A* and *B*. A different situation is present when two epithelially covered processes meet each other across a space (as happens in the development of the definitive palate), *C* and *D*. The epithelia of the two processes fuse. Subsequently, the epithelium in the fusion seam is broken down and continuity is established between the mesenchymal cores of the two processes.

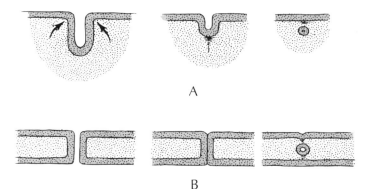

A

B

Fig. 7–14.   *A* in this figure should be compared with *A* and *B* in Fig. 7–13; *B* should be compared with *C* and *D* in Fig. 7–13. *A*, Several possible failures in the elimination of a groove between two adjacent facial processes are illustrated. In the left diagram, the facial processes have grown forward, but the groove area has not grown much if at all. In such a case, a complete facial cleft results. In the middle diagram, some groove elimination has taken place, but a small part of the groove persists. This results in an incomplete facial cleft. In the right diagram, the groove has been eliminated, but some epithelium was pinched off and has remained in the mesenchyme. Such an epithelial remnant may enlarge and develop into a developmental cyst in postnatal life. *B*, Failures in fusion between two epithelially covered processes, which approach each other across an open space, are illustrated. In the left diagram, the facial processes remain too short and never touch. This results in a complete cleft. In the middle diagram, the facial processes touch, but the epithelial seam is not broken down. During further development, such processes may be pulled apart and a complete cleft may result. In the right diagram, some epithelium has been broken down after fusion, but a large remnant remains. This remnant may be large enough to form a submucous cleft or it may develop into a cyst.

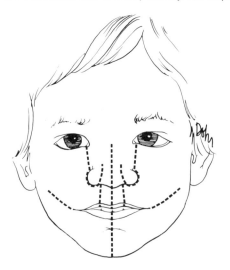

Fig. 7–15.   In this diagram of a face, the broken lines indicate the possible locations of facial clefts, formed if any of the events shown in Figure 7–14 *A* occur in any of these locations. The areas between the broken lines correspond with the areas formed by the original facial processes.

the external face of the embryo has begun to assume human features. The nasal pits have deepened and, at their deepest part, a degeneration of tissue has created an open communication between the primitive nasal cavities and the underlying oral cavity. In front of this open communication a horizontal strand of tissue separates oral and nasal cavities. This is the *primitive palate*. It is formed by the combined medial nasal processes and a small part of the maxillary processes. The primitive palate will become the upper lip, the incisor region of the alveolar arch of the upper jaw and the palate in front of the incisive foramen.

What remains to be formed is the *definitive palate*: the hard palate behind the incisive foramen and all of the soft palate. This is formed between weeks 6 and 12 of prenatal development.

The definitive palate is formed by two shelf-like processes, developing from those surfaces of the maxillary processes, which are *inside* the primitive oral cavity. The two *palatal processes* first grow downward, along the sides of the developing tongue. By the middle or the end of the eighth week, a combination of events occurs: the palatal processes have grown quite voluminous, the lower jaw and tongue have grown forward and downward, and the tongue muscles are contracting. As a result, the tongue is able to move out of the way of the palatal processes. These are now released from their

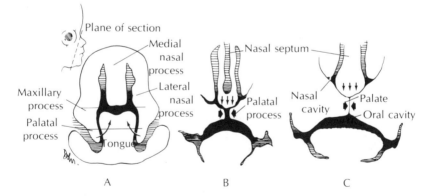

Fig. 7–16. The development of the definitive palate in the seventh and eighth weeks of human embryonic development is shown in oblique, nearly vertical sections through the facial region (at the level indicated in the diagram at the far left), at three consecutive stages. Initially, the two palatal processes grow downward, alongside the tongue, growing out vertically from the inside surfaces of the maxillary processes, A. Subsequently, the tongue moves out of the way, and the palatal processes flip up into a horizontal position (*arrows*). The three epithelially lined processes (combined medial nasal processes and two palatal processes) then are fused, B, and C, in the manner shown in Figure 7–13 C and D.

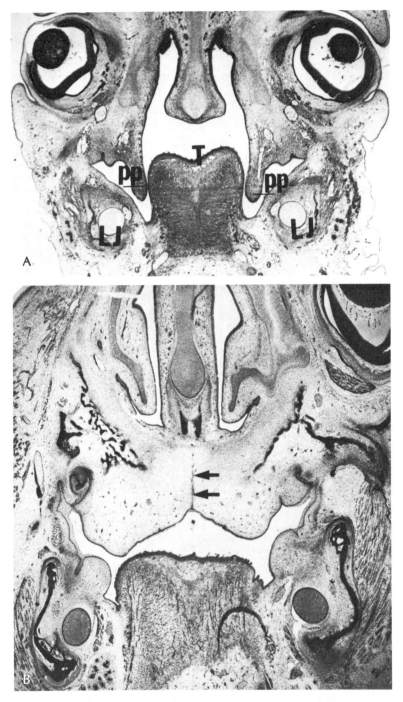

Fig. 7–17. *A,* Vertical section through the facial region of a 7-week-old human embryo. The 2 darkly staining eyes are included in the section. The tongue (T) and the palatal processes (PP), growing downward vertically along its sides, are clearly visible. LJ = lower jaw complex. Original magnification × 5. *B,* Oblique, nearly vertical section through the facial region of an 8.5-week-old human fetus. The palatal processes have moved up and have become fused with each other and with the nasal septum in a horizontal position. Some epithelial remnants (arrows) are still present in the midline seam between the palatal processes. Original magnification × 5.

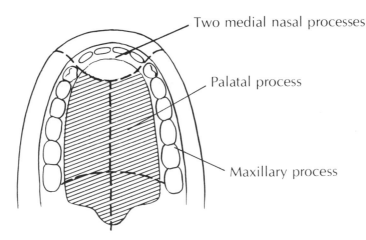

Two medial nasal processes

Palatal process

Maxillary process

Fig. 7–18. A diagram of the hard and soft palates, as they appear viewed from below. The area of the front teeth corresponds with the primitive palate, formed largely by the two medial nasal processes. The shaded part of the palate (part of the hard palate in front, and the soft palate in the back) is formed by the two palatal processes, which come together and fuse in the midline. Clefts are possible at all "seams" between the medial nasal processes and the palatal processes and in the midline between the two palatal processes.

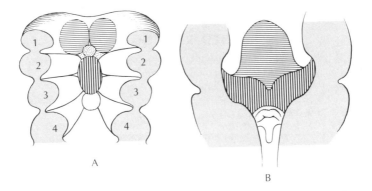

A

B

Fig. 7–19. Several originally independent swellings on the inside surfaces of the first (mandibular) through fourth arches in the embryo's neck region, participate in the formation of the tongue. The swellings are shown in a 3-dimensional view (from the inside) of the 4 arches in a 4-week-old embryo, A. At a somewhat later stage, B, the individual arches are no longer manifest, and the grooves between the adjacent swellings have been eliminated. Some swellings have overgrown others, and a recognizable tongue is formed. Corresponding parts in the 2 diagrams are shaded identically.

vertical position and flip up into a horizontal position. Their edges establish contact with each other, first in the front of the oral cavity and then gradually further backward (Figs. 7–16 and 7–17).

Fusion takes place between the touching edges of the palatal processes and the lower border of the nasal septal tissues, formed by the combined medial nasal processes. Fusion involves a "glueing together" of the touching epithelia of these three structures. A cellular glue is produced by the epithelial cells covering the edges. Subsequently, these epithelial cells break down, so that the epithelial "seams" disappear and the mesenchymal cores become continuous. The process of fusion is shown schematically in Figure 7–13, C, D.

Fusion of the palate occurs in a zipper-like fashion from the front to the back, from 8 weeks until 12 weeks, when the last part of the soft palate fuses. If fusion fails to occur, or if the epithelium fails to break down, or if either occurs incompletely, a cleft palate may result. Cleft palate may be found isolated or associated with a cleft lip. It may be unilateral or bilateral (Fig. 7–18).

DEVELOPMENT OF THE TONGUE. During the development of the external face, the tongue forms from five independent swellings on the inside surfaces (pharyngeal surfaces) of the first (mandibular) through the fourth arches.

The grooves between these individual swellings of the tongue are eliminated in a manner similar to the groove elimination of the external face (Fig. 7–19).

The body of a fully developed tongue is formed by contributions from arches 1 and 2. The root or base of the tongue is formed by contributions from arches 3 and 4.

SELECTED READING LIST

Hinrichsen, K.: The early development of morphology and patterns of the face in the human embryo. Adv. Anat. Embryol. Cell. Biol., *98*:1, 1985.

Kraus, B.S., Kitamura, H., and Lathman, R.A.: *Atlas of Developmental Anatomy of the Face. With Special Reference to Normal and Cleft Lip and Palate.* New York, Harper & Row, 1966.

Le Douarin, N.M.: *The Neural Crest.* Cambridge, Cambridge University Press, 1982.

Moss-Salentijn, L.: Anatomy and Embryology. In *Surgery of the Paranasal Sinuses.* Edited by A. Blitzer, W. Lawson, and W.H. Friedman. Philadelphia, W.B. Saunders Co., 1985.

Nishimura, H., et al.: *Prenatal Development of the Human with Special Reference to Craniofacial Structures: An Atlas.* Bethesda, MD, DHEW Publication No (NIH) 75-546, 1973.

Noden, D.M.: Origins and patterning of craniofacial mesenchymal tissues. J. Craniofac. Genet. Dev. Biol., *Suppl.2*:15, 1986.

O'Rahilly, R., and Müller, F.: *Developmental Stages in Human Embryos.* Washington, D.C., Carnegie Institution of Washington, Publication 637, 1987.

Sperber, G.H.: *Craniofacial Embryology.* 4th Ed. Dental Practitioners Handbook #15. London, Wright, 1989.

Tuchmann-Duplessis, H., David, G., and Haegel, P.: *Illustrated Human Embryology. Vol. I. Embryogenesis.* New York, Springer Verlag, 1972.

Waterman, R.E., and Meller, S.M.: Alterations in the epithelial surface of human palatal shelves prior to and during fusion: A scanning electron microscopic study. Anat. Rec., *180*:111, 1974.

Dental and Periodontal Tissues

8

Introduction to Part II

In the second part of this book, Chapters 9 through 14, we will introduce the tissues of the tooth—enamel, dentin, pulp, and cementum—and the tissues surrounding the tooth—alveolar bone, periodontal ligament, and dentogingival junction.

When inspecting your own teeth in front of a mirror, try again to identify incisors, canines, premolars, and molars. That part of a tooth which is visible inside the oral cavity is called the *crown* or, more precisely, the *clinical crown* of the tooth.

Another part of the tooth, which cannot be seen during inspection, is the *clinical root.* This is covered with gingiva and bone. Clinical roots may be seen in radiographs only.

The clinical crowns are shorter in young people than in older people because, with age, some of the bone is lost and the gingiva recedes, exposing more of the tooth to the oral cavity.

The tooth is a *complex* structure, consisting of four different "dental tissues": enamel, dentin, pulp, and cementum.

The pulp is located in the center of a tooth, and it is surrounded by a dentin shell. Dentin is found in both the (anatomical) crown and the root of the tooth. The dentin in the crown is covered by an enamel cap; the dentin in the root is covered with cementum. The borderline between enamel and cementum is located at the neck or *cervix* of the tooth. This is also the borderline between *anatomical root and crown* (Fig. 8–1).

The part of the tooth that is covered with enamel is the anatomical crown; the part covered with cementum is the anatomical root. Notice that anatomical crown and root are not necessarily identical with clinical crown and root.

Between the gingiva and the surface of the tooth, a special junction, the *dentogingival* junction, is present. In young individuals, this junction is located entirely on the enamel surface. With age and recession of the gingival tissues, the junction moves slowly onto the cementum, exposing more of the height of the tooth.

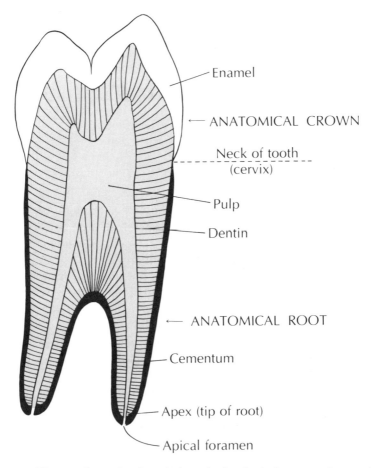

**Fig. 8–1.   Diagram of a section through the entire length of a human tooth (premolar).
The anatomical crown is the part of the tooth that is covered with enamel. The anatomical
root is the part of the tooth that is covered with cementum. The neck (cervix) of the tooth
is found where the anatomical crown meets the anatomical root. Both anatomical crown
and root have a central core of dental pulp (uncalcified, loose connective tissue) surrounded by a shell of dentin. The tip of a dental root is the apex. At the apex, an apical
foramen gives access to the pulp chamber.**

Thus, in young individuals the clinical crown (the part of the tooth
that is exposed) is *shorter* than the anatomical crown (the part of the
tooth that is covered with enamel). With recession of the gingiva,
the clinical crown becomes taller, first reaching the same height as
the anatomical crown, and subsequently becoming taller than the
anatomical crown (Fig. 8–2).

Enamel is a calcified tissue that is deposited by epithelial (ectodermal) cells. After enamel has been formed, these epithelial cells
are lost and enamel becomes a tissue without cells. This means that

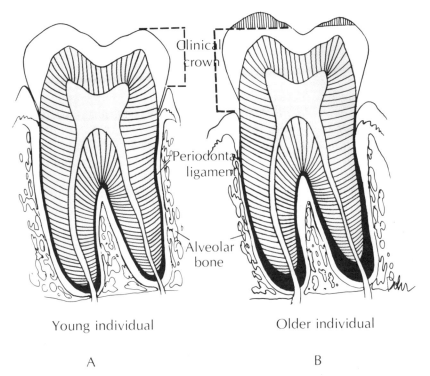

Young individual   Older individual

A   B

Fig. 8–2. Diagrams of sections of human molar teeth and the surrounding tissues in a young individual, *A,* and in a much older individual, *B.* Each tooth is suspended in a socket of alveolar bone, to which it is attached by means of a periodontal ligament. *A,* The height of the clinical crown (the exposed part of the tooth) is shorter than the height of the anatomical crown, because the latter is still partially covered with gingival tissue (free and attached gingiva). *B,* The gingival tissues and the upper rim of the alveolar bone socket have receded in the direction of the apices. This exposes all of the anatomical crown and even a small part of the anatomical root. The entire exposed part of the tooth is the clinical crown, which at this stage, is of greater height than the anatomical crown. Other age changes include wear of the enamel cap (and sometimes some dentin as well); increased thickness of dentin, and thus a decreased size of the pulp; and a thicker layer of cementum, especially near the apices.

enamel, once formed, changes little. It does not increase in thickness and has no healing ability to repair damages of caries and wear.

Dentin and cementum are both *calcified connective tissues.* Dentin is capable of continued appositional growth in an inward direction. This does not affect the external dimensions of a tooth, but it does encroach upon the centrally located pulp tissue. With age, the dentin layer becomes thicker and the pulp chamber correspondingly smaller.

Cementum is also capable of continued appositional growth in an outward direction. Thus, with age, the cementum layer becomes thicker, especially near the tip, or *apex,* of the root.

Pulp is an uncalcified, *loose connective tissue*. It contains the blood vessels and nerves necessary for the vitality of the tooth. The pulp is enclosed almost entirely by dentin. Only at the apex, through the *apical foramen,* is the pulp in contact with other connective tissues.

The borderline between dentin and enamel in the anatomical crown is called the *dentino-enamel junction.* The borderline between dentin and cementum in the anatomical root is called the *dentino-cementum junction*. These two junctions can be seen only in sectioned teeth. The borderline between cementum and enamel at the cervix of the tooth is called the *cemento-enamel junction.*

We distinguish three "periodontal tissues": dentogingival junction (epithelium), alveolar bone and periodontal ligament (connective tissue).

The anatomical root of a tooth is suspended in an individual bone socket or *alveolus.* The root is attached to this socket by means of a *dense connective tissue*, consisting primarily of highly organized, tendon-like collagen fiber bundles. This is the *periodontal ligament.* The periodontal ligament forms a specialized *joint* between the tooth and the alveolar bone, somewhat comparable to a suture.

In the following chapters, we will describe each of these dental and periodontal tissues in greater detail.

9

Tooth Development and Eruption

Tooth development takes place over a long period of time. It begins in the seventh week of embryonic life (primary dentition), and it continues well into the teenage years (third molar of the secondary dentition).

The following occurs during this period: (1) a *primary* dentition (milk dentition, deciduous dentition), consisting of 20 teeth, develops, erupts, functions, and is shed; and (2) a *secondary* dentition (permanent dentition), consisting of 32 teeth, develops, erupts (replacing all teeth of the primary dentition and adding molar teeth) and becomes functional.

From a clinical point of view, there are two important facts that require an understanding of tooth development:

1. Young children and teenagers who are seen in the dental office have teeth that are in several different stages of development. Clinically visible teeth may be part of a *mixed* dentition (teeth of both primary and secondary dentitions are functional simultaneously). Other teeth are not visible, but are still in the process of developing in the underlying tissues of the jaw. You should be prepared to recognize such teeth clinically as well as radiographically. From the standpoint of prevention, if developing teeth are present in the jaw, nutritional counseling and the restricted use of certain drugs, such as tetracyclines (see Chap. 10) are desirable to prevent developmental anomalies in the developing teeth.

2. You should also be aware that the presence of many developing teeth leaves little space for bone tissue in a child's jaw and can result in a weakening of the jaw structure, making it more responsive to trauma, i.e., fractures (Fig. 9–1).

At the end of this chapter, timetables for the emergence of the various teeth into the oral cavity, as well as reviews of the various developmental stages of the 2 dentitions, may be found. But first we will discuss the principal events in the process of tooth development.

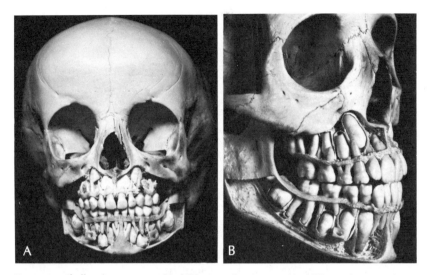

Fig. 9–1. Skulls of a 4½-year-old-child, *A*, and a 9-year-old child, *B*. The outer bone layers of upper and lower jaws have been removed to expose the teeth of the secondary dentition, which have not yet erupted and become functional. *A*, Only the teeth of the primary dentition are functional. The upper and lower jaws are filled with developing teeth of the secondary dentition, leaving little space for bone tissue. *B*, The incisors and the first molars of the secondary dentition have become functional. Secondary canines, premolars, and second molars are still developing inside the jaws, the canines and premolars beneath the roots of their primary predecessors.

TOOTH DEVELOPMENT

As noted in Chapter 8, a tooth is a complex structure, consisting of four tissues: three *calcified* tissues (enamel, dentin and cementum) and one *uncalcified* tissue (dental pulp).

Two embryonic tissues are responsible for the development of a tooth: (1) embryonic *connective tissue* (mesenchyme) of the jaw, derived from neural crest, and (2) oral *epithelial* tissue, derived from ectoderm.

Dentin, dental pulp and cementum are formed by cells of the embryonic connective tissue and are classified as *connective tissues.* Enamel is formed by the epithelial cells and may be classified as an *epithelial product.*

The embryonic connective tissue and epithelium continuously interact with each other during tooth development. For each successive step of the developmental process specific interactions are needed. If this sequence of interactions is interrupted, the process of tooth formation is interrupted.

In tooth development, two principal events must occur: (1) the establishment of the particular tooth *shapes* by a process called *morphodifferentiation*; and (2) the *differentiation* of special groups of cells into dentin-forming cells *(odontoblasts)*, enamel-forming cells *(ameloblasts)*, cementum-forming cells *(cementoblasts)* and pulp-forming cells *(fibroblasts)*, by a process called *cytodifferentiation.*

Morphodifferentiation

The main stages of morphodifferentiation, for both primary and secondary tooth development, are bud stage, cap stage, and bell stage (Fig. 9–2).

The differential growth of the oral epithelium into the underlying mesenchyme of the jaw is responsible for the outline of the tooth. Initially, the oral epithelium forms a horseshoe-shaped thickening along the surfaces of both future dental arches. An increased number of cell divisions in this thickened oral epithelium causes it to proliferate into the underlying mesenchyme.

As a result of the different rates of growth in the various parts of the proliferating epithelium, the ingrowth locally becomes thickened into *buds (bud stage)*, nearly spherical balls of epithelial cells. Each epithelial sphere is associated with a sphere of *condensed mesenchyme* (Fig. 9–3).

The buds form only in areas where the teeth will develop. There are, therefore, 10 buds in the upper jaw and 10 buds in the lower jaw, which go on to form the teeth of the primary dentition. Later 16 buds in the upper jaw and 16 buds in the lower jaw initiate the development of the teeth of the secondary dentition. Between the buds, the epithelium does not proliferate further downward and remains just a thickened band.

The epithelial cells of the buds continue to proliferate but not all at the same rate. This rapidly changes the shapes of these structures into *caps* (*cap stage*; Fig. 9–4). In this stage the future shape of the tooth becomes evident. With continued growth and differentiation the caps become highly specialized epithelial organs: *enamel organs.* These enamel organs reach full morphodifferentiation during the next stage, the *bell stage* (Fig. 9–5).

The bell stage is the final stage of morphodifferentiation. During this stage a specialization occurs of cells of the enamel organ itself, resulting in the establishment of four distinct epithelial layers: outer enamel epithelium, stellate reticulum, stratum intermedium, and inner enamel epithelium (Fig. 9–6).

Let us have a closer look at the developing tooth in the bell stage. A developing tooth, or *tooth germ,* consists of two components: the *epithelial* and the *mesenchymal.*

The *epithelial component* (enamel organ), in the bell stage undergoes specialization into the four distinct layers already mentioned. The innermost layer, the inner enamel epithelium, which

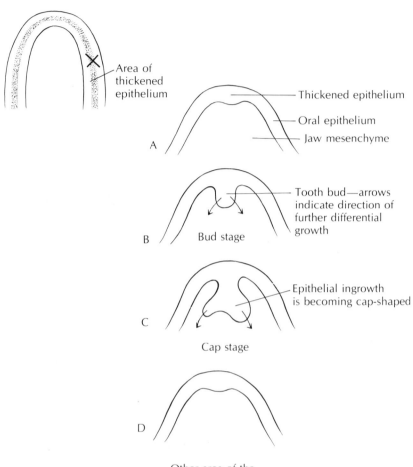

Fig. 9–2. Early stages in the morphodifferentiation of developing teeth. The diagram at top left shows the oral surface of a jaw. A horseshoe-shaped thickening of oral epithelium (stippled) is formed along this surface. The epithelium grows into the underlying mesenchyme. x indicates the plane of section through the jaw, shown in diagrams *A* through *C*. *A*, The first development of thickened epithelium. At a slightly later stage, *B*, bud-like thickenings have formed in specific areas, corresponding with the locations of future teeth. Differential growth of the epithelium in each of these buds leads to the formation of epithelial caps in the next phase of development, *C*. The arrows indicate the preferential directions of epithelial growth, leading to the formation of the cap-shape. The caps remain attached for a while to the oral epithelium by an epithelial sheet (shown as a strand in cross section): the dental lamina. *D*, Section through the jaw (at the same phase of development as shown in *C*) in an area between the locations of developing teeth. Here, no further development takes place beyond the stage of thickened epithelium.

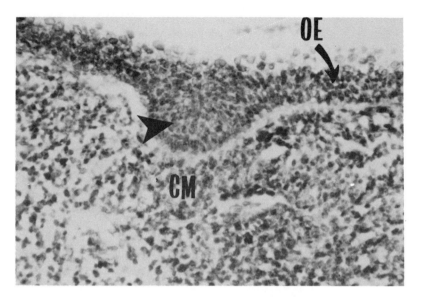

Fig. 9–3. Tooth development in the bud stage. The thickened epithelial bud is indicated with an arrowhead. OE = oral epithelium. CM = condensed mesenchyme. Original magnification ×125.

lines the concave inner surface of the enamel organ, will be responsible for the formation of enamel. The stratum intermedium, stellate reticulum and outer enamel epithelium will support and assist the inner enamel epithelium in this future function.

The *mesenchymal component* is further subdivided into the *dental papilla* and the *dental sac.*

The *dental papilla* is condensed mesenchyme located in the concavity of the enamel organ. The peripheral cells will form dentin, while the central part of the dental papilla will further develop into the dental pulp.

The *dental sac* (dental follicle) also is condensed mesenchyme. It is continuous with the dental papilla and its proliferating cells form a thin layer surrounding the convex surface of the enamel organ. It supplies the cells that will form cementum, the periodontal ligament and part of the alveolar bone socket of the tooth.

The epithelial strand, which still connects the enamel organ with the oral epithelium, is the *dental lamina.* It has no further role once tooth development has progressed this far, and eventually it will fall apart. However, some epithelial cells of the dental lamina may stay behind as strands or as clumps. These cell remnants may undergo further mitoses and occasionally even some central keratinization. If that occurs, they may enlarge and become visible as little white bumps beneath the oral mucosa of a baby. Usually no complications

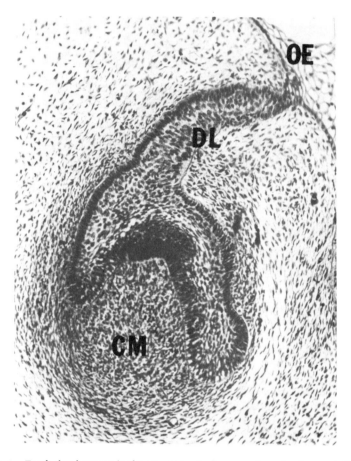

Fig. 9–4. Tooth development in the cap stage. A clear cap-shape has been established by the ingrowing epithelium. Spaces have begun to develop between the epithelial cells in the center of the cap. OE = oral epithelium; DL = dental lamina; CM = condensed mesenchyme. Original magnification × 20.

result, and these structures are lost during the process of tooth eruption, when the tooth emerges through the epithelium into the oral cavity.

DEVELOPMENTAL INTERACTIONS. As we stated before, in order for a tooth to develop, the presence of both epithelial and mesenchymal components is essential. The reason for this is that these 2 tissues continuously communicate with each other, *both* during morphodifferentiation *and* during cytodifferentiation. Messages move in alternate directions across the *basal lamina*, the boundary between epithelium and mesenchyme.

The first communication comes from the mesenchyme in the earliest stages of morphodifferentiation. This message, on reaching the

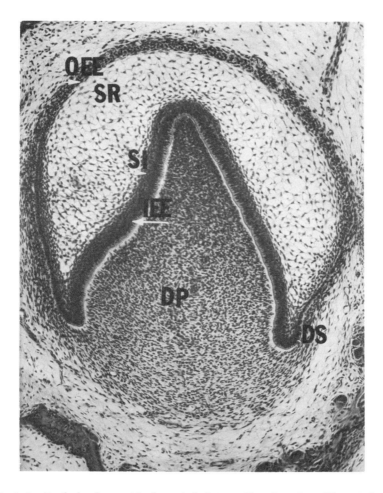

Fig. 9–5. Tooth development in the early bell stage. There is a clear differentiation in the epithelial enamel organ between the cells of the outer enamel epithelium (OEE), stellate reticulum (SR), stratum intermedium (SI) and inner enamel epithelium (IEE). The condensed mesenchyme inside the enamel organ is the dental papilla (DP). The condensed mesenchyme around the enamel organ is the dental sac (DS). Around the tooth germ, a much-less-condensed mesenchyme is visible and some of the developing bone of the jaw (darkly staining). No dental lamina is visible because this section is somewhat off-center through the enamel organ. Original magnification × 20.

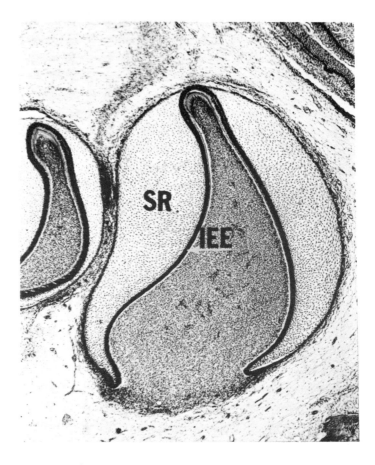

Fig. 9–6.   Two tooth germs (incisors of the primary dentition) in the late bell stage of development. At the end of the bell stage and during the earliest deposition of the hard dental tissues, the shaping process of the dentino-enamel junction (in the anatomical crown) by the inner enamel epithelium (IEE) is nearly completed. The stellate reticulum (SR) is extensive. A very thin layer of dentin has been deposited near the incisal edges. The tooth germ of the incisor at the left is somewhat tilted. This results in a sectioned, image, resembling the section through the side of a bowl (Appendix III). Original magnification ×6.

oral epithelium, instructs the epithelium to grow downward into the mesenchyme and shape the tooth.

It is now clear that the mesenchyme is the important determinant for the *initiation* of tooth development and for the specific *type* of tooth (incisor vs. molar for instance). The precise nature of the message is not known at this time. It is possible that the mesenchymal cells produce a substance that serves as a message for the initiation of tooth development. If the message in fact consists of such a substance, it must move through the basal lamina from the mesenchymal cells to the epithelial cells, become attached to specific receptors on the epithelial cell membranes, and stimulate these cells to undergo the greater numbers of mitoses that are necessary for *morphodifferentiation*. Alternately, the only message given by the mesenchyme

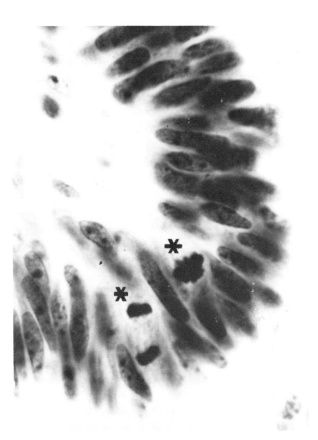

Fig. 9–7. Histologic section through the cervical loop of an enamel organ in the bell stage. At this loop, inner and outer enamel epithelia meet. Two mitotic figures are visible *(asterisks)*, evidence that this part of the enamel organ is characterized by very active growth. Original magnification × 500.

may be the creation of a three-dimensional spatial environment, that permits morphodifferentiation of the epithelium.

Before discussing *cytodifferentiation*, we should make two important points:

1. *Overlap* of morphodifferentiation and cytodifferentiation periods. You may have noticed in Figures 9–5 and 9–6, depicting tooth development, that the shaping of a tooth, is a gradual process. The first part of a tooth to be shaped is the part nearest the oral epithelium: the future cusps of a molar or the incisal edge of an incisor. The rest of the crown is gradually shaped further in an *occlusocervical direction*, and only when the shape of the crown is established fully will the root be shaped.

The structure responsible for this continued shaping process is the *cervical loop* (Fig. 9–7). The cervical loop is the cervical-most rim of the enamel organ, where outer and inner enamel epithelia meet. Mitoses of the epithelial cells in this rim are responsible for the continued growth of the cervical loop, thereby shaping first the rest of the crown and later the root.

This process of continued *morpho*differentiation takes place while in the occluso-incisal region *cyto*differentiation is well under way. Therefore, the oldest part of the tooth, with respect to both morphodifferentiation and cytodifferentiation, is its incisal edge or cusp; the youngest part of a tooth is the tip, or apex, of its root.

2. The *precise* part of the future tooth, which is shaped by the differential growth of the epithelial enamel organ. On the preceding pages we have indicated that the inner enamel epithelium establishes the shape of the tooth. The exact part of the tooth to be shaped by the epithelium is the *borderline* between dentin and enamel, the dentino-enamel junction. This borderline reflects the exact position of the borderline between dental papilla and inner enamel epithelium at the conclusion of the morphodifferentiation process and the beginning of the cytodifferentiation process (Fig. 9–8).

Cytodifferentiation of Odontoblasts and Ameloblasts

Cytodifferentiation is the result of a series of *cellular interactions* between epithelial and mesenchymal components of the tooth germs.

Following the developmental interactions that resulted in morphodifferentiation, the second series of messages resulting in cytodifferentiation, are exchanged between the cells of the inner enamel epithelium and the peripheral cells of the dental papilla. Again, it should be remembered that this is a *sequential* process. Cytodifferentiation begins occlusally or incisally and moves in a gradual wavelike fashion toward the cervix of the tooth (Figs. 9–9 and 9–10).

The cells of the inner enamel epithelium give a message to the

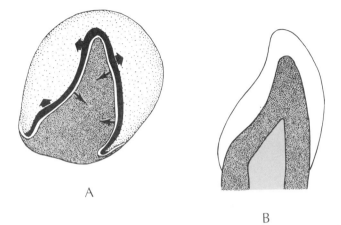

A

B

Fig. 9–8. Diagrams showing a tooth germ in the bell stage, A, and the anatomical crown of a fully formed tooth, B. The dentino-enamel junction is shaped by the inner enamel epithelium (dark band in A). During the deposition stage, the inner enamel epithelial cells move backward (large arrows) while depositing enamel (blank in B). At the same time, the mesenchymal cells of the dental papilla move backward (small arrows) while depositing dentin (stippled in B). Thus, the location of the inner enamel epithelium in the bell stage is preserved as the interface between enamel and dentin (the dentino-enamel junction) in the fully formed tooth.

peripheral cells of the dental papilla, which results in the cytodifferentiation of the latter. In order to give this message to the mesenchymal cells, the cells of the inner enamel epithelium must have completed the process of morphodifferentiation at their level in the tooth. This means that the inner enamel epithelium cells have stopped dividing. They grow taller and more columnar, and their nuclei move from the central position to that part of the cell, which faces away from the basal lamina. In this way a *polarity* is established in the inner enamel epithelial cells.

All these changes are the result of the development of large amounts of protein-synthesizing organelles in these cells. The elongated epithelial cells are now called *pre-ameloblasts,* and the first product they synthesize is secreted into the basal lamina. The basal lamina is composed of a basal-lamina-specific collagen (Type IV) and associated proteoglycans and glycoproteins, most of which are epithelial products. We do not know which of these products, alone or in combination, provides the interactive message for the peripheral cells of the dental papilla to become odontoblasts. It is clear, however, that the critical communication occurs when the cell processes of the future odontoblasts touch the basal lamina. The cell-basal lamina contact is necessary for *odontoblast cytodifferentiation.*

The differentiating odontoblasts line up in a single layer along the basal lamina. Their cytodifferentiation involves the formation of

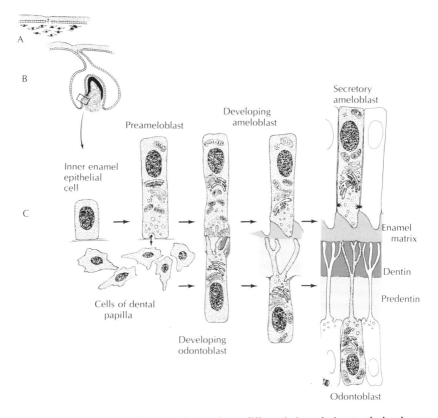

Fig. 9–9. Sequence of cell interactions and cytodifferentiations during tooth development. *A*, The initiation of tooth development. A message crosses the basal lamina from mesenchyme to epithelium. The epithelium responds by downgrowth and differentiation into an enamel organ. *B*, The outline of an enamel organ is shown. The dental papilla is stippled. A dark strip of dentin is present in the incisal region. A small area is shown in greater detail in C. While all stages of cytodifferentiation illustrated in C can be found simultaneously in a single tooth germ at this stage of development, it should be remembered that each epithelial cell and each odontoblast undergo all these stages of development sequentially. Initially, the inner enamel epithelial cell becomes a taller preameloblast. This preameloblast produces a substance that is transmitted through the basal lamina *(arrow)* and reaches some of the mesenchymal cells of the dental papilla. These cells now develop into tall odontoblasts and begin to synthesize predentin. The basal lamina disappears and the cell processes of the developing odontoblast come in close contact with the cell processes of the preameloblast. Subsequently, the preameloblast differentiates into an ameloblast and starts producing enamel matrix. Because the odontoblast starts its productive activities some time before the ameloblast, the dentin layer in any location in a developing tooth is thicker than the corresponding layer of enamel matrix.

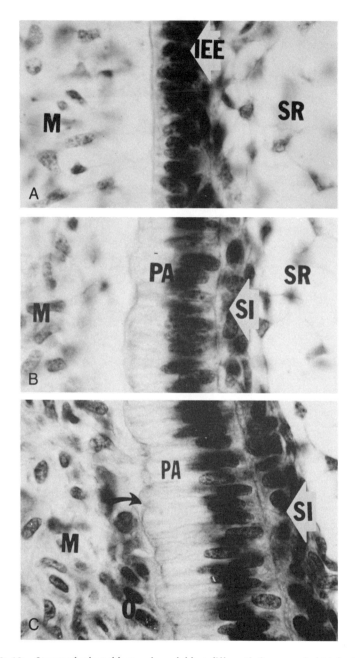

Fig. 9–10.   Stages of odontoblast and ameloblast differentiation, seen in histologic section. *A*, Inner enamel epithelial cells face the undifferentiated mesenchymal cells of the dental papilla. A basement membrane intervenes between the two. *B*, Elongation of inner enamel epithelial cells into preameloblasts. Stellate reticulum and stratum intermedium are visible. *C*, Alignment of the mesenchymal cells along the basal lamina (starting at the level of the asterisk). Differentiation of the odontoblasts begins. (Cont'd p. 178)

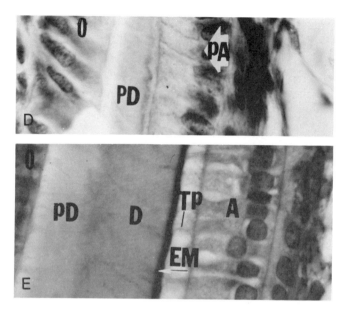

Fig. 9–10 (Cont'd).   *D,* First (uncalcified) dentin deposition by the newly differentiated odontoblasts. The preameloblasts differentiate further, but will not become secretory cells until the first-formed dentin begins to calcify. *E,* Ameloblasts, with Tomes' processes, are engaged in enamel matrix deposition. Calcified dentin and uncalcified predentin are visible. Key to abbreviations: IEE = inner enamel epithelium: SI = stratum intermedium; SR = stellate reticulum; M = mesenchymal cells; PA = preameloblasts; A = ameloblasts; O = odontoblasts; PD = predentin; D = dentin; EM = enamel matrix; TP = Tomes' process. Original magnification ×125.

large numbers of organelles, which will eventually synthesize the components of the fibrous matrix and the ground substance of dentin.

The odontoblasts elongate during their differentiation, and their nuclei move away from the basal lamina (polarization). Differentiated odontoblasts are no longer able to undergo mitoses.

As soon as the odontoblasts have differentiated and have begun to produce dentin matrix, another communication is needed for the *cytodifferentiation of the ameloblasts* (Figs. 9–9 and 9–10). Once again, it is the turn of the mesenchyme, now the differentiated odontoblasts, to give the message to the epithelium now the pre-ameloblasts. In this stage, the basal lamina between these two cell types breaks down, allowing cell extensions of odontoblasts and pre-ameloblasts to contact each other *temporarily.* It is possible that, during this brief period of actual cell–cell contact, the odontoblasts convey an interactive message to the pre-ameloblasts, permitting the latter to become ameloblasts and, after calcification of the first produced dentin, begin enamel matrix production.

We should emphasize here that each of the aforementioned interactions between epithelial and mesenchymal cells is a prerequisite for the further development of the tooth. If the pre-ameloblasts fail to give a message to the odontoblasts, the next interaction, the communication between odontoblasts and pre-ameloblasts (for the cytodifferentiation of the ameloblasts) cannot occur either.

Dentin and Enamel Formation

There are some similarities between the processes of enamel and dentin formation, and some differences.

SIMILARITIES. Both odontoblasts and ameloblasts are *polarized* cells. With their secretory sides they face the basal lamina, while the nuclei are located in the opposite ends of the cells. During dentin and enamel production, the odontoblasts and the ameloblasts both move away from their original positions next to the basal lamina, leaving their products behind. Since ameloblasts and odontoblasts are located on opposite sides of the basal lamina, they move away from this structure, the future dentino-enamel junction, in *opposite directions* (Fig. 9–11).

In the absence of serious complications, the production of dentin and enamel is an orderly process. The cellular sheets, formed by the layer of odontoblasts and the layer of ameloblasts, behave as 2 coordinated units. This is possible because of the presence of gap junctions and tight junctions, which allow odontoblasts to communicate freely with neighboring odontoblasts, and ameloblasts to communicate similarly with neighboring ameloblasts.

Depending on their location in a particular tooth, odontoblasts and ameloblasts produce, on the average, about 4 μm, respectively, of dentin and enamel daily.

DIFFERENCES. (1) The *odontoblasts* produce a *connective tissue* product that resembles bone. The product consists of a collagenous fibrous matrix and a proteoglycan and glycoprotein-rich ground substance. The *ameloblasts,* on the other hand, are epithelial cells and they produce a rather distinct and unique *epithelial product*: an enamel matrix consisting of two classes of glycoproteins: amelogenins and enamelins.

(2) At some distance from the receding odontoblasts, the *dentin matrix* begins to undergo calcification. Hydroxyapatite salts are deposited in this matrix. Between the odontoblasts and the calcification front, a strip of uncalcified *predentin* (like the osteoid seam in bone) is present (Fig. 9–12).

The *enamel matrix*, produced by the ameloblasts, contains a small amount of hydroxyapatite, almost from the moment it is laid down; therefore, *no* wide strip of uncalcified enamel matrix is present. The small crystals of hydroxyapatite salt, *hydroxyapatite crystallites,* are

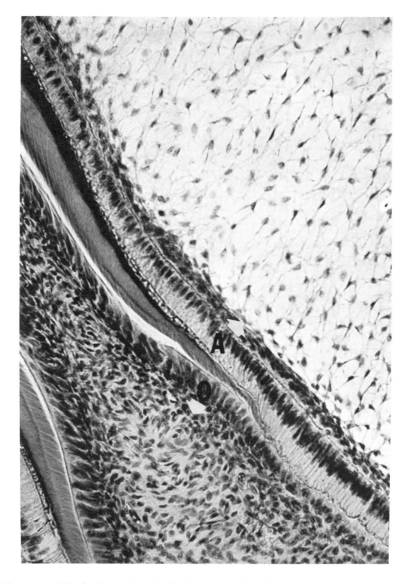

Fig. 9–11. Histologic section of a developing tooth at the time of enamel and dentin formation. The arrows indicate the directions in which ameloblasts (A) and odontoblasts (O) move, while depositing their products. The darkest staining layer is enamel matrix; the somewhat lighter staining tissue next to it is the dentin. At the bottom right of this picture, the odontoblasts are just differentiating. Original magnification ×50.

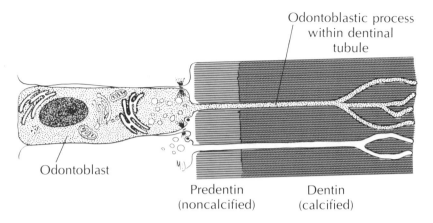

Odontoblastic process
within dentinal
tubule

Odontoblast

Predentin   Dentin
(noncalcified)   (calcified)

Fig. 9–12.   Diagram of an odontoblast, actively engaged in dentin formation. The various organelles associated with protein synthesis are found in the odontoblastic cell body. Each odontoblast leaves an odontoblastic process behind inside a dentinal tubule. The layer of most recently formed dentin is noncalcified predentin. It undergoes calcification and becomes dentin at a short distance from the retreating odontoblasts.

delicate, and a relatively large amount of enamel matrix is found between them. Once deposited, the enamel matrix continues to undergo further calcification, sometimes called *maturation*. During this process it becomes the most heavily calcified tissue of the body. The maturation consists of an *enlargement* of the hydroxyapatite crystallites that are already present in the enamel matrix. This enlargement occurs at the expense of the matrix, specifically the amelogenins, which are broken down and *removed* by the same ameloblasts that originally deposited this matrix. The ameloblasts have, therefore, first a predominantly synthetic stage, with some early digestion, followed by a digestive stage (characterized by lysosomal activities) (Figs. 9–13 and 9–14).

(3) When the *odontoblasts* move backward and produce dentin matrix, they do not ordinarily become enclosed in this matrix (unlike the osteoblasts, which may become osteocytes). However, each odontoblast leaves one long, cytoplasmic cell extension, an *odontoblastic process*, behind in the dentin matrix. This dentin matrix encloses the odontoblastic processes in individual tubes or *dentinal tubules*. Throughout the life of the tooth, the odontoblasts and their processes remain a vital part of the dentin tissue that they produced.

The *ameloblasts*, on the other hand, are lost when the tooth emerges into the oral cavity during eruption. Since no cells are associated with the mature enamel, strictly speaking, enamel is not a true tissue, although it is usually called a tissue. It is a secretion product, incapable of repair once it is formed. During the period of enamel matrix production, the ameloblasts have a shovel-shaped

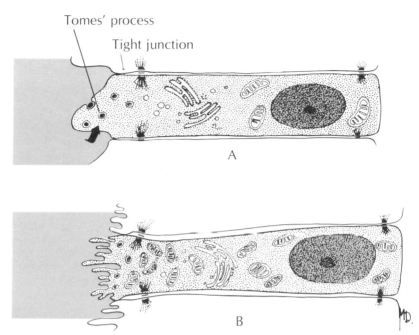

Fig. 9–13. The appearance of an ameloblast during its synthetic (secretory) stage, A, and during its digestive (back resorptive) stage, B, which occurs later. A, The ameloblast has the typical organelles associated with synthetic activities. Secretory granules are released from a typical, somewhat conical, cell extension: the Tomes' process. This process is present only during the secretory stage. The small arrow indicates that a limited digestive activity does take place on part of the Tomes' process surface, modifying the newly deposited enamel matrix for its calcification. B, During the digestive phase, the ameloblasts alternate between the state shown here (with ruffled border facing the enamel matrix and typical organelles associated with digestive activities) and a state during which a smooth-surfaced membrane replaces the ruffled border. These alternating states reflect alternating functional periods of matrix digestion and further calcium-salt deposition.

Fig. 9–14. Decalcified histologic section, A, ground section, B, and radiograph of a ground section, C, of the same primary tooth and its secondary successor. Notice that the enamel of the primary tooth is absent in the decalcified section, present in the ground section, and very radiopaque (white) in the radiograph. This reflects the fact that mature enamel is highly calcified, with so little enamel matrix that the matrix disintegrates during decalcification. In the developing tooth, the most recently deposited enamel matrix (near the cervix) is still present in the decalcified section; but near the incisal edge, the older enamel is maturing (acquiring more mineral and losing matrix components). The radiograph shows also that more mineral is present near the incisal edge along the dentino-enamel junction than in the remainder of the developing enamel. Original magnification A and B, ×2; C, ×4. (Courtesy the late Dr. E. Applebaum.)

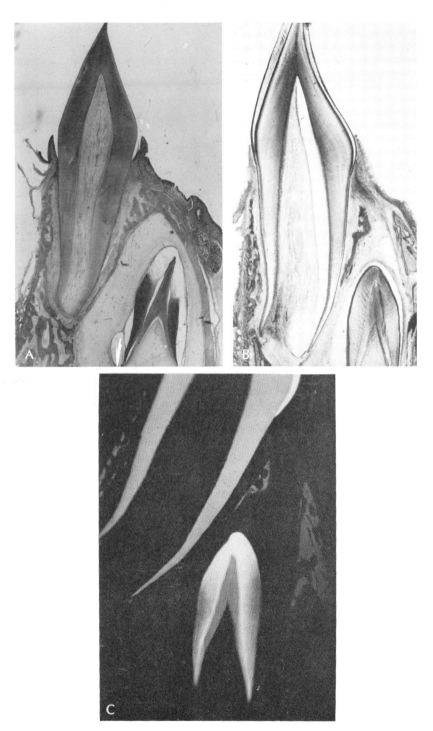

Fig. 9–14.   See legend on facing page.

cytoplasmic extension with a wide base and a thin outer edge at their secretory surface. As we shall see later, this extension (Tomes' process) is responsible for the particular pattern in which enamel matrix is laid down.

(4) Both dentin and enamel formation begin at the dentino-enamel junction of the cusps or incisal edges of the various teeth. Since the odontoblasts undergo cytodifferentiation somewhat earlier than the ameloblasts in corresponding locations, dentin formation is somewhat further advanced in a cervical direction than enamel formation at any given time during dental crown development.

Root Development

Root development begins when the enamel organ has shaped the crown completely and when the developing tooth has started its eruptive movement.

MORPHODIFFERENTIATION. The root is shaped by further epithelial downgrowth. Remember that during the morphodifferentiation of the crown, the occlusal/incisal surfaces are shaped first, and that the continued downgrowth of the cervical loop is responsible for further shaping of the rest of the crown. When the entire crown is shaped, the *outer* and *inner* enamel epithelia, which meet at the cervical loop, begin to proliferate further apically. These two layers of epithelium form the *epithelial root sheath* (Hertwig's sheath). Its function is the shaping of the root or roots, and the induction of the odontoblasts, to deposit the dentin of the roots.

The epithelial root sheath does *not* shape the outer surface of the root, but rather the *dentino-cementum junction.* The epithelial root sheath proliferates apically at approximately the same rate at which the developing tooth is erupting. As a result, the growing tip of the root remains in about the same position within the jaw, while the root becomes longer (Figs. 9–15, 9–16, and 9–17).

The inner enamel epithelium of the root sheath faces the dental papilla, from which it is separated by a basal lamina. The outer enamel epithelium faces the dental sac, from which it is separated by a basal lamina, which is continuous with the basal lamina between inner enamel epithelium and dental papilla.

CYTODIFFERENTIATION OF ODONTOBLASTS. The inner enamel epithelium of the root sheath induces the peripheral cells of the dental papilla to differentiate into odontoblasts. This occurs in a manner that is similar to what takes place in the crown. When the odontoblasts are differentiated and begin to deposit dentin, the basal laminae on both sides of the epithelial root sheath break down and the continuity of the root sheath itself is lost.

In contrast to the events in the crown, the inner enamel epithelial

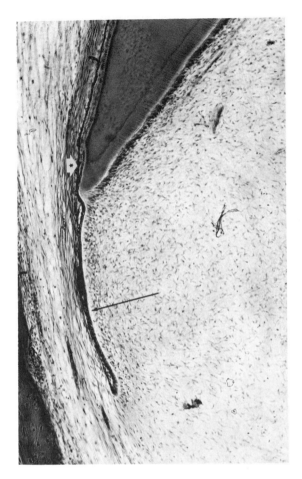

Fig. 9–15. During early morphodifferentiation of a dental root, an epithelial root sheath *(arrow)* grows apically, shaping the future dentino-cementum junction by inducing the odontoblasts, which will form the root dentin. At the level of the asterisk, cells from the dental sac have moved between the remnants of the root sheath and the surface of the dentin, where they will differentiate into cementoblasts. Original magnification ×40.

cells of the root sheath do *not* undergo any further differentiation after they have induced the odontoblasts, and they do not seem to have any further function.

   CYTODIFFERENTIATION OF CEMENTOBLASTS. The breakdown of the epithelial root sheath at the levels of the developing root at which dentin production has begun, allows the undifferentiated mesenchymal cells of the dental sac to move toward the surface of the root dentin. In doing so, they displace the epithelial remnants of the root sheath (cell rests of Malassez), away from the root dentin. Some components of the recently deposited dentin matrix probably

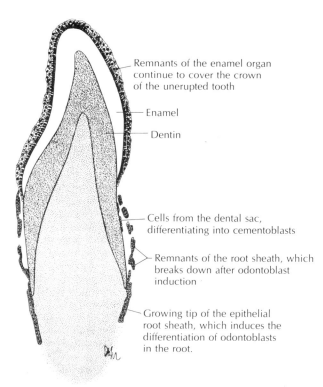

Remnants of the enamel organ
continue to cover the crown
of the unerupted tooth

Enamel

Dentin

Cells from the dental sac,
differentiating into cementoblasts

Remnants of the root sheath, which
breaks down after odontoblast
induction

Growing tip of the epithelial
root sheath, which induces the
differentiation of odontoblasts
in the root.

Fig. 9–16. Diagram of root development. The growing tip of the epithelial root sheath continues to proliferate apically, further shaping the dentino-cementum junction of the anatomical root. Once the first root dentin has been deposited, the root sheath breaks down. Between the epithelial remnants, cells of the dental sac move to the root dentin surface, where they will differentiate into cementoblasts. While all these stages can be seen in one developing tooth, they will all take place in sequence, at all points along the growing root from cervix to apex.

are responsible for the inductive message, which leads to the differentiation of the dental sac cells into *cementoblasts.* This involves the development of extensive rough endoplasmic reticulum and Golgi systems.

Calcification of the first formed dentin is a requirement for the newly differentiated cementoblasts to begin depositing cementum on the dentin surface of the root (Fig. 9–18). Cementum is first laid down as an uncalcified matrix (*cementoid*, similar to osteoid or predentin), which calcifies at some distance from the receding cementoblasts.

Little cementum is deposited before and during the emergence of the tooth in the oral cavity. Only after the tooth reaches functional occlusion is cementum deposited in substantial amounts. Some cementoblasts become enclosed by their product and are then called

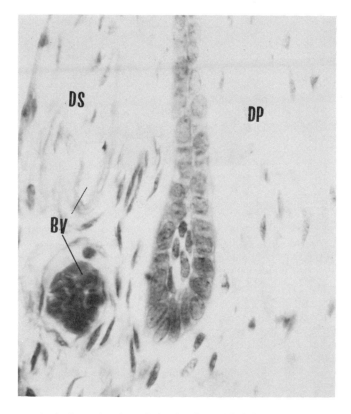

Fig. 9–17.   Histologic section through the tip of an epithelial root sheath. This structure essentially consists of two layers of epithelial cells, one of which is continuous with the outer enamel epithelium, while the other is continuous with the inner enamel epithelium of the enamel organ. DP = dental papilla; DS = dental sac with cross sections through two blood vessels (BV). Original magnification ×400.

cementocytes. Cementoblasts and cementocytes remain associated with the tissue they produced, and cementum may be deposited throughout the functional life of the tooth.

Multirooted Teeth

In teeth with a single root, the epithelial root sheath simply grows apically, as an epithelial cylinder, from the cervical edge of the enamel organ. In teeth with two or three roots, the single cervical opening, bordered by the cervical edge of the enamel organ, must first be subdivided into two or three openings. This subdivision is done by the horizontal outgrowth of two or three epithelial flaps across the cervical opening. These flaps, consisting usually of two

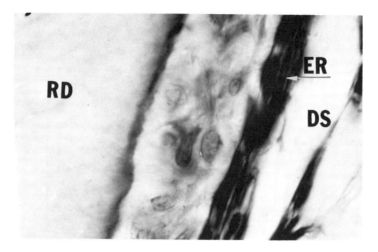

Fig. 9–18.   Histologic section through the future dentino-cementum junction of a developing tooth. RD = root dentin; DS = dental sac; ER = large epithelial remnant of
the epithelial root sheath. Between the epithelial remnant and the root dentin, several
dental sac cells have lined up along the dentin surface and have differentiated into cementoblasts. Early cementum deposition is taking place. Original magnification ×500.

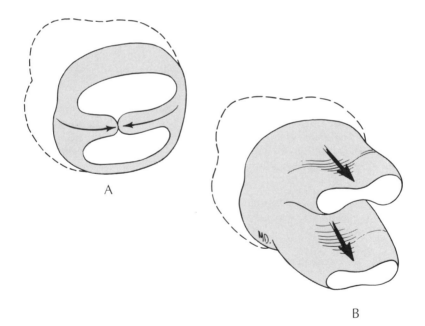

Fig. 9–19.   Diagram of the development of a tooth with two separate roots. The broken
outline reflects the anatomical crown region. The developing tooth is tilted on its side.
A, The outgrowth of two epithelial flaps *(arrows)* from the cervical loop subdivides the
single cervical opening into two separate openings. From the edges of both these openings,
epithelial root sheaths grow apically, B, *(arrows)*, shaping two separate roots.

cell layers (inner and outer enamel epithelium, like the epithelial root sheath), meet in the center of the cervical opening, where they fuse. Now from the edges of these newly formed, smaller openings, two or three cylindrical root sheaths grow apically, shaping two or three separate roots (Figs. 9–19 and 9–20).

Occasionally a tooth has a single root with 2 separate root canals in it. This situation is produced as follows: a single epithelial root sheath is present. A cross section through this root sheath reveals a gradual change from a circular to an oval outline, with central indentations (Fig. 9–21). The odontoblasts, differentiated within this outline, produce dentin in a central direction, all at about the same rate. This leads to a rapid obliteration of the dental papilla in the central, indented region and to the establishment of two separate canals for the root pulp.

Bony Compartments and Crypts

During the early stages of dental development, intramembranous ossification is taking place in the upper and lower jaw regions. Soon, a delicate network of bone is formed, which partially surrounds the tooth germs. No bone forms in the spaces occupied by the enamel organs, their dental sacs, dental papillae, dental lamina or its remnants.

In these early stages, the individual tooth germs are all located in a common bony groove, whose outer edges curve gently inward, seemingly preventing the tooth germs from "falling out" of the bony groove. Subsequently, as growth continues and the teeth come to lie somewhat further apart, this common groove is subdivided into individual *compartments* (Fig. 9–22; see also 9–26A), or *bony crypts* in the case of secondary teeth (see Fig. 9–26B).

Innervation and Vascularization

Tooth development is an active metabolic process, requiring a great deal of energy. From the earliest stages of epithelial ingrowth, a large number of *capillaries* surrounds the spherical mass of condensed mesenchyme of the tooth germ.

In the cap and bell stages of tooth development, these capillaries invade the dental papilla and the dental sac. The future ameloblasts and odontoblasts initially both receive their nutrition from the capillaries in the dental papilla. When the odontoblasts have differentiated and are depositing dentin, the capillary network becomes even richer. Many capillaries lie in and immediately underneath the odontoblast layer.

However, the very deposition and calcification of dentin and

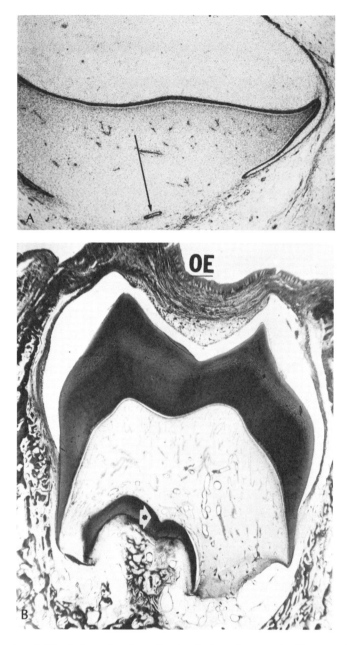

Fig. 9–20. *A*, Histologic section through a developing primary molar. The enamel organ is cut slightly off-center, so that the processes of dentin and enamel formation, which are taking place in the cusp region, are not visible. A cross section through a small epithelial flap, which is growing across the cervical opening, is visible. This is the first stage in the root development of a multi-rooted tooth. Original magnification ×10. See Appendix III, Fig. A–4, for a computer-aided three-dimensional graphic reconstruction of a developing molar in this stage. *B*, Histologic section through a developing primary molar, just before the tooth emerges into the oral cavity (OE = oral epithelium). This is a later stage in the development of two separate roots. The dentin, marked with an asterisk, has been produced by the odontoblasts, which were induced by the epithelial flaps subdividing the cervical opening. Original magnification ×2.

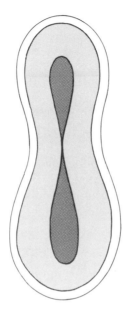

Fig. 9–21.   The development of two separate root canals in a single root is shown in this diagram of a cross section through the root. When the root sheath has central indentations, subsequent even dentin production leads to a central obstruction and two separate root canals.

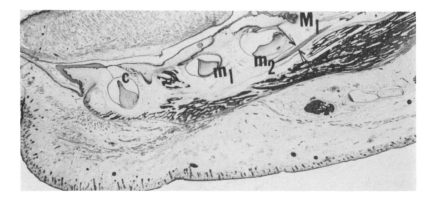

Fig. 9–22.   Histologic section through the molar region in the lower jaw of a human fetus (second trimester of pregnancy). Developing primary canine (c), first and second primary molars (m_1 and m_2) and the enamel organ (cap stage) of the first molar of the secondary dentition (M_1) are visible. Most developing teeth still lie in a common bony groove, together with the major nerves and blood vessels of the lower jaw *(arrows)*. No subdivision into individual bony compartments (and canal) has taken place yet. Original magnification × 2. (Courtesy the late Dr. E. Applebaum.)

enamel matrix cuts off the ameloblasts from their source of nutrition in the dental papilla. Suddenly, the rich capillary network in the dental sac, outside the outer enamel epithelium, becomes their source of metabolic exchange. These vessels come even closer to the ameloblasts because of the gradual *collapse* of the enamel organ, during the phase of enamel matrix deposition.

In addition to small capillaries, delicate nerve fibers are present in the dental papillae and the dental sacs as early as the cap and bell stages of dental development. The nerves in the dental papillae eventually grow toward the odontoblastic cell layer. But only *after* the odontoblasts have deposited a thick layer of dentin (about two thirds of its future thickness) do the nerve fibers terminate on some of the odontoblasts.

TOOTH MOVEMENTS AND TOOTH ERUPTION

Throughout their development, the tooth germs move relative to each other and relative to the developing bone of the jaw. Most of these motions appear to be somewhat random, the results of differential growth patterns inside the tooth germs.

Once most of the tooth crown has been formed and all crown odontoblasts and ameloblasts have differentiated, eruptive movements begin. *Eruptive movements* of a tooth consist of movements in a predominantly vertical direction, during which the crown of the tooth moves from its site of development inside the jaw to a position of functional occlusion in the oral cavity.

At some time during this eruption the tooth crown *emerges* through the oral epithelium into the oral cavity. This is what is clinically called tooth *eruption*. However, you should understand that eruption takes place over a long period of time and that the actual *emerging* of the tooth is only one episode in the stages of eruption.

The eruption from the developmental position inside the jaw to a position of functional occlusion inside the oral cavity is the result of real movements of the tooth relative to its environment and is called *prefunctional, active eruption*.

However, after the tooth has reached occlusion, wear of the occlusal or incisal surfaces may occur, and the tooth has to erupt a little bit more to maintain occlusal contact. This (minor) eruptive movement is called *functional, active eruption*.

Finally, with age, the gingiva recedes usually exposing more of the tooth (clinical crown) than was originally exposed. Although the tooth seems to move up relative to the gingiva, the actual movement is done by the gingiva, while the tooth remains in the same position. Such "eruption" of the tooth is called *passive eruption*.

While we are able to *describe* the appearances of the various stages of eruption, until now no satisfactory explanation has been given for questions such as: "What makes a tooth erupt?" and "What constitutes the mechanism of the eruptive movements?"

Answers that have been considered are: the expansion of the dental papilla, the growth of the epithelial root sheath, bone deposition on the floor of the bony crypt, and the growth activities of the dental sac. At present, we believe that the answer to this question should be sought in some property of the dental sac.

At the start of the prefunctional, active eruption, the situation is as follows. The developing tooth is located in a bony compartment, which is a subdivision of the original, common, bony groove. All crown odontoblasts and all ameloblasts have differentiated, and the more cervical of these cells are still involved in the deposition of dentin and enamel. In the incisal/occlusal part of the crown, dentin and enamel deposition are largely completed.

The outer enamel surface is covered with the collapsed remnants of the enamel organ, which *together* are called the *reduced enamel epithelium*. Cervically, the epithelial root sheath begins to proliferate, to start shaping the root.

As the tooth crown begins to move toward the oral epithelium, the inwardly curved edges of the bony compartment undergo bone resorption. This will allow the tooth crown to move freely out of the bony compartment. Once the bone opening is wide enough for the tooth to pass through, bone deposition takes place in a vertical direction (toward the oral mucosa) at the edges of the bone. This is the beginning of the formation of the alveolar bone socket, which will hold the root(s) of the mature, functional tooth.

Vertical movements of the crown toward the oral epithelium are possible, because the connective tissue between the oral epithelium and the reduced enamel epithelium is broken down and digested by the cells of the reduced enamel epithelium (Fig. 9–23).

Once the oral epithelium and the reduced enamel epithelium come together, fusion takes place between the two epithelia. The fused epithelia no longer have a blood supply, and as a result, the central cells perish, establishing an open path for the emergence of the tooth into the oral cavity.

When the tooth reaches its functional occlusion, the cervical part of the anatomical crown is still covered with reduced enamel epithelium. This epithelium is fused orally with the gingival epithelium. For some time after the tooth has started functioning, this remnant of the reduced enamel epithelium forms the first junction between the tooth and the gingiva. Only later will these epithelial cells be replaced by cells of the oral epithelium (Chap. 14).

Proliferation of the epithelial root sheath generally coincides with the eruptive movements of the tooth. Since the speed of the apical

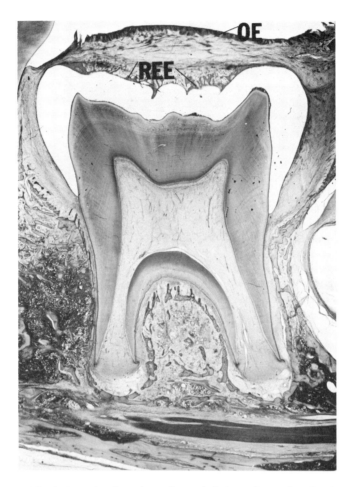

Fig. 9–23.   Histologic section through a molar tooth during active, prefunctional eruption. The reduced enamel epithelium (REE) has approached the oral epithelium (OE) closely, at the expense of the intervening tissues. (From Sicher, H., and DuBrul, D.L.: *Oral Anatomy.* 6th Ed. St. Louis, The C.V. Mosby Co., 1975.)

proliferation of the root sheath is approximately the same as the speed of the occlusal eruptive movements, the proliferating tip of the root sheath remains in about the same position, relative to the jaw bone.

When the speed of the eruptive movements exceeds that of the root sheath proliferation (usually temporarily), the entire developing tooth, including the tip of the root sheath, undergoes a net movement in occlusal direction. In such a case bone deposition on the floor of the bony compartment fills in the area vacated by the root tip.

When the speed of root sheath proliferation exceeds (temporarily) that of the eruptive movements, the root sheath proliferates deeper (further apically) into the bone of the jaw. Under those circumstances the bony compartment has to be enlarged, and this is accomplished by resorption of bone in the floor of the compartment.

As we mentioned before, once the epithelial root sheath has shaped the root and has induced the differentiation of odontoblasts to form root dentin, the sheath falls apart into small rests of *Malassez,* without any further, apparent function. Some dental sac cells move between these cell rests and the root dentin, where they differentiate into cementoblasts.

Other cells of the dental sac differentiate into osteoblasts and begin to form inner walls of the alveolar socket of the tooth. The remaining dental sac cells differentiate into fibroblasts and begin to form the collagen fibers of the periodontal ligament.

When the tooth reaches functional occlusion, about two-thirds of the length of its root(s) has (have) been formed. The root is still wide open apically; a thin layer of cementum has been deposited on its outer surface. Only the most cervical part of the periodontal ligament has been formed. The remainder of the root, its apical foramen, most of the cementum, the periodontal ligament and the alveolar bone are formed *after* the tooth has begun functioning.

Depending on the type of tooth, this may last another 1.5 to 3.5 years after functional occlusion has been reached (see timetables at the end of this chapter).

DEVELOPMENT AND ERUPTION OF THE SECONDARY DENTITION

Thus far we have discussed tooth development and eruption, limiting ourselves mainly to the developing primary dentition. Although the development and eruption of the teeth of the secondary dentition resemble these processes for the teeth of the primary dentition, a few differences should be noted.

The incisors, canines and premolars of the secondary dentition, which will replace elements of the primary dentition, first develop from tooth buds growing off the dental lamina, at the level of the tooth germs of the primary dentition, which are at that time in the bell stage. The secondary enamel organs remain temporarily attached to this parent dental lamina by a *successional dental lamina.* The secondary tooth germs form *lingual* to the primary tooth germs (Fig. 9–24).

The molars of the secondary dentition have *no* primary predecessors. Their enamel organs develop from a blind extension of the dental lamina of the primary dentition. This blind extension grows backward in the jaw, underneath the oral mucosa, from the dental lamina of the second molars of the primary dentition. This extension

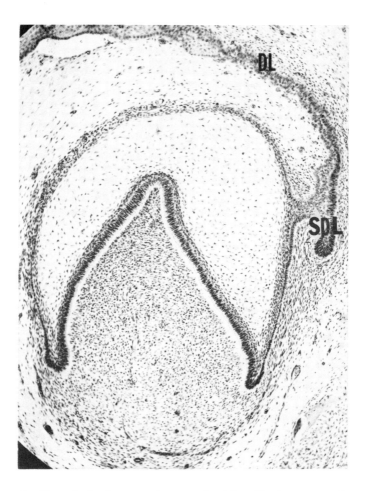

Fig. 9–24.   The early development of a successional dental lamina (SDL), as it appears in a histologic section, located lingual to the enamel organ (bell stage) of the primary tooth. DL = dental lamina. Original magnification ×20.

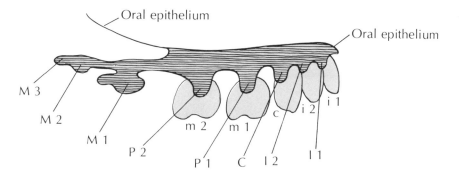

Fig. 9–25.   A highly theoretical diagram (all components are not present at the same time) of the dental lamina and all enamel organs of primary and secondary dentitions in the left lower jaw, seen from the lingual side (inside). The primary enamel organs form after direct downgrowth of the dental lamina (darkly shaded) from the oral epithelium (indicated by a single line). The secondary successors of the primary teeth form from separate successional dental laminae (localized further outgrowths of the dental lamina), lingual to the enamel organs of the primary teeth. The secondary molars develop from an extension of the dental lamina, growing backward underneath the oral epithelium.

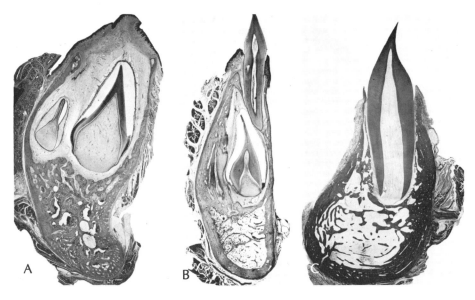

Fig. 9–26.   Relative positions, at various stages of development of a lower primary incisor and its secondary successor. A, Both teeth are located within a common bony compartment, at approximately the same vertical level. B, The primary tooth has become functional. Its root is located in a bony socket, while the secondary tooth is located in a separate bony crypt. During eruption of the secondary tooth, which is about to begin at this stage, the intervening connective tissues, the bone plate, which separates the crypt from the socket, and the root of the primary tooth must be resorbed. C, A newly erupted secondary incisor (the section has been reversed, so that the lingual side is now to the right). Bone remodeling has taken place to adapt the bony socket to this large new tooth. Original magnification A, ×2; B and C, ×1.

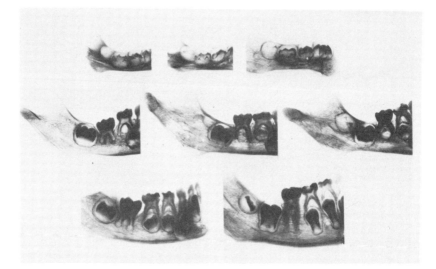

Fig. 9–27.   A series of positive prints of radiographs of part of the lower jaw at various stages of development of the primary and secondary dentitions. What would be white in a radiograph is black in these prints. In the top row (late fetal and early neonatal period), the developing primary teeth are still located in the bony compartments within the jaw. In the middle row (2 to 4 years of age), the second molar of the primary dentition has just erupted. The bottom row, representing the age of 6 to 7 years, shows the first molar of the secondary dentition emerging. The second molar is still located in its bony crypt. The central incisor, not visible in these radiographs, is erupting as well. Once some of the secondary teeth have emerged, we speak of a mixed dentition. Both primary and secondary teeth are present simultaneously. This condition lasts until about the age of 12 to 13 years.

gives rise, in succession, to the enamel organs of the first, second and third molars of the secondary dentition (Fig. 9–25).

   Once the tooth development of elements of the secondary dentition has been initiated, the development is essentially similar to that of the primary dentition.

   Initially, the teeth of both dentitions develop at about the same vertical level: the primary teeth on the "outside," nearer the lips and cheeks, and the secondary teeth on the "inside," nearer the palate and the tongue. Also, all teeth are located within the same bony groove for a while, and later each primary tooth and its secondary successor share the same bony compartment (Fig. 9–26).

   Once the primary teeth have erupted, the crowns of the secondary teeth are located on the lingual sides of the primary roots and, in some cases, even underneath these roots. Further bone development leads to the formation of separate bony sockets for the roots of the primary teeth and bony crypts for the crowns of the secondary teeth.

   While the secondary teeth are more completely enclosed by their bony crypts than the primary teeth ever were, a small occlusal open-

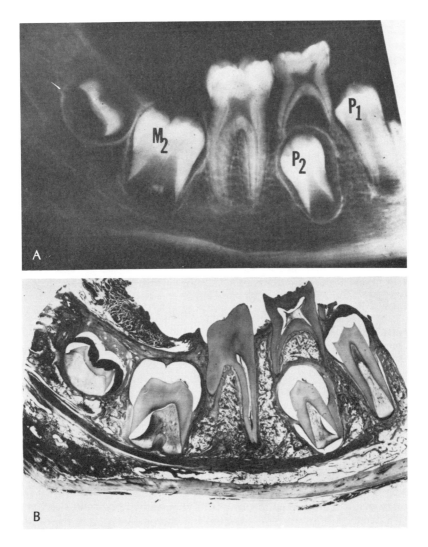

Fig. 9–28.   Comparison of a radiograph *(A)* of the premolar-molar region and a histologic section *(B)* through the same region in the lower jaw of a child about 12 years of age. Notice especially the appearance of the developing roots in first and second premolars (P₁ and P₂) and in the second molar (M₂) of the secondary dentition. Note also the radiopaque (white) outline of the walls of the bony crypts around the developing second premolar and the second and third molars. Original magnification ×1.

ing is always present in the bony crypt wall containing the remnants of the successional dental lamina.

When the secondary teeth, except the molars, start their *eruption*, they not only have to remove some bone, connective tissue and epithelial cells, but also a more complete bony wall, a periodontal ligament and the root(s) of their predecessor. This is done not only by the digestive abilities of the reduced enamel epithelium of the secondary teeth but also by the differentiation of bone-resorbing cells *(osteoclasts)* and cementum and dentin-resorbing cells (multinucleated cells, resembling the osteoclasts in both appearance and function).

This process of resorption takes place slowly. First the wall of the bony crypt and part of the socket of the primary tooth are broken down. Cementum resorption at the surface of the root of the primary tooth follows, first and mostly on the side that faces the erupting secondary tooth.

The eruption of the secondary tooth is *not* continuous once it has started. There are long rest periods during which the secondary tooth may even move somewhat backward, allowing some repair-cementum to be formed in the resorption cavities of the primary root. Ultimately, however, the secondary tooth returns and more resorption of the primary root takes places.

These alternating periods of resorption, rest and repair, and new resorption continue until the entire root of the primary tooth has been resorbed. The crown of the primary tooth now falls out (the tooth is "shed") and the secondary tooth is able to erupt without further obstacles (Fig. 9–26).

TIMETABLES

Tables 9–1, 9–2, and 9–3 show the development and eruption of primary and secondary dentitions. Please remember that these dates are averages and that individuals may show a certain amount of variation without being abnormal. Nevertheless, these timetables, which should *not* be memorized, should give you some basic reference list to judge the state of development of dentition in the dental practice (Figs. 9–27 and 9–28).

Table 9–1.   Stages in the Development of the Primary Dentition

Tooth		Enamel organ in the bell stage, just prior to dentin deposition. (Age in weeks after conception)	Crown formation completed. (Age in months after birth)	Root formation completed. (Age in years/months after birth)
i_1	upper	10	1.5	2/9
	lower	11	2.5	2/9
i_2	upper	12	2.5	2/9
	lower	12	3	2/6
c	upper	14	9	3/7
	lower	14	8–9	3/7
m_1	upper	13–14	6	3/1
	lower	13–14	5–6	2/10
m_2	upper	15–16	11	3/11
	lower	15–16	8–11	3/6

Table 9–2.   Stages in the Development of the Secondary Dentition

Tooth		Enamel organ in the bell stage, just prior to dentin deposition. (Age in months after conception)	Crown formation completed. (Age in years after birth)	Root formation completed. (Age in years after birth)
I_1	upper	7.0	3.3–4.1	8.6–9.8
	lower	7.0	3.4–5.4	7.7–8.6
I_2	upper	7.0	4.4–4.9	9.6–10.8
	lower	7.0	3.1–5.9	8.5–9.6
C	upper	7.0	4.5–5.8	11.2–13.3
	lower	7.0	4.0–4.7	10.8–13.0
P_1	upper	7.0	6.3–7.0	11.2–13.6
	lower	7.0	5–6	11.0–13.4
P_2	upper	7.0	6.6–7.2	11.6–14.0
	lower	7.0	6.1–7.1	11.7–14.3
M_1	upper	5.5	2.1–3.5	9.3–10.8
	lower	5.5	2.1–3.6	7.8–9.8
M_2	upper	6 months after birth	6.9–7.4	12.9–16.2
	lower	6 months after birth	6.2–7.4	11.0–15.7
M_3	upper	6 years after birth	12.8–13.2	19.5–19.6
	lower	6 years after birth	12.0–13.7	20.0–20.8

Table 9–3.   Clinical Emergence of Teeth in the Oral Cavity

Primary teeth:	i_1	upper :	9.1–10.6 months after birth			
		lower :	7.3– 8.7	"	"	"
	i_2	upper :	10.4–12.3	"	"	"
		lower :	13.0–14.4	"	"	"
	c	upper :	18.9–20.2	"	"	"
		lower :	19.3–20.2	"	"	"
	m_1	upper :	14.4–16.1	"	"	"
		lower :	15.6–16.4	"	"	"
	m_2	upper :	24.8–29.4	"	"	"
		lower :	23.4–27.1	"	"	"
Secondary teeth:	I_1	upper :	6.7– 8.1 years after birth			
		lower :	6.0– 6.9	"	"	"
	I_2	upper :	7.0– 8.8	"	"	"
		lower :	6.8– 8.1	"	"	"
	C	upper :	10.0–12.2	"	"	"
		lower :	9.2–11.4	"	"	"
	P_1	upper :	9.6–10.9	"	"	"
		lower :	9.6–11.5	"	"	"
	P_2	upper :	10.2–11.4	"	"	"
		lower :	10.1–12.1	"	"	"
	M_1	upper :	6.1– 6.7	"	"	"
		lower :	5.9– 6.9	"	"	"
	M_2	upper :	11.9–12.8	"	"	"
		lower :	11.2–12.2	"	"	"
	M_3	:	17.0–19.0	"	"	"

SELECTED READING LIST

Gaunt, W.A., and Miles, A.E.W.: Fundamental aspects of tooth morphogenesis. In *Structural and Chemical Organization of Teeth. Vol. I.* Edited by A.E.W. Miles. New York, Academic Press, 1967.

Kollar, E.J.: Epithelial-mesenchymal interactions in the mammalian integument: tooth development as a model for inductive interaction. In *Epithelial Mesenchymal Interactions In Development.* Edited by R.H. Sawyer and J.F. Fallon. New York, Praeger, 1983.

Kollar, E.J., and Lumsden, A.G.S.: Tooth morphogenesis; the role of innervation during induction and pattern formation. J. Biol. Buccale, *7*:49, 1979.

Kraus, B.S., and Jordan, R.E.: *The Human Dentition Before Birth.* Philadelphia, Lea & Febiger, 1965.

Linde, A.: Calcium metabolism in dentinogenesis. In *The Role of Calcium in Biological Systems.* Edited by L.J. Anghileri and A.M. Tuffet-Anghileri. Boca Raton, CRC Press, 1982.

Linde, A.: *Dentin and Dentinogenesis. Vols. I and II.* Boca Raton, CRC Press, 1984.

Nery, E.R., Kraus, B.S., and Croup, M.: Timing and topography of early human tooth development. Arch. Oral. Biol., *15*:1315, 1970.

Oöe, T.: *Human Tooth and Dental Arch Development.* Tokyo, Ishiyaku Publishers, 1981.

Provenza, D.V., and Sisca, R.F.: Electron microscopic study of human dental primordia. Arch. Oral. Biol., *16*:121, 1971.

Reith, E.J., and Boyde, A.: The arrangement of ameloblasts on the surface of maturing enamel of the rat incisor tooth. J. Anat., *133*:381, 1981.

Reith, E.J., and Boyde, A.: Autoradiographic evidence of cyclical entry of calcium into maturing enamel of rat incisor tooth. Arch. Oral. Biol., 26:983. 1981.

Ruch, J.V.: Odontoblast differentiation and the formation of the odontoblast layer. J. Dent. Res., 64:489, 1985.

Ruch, J.V., et al.: Epithelial-mesenchymal interactions in tooth germs: mechanisms of differentiation. J. Biol. Buccale, 11:173, 1983.

Sasaki, T.: Endocytotic pathways at the ruffled borders of rat maturation ameloblasts. Histochemistry, 80:263, 1984.

Sasaki, T.: Tracer, cytochemical, and freeze-fracture study on the mechanisms whereby secretory ameloblasts absorb exogenous proteins. Acta Anat., 118:23, 1984.

Saxen, L., et al.: Inductive tissue interactions. In The Cell Surface in Animal Embryogenesis and Development. Edited by G. Poste and G.L. Nicolsen. Amsterdam, Elsevier/North Holland Biomedical Press, 1976.

Slavkin, H.C.: Embryonic tooth formation. A tool for developmental biology. Oral Sci. Rev., 4:1, 1974.

Takano, Y., Crenshaw, M.A., and Reith, E.J.: Correlation of ⁴⁵Ca incorporation with maturation ameloblast morphology in the rat incisor. Calc. Tiss. Int., 34:211, 1982.

Thesleff, I., Lehtonen, E., Wartiovaara, J., and Saxen, L.: Interference of tooth differentiation with interposed filters. Dev. Biol., 58:197, 1977.

Thesleff, I., Jalkanen, M., Vainio, S., and Bernfield, M.: Cell surface proteoglycan expression correlates with epithelial-mesenchymal interaction during tooth morphogenesis. Dev. Biol., 129:565, 1988.

Thylstrup, A., Leach, S.A., and Qvist, V. (eds.): Dentine and Dentine Reactions in the Oral Cavity. Oxford, IRL Press, 1987.

Tominaga, H., Sasaki, T., and Higashi, S.: Ultrastructural changes in odontoblasts during early development. Bull. Tokyo Dent. Coll., 25:9, 1984.

Van der Linden, F.P.G.M., and Duterloo, H.S.: Development of the Human Dentition. An Atlas. Hagerstown, MD, Harper & Row, 1976.

Weinstock, A., and LeBlond, C.P.: Elaboration of the matrix glycoprotein of enamel by secretory ameloblasts of the rat incisor as revealed by radioautography after galactose² injection. J. Cell. Biol., 51:26, 1971.

The Timetables of Dental Development (Tables 9–1, 9–2, and 9–3) were based on data from the following:

Fass, E.N.: J. Dent. Child., 36:391, 1969.

Haavikko, K.: Suom. Hammaslääk. Toim., 66:107, 1970.

Hurme, V.O.: J. Dent. Child., 16:11, 1949.

Knott, V.B., and Meredith, H.V.: Angle Orthod., 36:68, 1966.

Lunt, R.C., and Law, D.B.: J. Am. Dent. Assoc., 89:872, 1974.

Lysell, L., Magnusson, B., and Thilander, B.: Odont. Revy, 13:217, 1962.

Moorrees, C.F.A., Fanning, E.A., and Hunt, E.E.: Am. J. Phys. Anthrop., 21:205, 1963.

Moorrees, C.F.A., Fanning, E.A., and Hunt, E.E.: J. Dent. Res., 42:1490, 1963.

Nomata, N.: Bull. Tokyo Med. Dent. Univ., 11:55, 1964.

Robinow, M., Richards, T.W., and Anderson, M.: Growth, 6:127, 1942.

Röse, C.: Dtsch. Monatschr. Zahnheilk., 27:553, 1909.

Schopf, P.M.: Fortschr. Kieferorthop., 31:39, 1970.

Scott, J.H., and Symons, N.B.B.: Introduction to Dental Anatomy. 8th Ed. Edinburgh, Churchill Livingstone, 1977.

Stones, H.H., Lawton, F.E., Bransby, E.R., and Hartley, H.O.: Br. Dent. J., 90:1, 1951.

Tegzes, E.: Acta. Paed. Hung., 1:289, 1960.

Turner, E.P.: Arch. Oral Biol., 8:523, 1963.

10

Pulp and Dentin

Developmentally and functionally, pulp and dentin are closely related, as they are both products of the *dental papilla* (which, in turn, is derived from neural crest cells).

During tooth development, the peripheral cells of the dental papilla differentiate to become odontoblasts. These cells produce dentin while retreating from the dentino-enamel junction toward the center of the dental papilla. Whatever remains of the dental papilla after the dentin has been formed is transformed into the dental pulp.

Dentin and pulp form the core of any tooth. The *pulp,* a loose connective tissue with some unusual characteristics due to its unique location (Fig. 10–1), is the most centrally located tissue. It is enclosed entirely within the dentin, except at the *apical foramen.* The blood vessels and nerves of the pulp enter through this foramen, thus allowing some communication between the pulp and the tissues surrounding the tooth.

Clinically, this contact is important. A disease of the pulp tissue, most commonly inflammation, may spread through the apical foramen to the tissues of the periodontal ligament and to part of the alveolar bone. If the bone is affected, it will be resorbed. In radiographs the effect of such resorption is visible as a dark (radiolucent) area around the root tip.

However, the patient usually has sought help before the problem gets this far. The pulp has the ability to cause excruciating pain. Because of this, people sometimes call the pulp the nerve(s) of the tooth, although in fact only a small part of the volume of the pulp consists of nerves.

Any time dentin is exposed to the oral cavity, an open connection is established between the oral cavity and the pulp tissue, via a large number of open *dentinal tubules.* All stimuli reaching the pulp (heat, cold, pressure) are translated as *pain* by this tissue.

In young healthy teeth *dentin* is *not* ordinarily exposed to the oral cavity. There are, however, certain situations in which dentin may become exposed. On those occasions when this does occur, the experience can be a painful one.

204

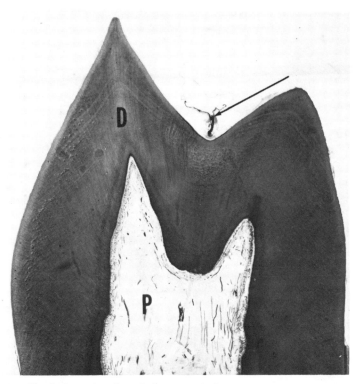

Fig. 10–1. Histologic section through the anatomical crown of a young, newly erupted premolar. The enamel cap has been lost during histologic processing. Only the organic contents of the occlusal fissure *(arrow)* remain. The darkly staining dentin (D) forms a shell of calcified tissue around the dental pulp (P) in the pulp chamber. The pulp is a highly vascularized, loose connective tissue (proper) organ. Original magnification × 5.

1. Dentin may be exposed as the result of *wear.* During occlusal function, enamel is gradually and slowly worn away at the cusps or incisal edges. Dentin, uncovered in this way, is generally *not* painful, because the wearing process is slow. This allows gradual changes to occur in the dentinal tubules and enables the tooth to produce *reactive dentin* (see section on aging phenomena in this chapter). The changes in the tubules lead to their partial or complete closure (they become filled with calcium salts), while reactive dentin seals off the pulpal openings of the dentinal tubules that are still patent, thus reducing the possibility of pain.

2. Dentin may be exposed as the result of *caries* or *trauma.* If the caries process is sufficiently slow, reactive dentin may be produced, minimizing the pain until the caries reaches the pulp and the pain becomes serious. When caries spreads rapidly or, in the case of trauma, when part of the tooth is broken off, the acutely exposed dentin will be exquisitely painful.

3. Some dentin may remain exposed because it is never covered with either enamel or cementum during *development.* This situation occurs at the cervix of approximately 18% of all teeth, with a somewhat higher incidence in the front teeth (see a more extensive description in Chap. 14). In a young individual such areas are covered with the tissues of the dentogingival junction, but as these tissues recede with age, the uncovered dentin is exposed to the oral cavity, causing frequently "painful necks of teeth" in older patients.

DENTAL PULP

The dental pulp is a *loose connective tissue* with components commonly found in connective tissues (Fig. 10–2):

1. *Cells*—fibroblasts and undifferentiated mesenchymal cells; other cell types required for the maintenance and defense of the tissue, specifically histiocytes and lymphocytes.

2. *Fibrous matrix*—predominantly Type I and Type III collagen fibers, randomly dispersed, but present in greater density around the bundles of blood vessels and nerves.

3. *Ground substance*—predominantly proteoglycans and glyco-

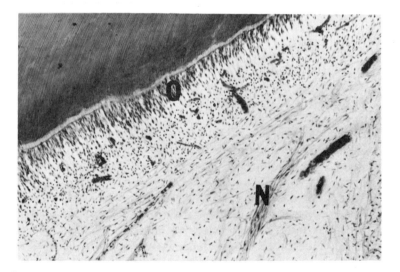

Fig. 10–2. Peripheral pulp tissue in the anatomical crown of a young, newly erupted premolar. At the periphery of the pulp, a layer of odontoblasts (O) is located, each with a cytoplasmic process extending into a dentinal tubule. The dentinal tubules appear as dark lines in the dentin. The darkly staining structures inside the pulp tissue are blood vessels filled with red blood cells. The finest branches of these vessels are near the odontoblast layer. A nerve (N) is visible in the delicate fibrous matrix of the pulp. The presence of a large number of cells is characteristic for young pulp tissue (see section on aging, this chapter). Original magnification × 40.

proteins. The ground substance contains large amounts of water and is chemically similar to the ground substance in other loose connective tissues, with only minor variations in the relative proportions of the ground substance components.

The dental pulp gives the (incorrect) impression of being a somewhat immature connective tissue. This is due to the relatively high proportion of delicate Type III collagen and to the small diameters of the Type I collagen fibers. No elastic fibers are present in the pulp, but a limited amount of randomly dispersed oxytalan fibers has been noted.

The cell population in the dental pulp consists, to a large extent, of *fibroblasts* and *undifferentiated mesenchymal cells.* The relatively large number of the latter enables the pulp to recruit newly differentiating cells to replace others when they are lost, specifically the odontoblasts. As we stated before, odontoblasts, once differentiated, no longer are capable of mitoses under normal conditions. If groups of odontoblasts are lost, undifferentiated cells must be mobilized to replace them.

Along the blood vessels *histiocytes* are found. These cells are capable of digestive activities. When they are well filled with ingested material, they are called *macrophages.*

Mast cells, commonly found in connective tissue proper, are difficult to demonstrate in dental pulps with most histologic techniques. However, with the proper technique their presence can be shown in both healthy and inflamed human pulp. These cells contain vesicles filled with heparin, histamine and a variety of other enzymes. They are capable of increasing vascular permeability (thereby promoting edema), phagocytosis, interference with blood clotting and collagen degradation.

Of the wandering cells, which may be present in connective tissues proper, the only group of cells frequently seen in dental pulps are the *lymphocytes.* When present, they tend to be localized near the odontoblast layer, at the periphery.

The presence in the pulp of monocytes, polymorphonuclear leukocytes, eosinophils and plasma cells generally is indicative of disease. *No fat cells* are found in the dental pulp.

Vascularization and Innervation

Both the vascularization and innervation patterns of the dental pulp (Fig. 10–3) underscore the primary function of this tissue: the *support* and *maintenance* of the *odontoblast layer* at its periphery. The odontoblasts, in turn, maintain the dentin.

Blood vessels accompanied by nerves enter the pulp via the apical foramen. One or more small arterioles enter and run in a fairly

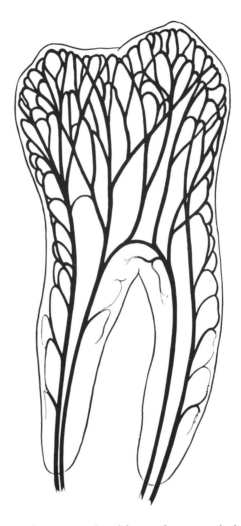

Fig. 10–3.   Diagrammatic representation of the vascular pattern of a dental pulp. A similar pattern exists for the nerves of the pulp. Arteries enter the pulp and veins leave the pulp via the apical foramen (as do the nerves). They run through the root canal, where they give off relatively few branches. In the pulp chamber of the crown, a profuse branching takes place. The microvasculature of the pulp is associated with the odontoblast layer. Similarly, the richly branching afferent nerves form a fine network (plexus) near the odontoblast layer.

straight course through the pulp of the root canal. Once they reach the pulp chamber in the crown, they branch out, forming a rich capillary network at the periphery immediately underneath, and occasionally within, the layer of odontoblasts. The odontoblast layer is active metabolically, and the capillaries near the odontoblasts have many pores (see Chap. 6); consequently there is extensive exchange of materials across the capillary wall.

Drainage from the capillary bed is by several small venules, which come together into two or three larger venules, running back toward the apical foramen.

It is difficult to demonstrate satisfactorily the presence of lymph capillaries in the dental pulp. A few investigators claim to have provided some morphologic evidence for such vessels. However, most would agree that no lymph capillaries are present in the dental pulp. If the latter claim is correct, fluid from the ground substance, which in most other tissues returns to the blood via the lymph capillaries, must take a different pathway in the pulp, perhaps directly back into the blood capillaries.

Two types of *nerve fibers* enter the dental pulp via the apical foramen: *autonomic* and *afferent.*

AUTONOMIC NERVE FIBERS. Only sympathetic autonomics are found in the pulp. The fibers consist of the cell processes of those neurons whose cell bodies are located in the superior cervical ganglion. These *unmyelinated* nerve fibers travel along with the blood vessels. Their function in the pulp is the innervation of the smooth muscle cells of the arterioles and thus the *regulation* of the *blood flow* in the *microvascular bed.*

AFFERENT (SENSORY) FIBERS. These fibers come from branches of the second and third divisions of the fifth cranial (trigeminal) nerve. These *mostly myelinated* fibers initially run along with the blood vessels into the pulp chamber of the crown. Some fibers terminate in the central pulp. Others branch out and break up into small, individual fibers, which form a rich network *(plexus of Raschkow)* underneath the odontoblastic layer. From this plexus, individual nerve fibers run peripherally toward the odontoblasts. These nerve fibers are no longer covered with a myelin sheath; they consist of axons, supported by Schwann cells.

The nerve fibers finally lose their Schwann cell support and terminate as *"free endings."* This is the only type of afferent nerve terminal found anywhere in the dental pulp, centrally or at the periphery, near the odontoblasts. Near the odontoblasts, the free ending may touch the cell body of an odontoblast, or it may run for a short distance inside the dentinal tubule and terminate on the odontoblastic process (Fig. 10–4). Most odontoblasts are *not* associated with such free nerve endings, but since the odontoblasts are connected

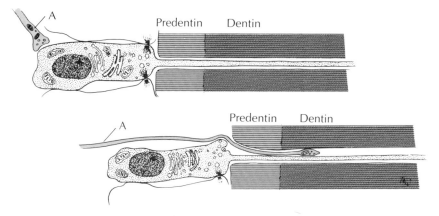

Fig. 10–4. This diagram shows afferent nerve endings on two odontoblasts. The axon (A) has lost its Schwann cell support, just before reaching the odontoblast layer. The axon may terminate in close association with the odontoblast's cell body (top), or it may run for a short distance inside a dentinal tubule and terminate on an odontoblastic process (bottom). The nerve terminals somewhat resemble a synapse.

with each other via gap junctions and/or tight junctions, a sheet of these cells can behave as a coordinated unit, so that individual innervation is not required. The presence of free nerve endings is held responsible for the perception of *pain* by the dental pulp of all stimuli, regardless of the nature of these stimuli (heat, cold, pressure).

DENTIN

Dentin, somewhat comparable to bone tissue, has the 3 components commonly found in connective tissues: *cells* (odontoblasts), *fibrous matrix* (Type I collagen fibers) and *ground substance* (mainly proteoglycans and glycoproteins, chemically rather similar to the ground substance of bone).

The dominant component of this tissue is the fibrous matrix. Dentin is calcified, which means that hydroxyapatite salts are present in the fibrous matrix and ground substance.

Morphologically, dentin is unique in that the odontoblasts do *not* become *enclosed* by their product, except for one long cell process, which each of these cells leaves behind in the dentin.

The cell bodies of the odontoblasts are located in the dental pulp at the inner (pulpal) surface of the dentin. Their long cell processes are surrounded by dentin matrix, which is calcified in the mature dentin and uncalcified in the immature predentin, so that each process lies in its individual *dentinal tubule.* All dentinal tubules run from the dentino-enamel junction to the dental pulp.

Once dentin is exposed by a carious lesion, trauma or otherwise, there is a direct contact between the outside world and the dental pulp via a large number of patent dentinal tubules. This contact is usually experienced as extremely unpleasant and painful.

Dentinal Tubules

It would be possible to fill several pages with the many histologic details of dentin, but from a clinical viewpoint the most important attributes of this tissue are its dentinal tubules.

COURSE OF THE DENTINAL TUBULES: S-SHAPED CURVATURES. As we stated before, the dentinal tubules are formed as the result of deposition of dentin *around* the odontoblastic cell processes which, during dentin formation, are left behind by the odontoblasts. Since the odontoblastic processes are left behind while the odontoblasts are moving away from their initial positions, the shapes of the odontoblastic processes and of the dentinal tubules in which they are located provide us with an accurate record of the path taken by the odontoblasts.

In analyzing a longitudinal section of a tooth, you will soon recognize that in a large part of the tooth the dentinal tubules are not straight, but rather gently curved in an S-shape.

The peculiar course of the dentinal tubules is explained when you realize that, during the deposition of the dentin matrix, the odontoblasts move toward the center of the dental papilla. This means that the cells start out on a larger surface (the future dentino-enamel junction) and end up on a much smaller surface. If both the initial surface and the final surface would be perfectly spherical or perfectly cylindrical, the cells would all move centrally in a straight line while becoming increasingly more densely packed.

However, the tooth while being somewhat cylindrically shaped, is closed on one end by the presence of cusps or an incisal edge. This forces the odontoblasts to move in a slightly more complicated manner. In the roots, which are fairly cylindrical, the dentinal tubules run relatively straight. In the crown, on the other hand, uneven and locally acute crowding patterns would develop if the odontoblasts would all try to move straight backward during their secretory activity.

They do so, but only for a short distance. Thereafter they move obliquely in an apical direction (Fig. 10–5), producing an S-shaped curve and thus making accommodations for the more occlusally/incisally located odontoblasts. In this way, while the odontoblasts do become densely packed, the crowding is at least evenly divided.

For survival, the odontoblastic cell bodies, which were arranged in a single layer at the start of their secretory activities, become stacked into several layers, up to 8 layers in the crown.

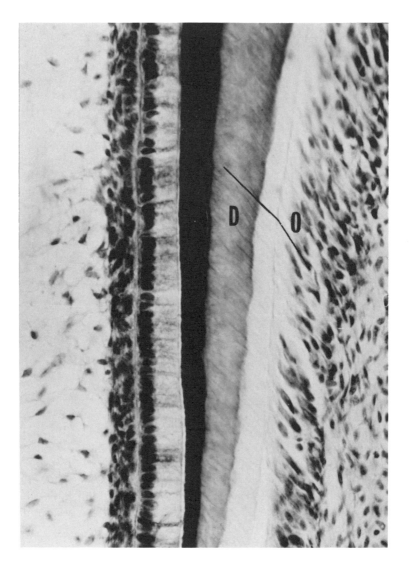

Fig. 10–5.   Early crowding patterns in the odontoblast layer (O) during dentin formation. The orientation of the odontoblastic cell bodies forms an angle with the orientation of the first-formed segments of the dentinal tubules in the dentin (D). Since the odontoblasts will move further backward in a direction corresponding with the orientation of their cell bodies, the first part of an (inverted) S-curve is about to be formed. Original magnification ×125.

The S-shaped curvature of the dentinal tubules in the crown and the cervical region of the tooth has clinical significance. Caries, or any other external insult that affects the peripheral dentin, may have a local effect in the dental pulp at a more apical level than the level at which the external insult occurred. Conversely, if a stained, pigmented endodontic filling has been placed above a certain level in the root canal, but still below the cervix, discoloration of the dentin in the crown may follow nonetheless, since the pigments travel in occlusal/incisal direction, upward along the S-shaped dentinal tubules (Fig. 10–6).

SECONDARY CURVATURES OF THE DENTINAL TUBULES. Careful microscopic study of the dentinal tubules may reveal the presence of a finer pattern of delicate curves, or *secondary curvatures,* along their course. These curvatures consist of small waves in the dentinal tubules, with crests about 4 µm apart. They probably reflect the minor changes in the direction of movement of the dentin-producing odontoblasts during successive 24-hour periods.

DENSITY AND BRANCHING OF THE DENTINAL TUBULES. An odontoblastic process and the tubule in which it lies reflect the path taken by the odontoblast during dentin deposition. Since the odontoblasts become progressively more crowded as they move toward the center of the dental papilla, it is easy to understand that in the mature dentin the dentinal tubules are closer together near the pulp than in the peripheral dentin. In fact, if one were to count the total number of cross-sectioned tubules in 1 mm^2 of a section of dentin as a measure of tubular *density,* this density would be 4 to 5 times higher in the dentin near the pulp than in the peripheral dentin.

At the dentino-enamel junction, however, the tubule density becomes suddenly higher than in the rest of the peripheral dentin. This is because the dentinal tubules are branched into two or three short, *terminal branches,* near the dentino-enamel junction. The higher tubular density in this most peripheral dentin makes it particularly sensitive on exposure, almost as sensitive as the dentin near the pulp.

The terminal branching of the dentinal tubule is produced during the earliest stages of dentin formation. At that time the odontoblasts have several cell processes, some of which contact the processes of the pre-ameloblasts across the broken-down basal lamina (see Chap. 9). As the odontoblasts recede, the original processes come together into one single odontoblastic process. The dentin is first deposited around the larger number of smaller processes and later around the single process, producing the terminally branched tubule.

Aside from the terminal branching, the dentinal tubules in the crown dentin are relatively unbranched (Fig. 10–7). In the root den-

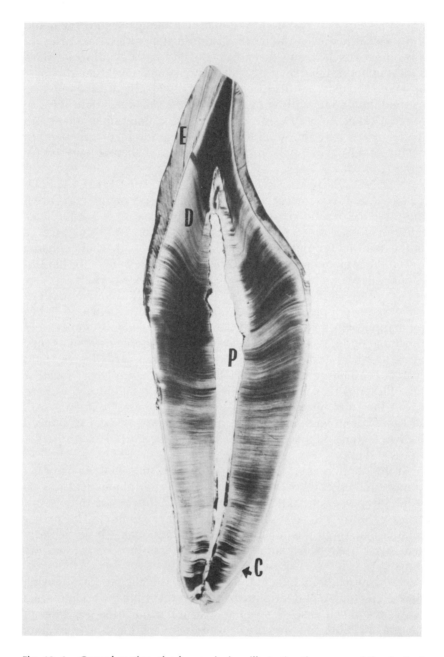

Fig. 10–6. Ground section of a human incisor illustrating the course of the dentinal tubules. In the crown dentin and the dentin near the cervix, the dentinal tubules run in an S-shaped course. This is well illustrated on the right side of the section. On the left side, a mirror image of an S-shaped curve may be seen. Further apically, in the root dentin, the tubules straighten out and become horizontal. E = enamel; D = dentin; P = pulp; C = cementum. Original magnification ×1.

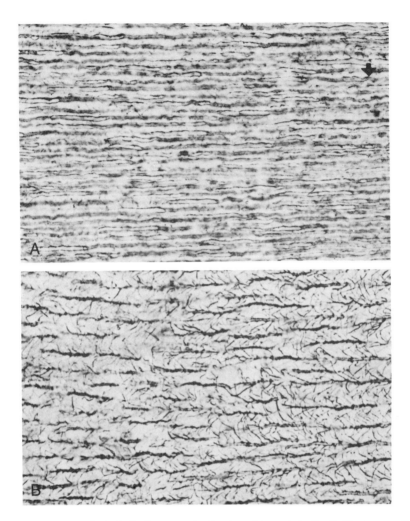

Fig. 10–7.   Dentinal tubules in crown dentin, *A,* and in root dentin, *B.* The inner walls of the tubules are stained darkly. The tubules in the crown dentin are relatively unbranched compared with the tubules in root dentin. The gentle waves in the course of the tubules represent secondary curvatures *(arrow).* Original magnification × 520.

tin, however, the tubules have many side branches, all along their lengths. These side branches are also produced during dentin formation, and they are the result of cell junctions between the adjacent odontoblasts or additional small cell processes, which become trapped in the forming dentin.

DIAMETERS AND CONTENTS OF THE DENTINAL TUBULES. When the dentinal tubules are first formed, during the process of dentin formation, they are wide, up to 4 μm in diameter. With further development, however, a small amount of dentin is added to the inner surfaces of the tubular walls. This reduces the diameter of these tubules somewhat.

The tubule diameter near the dentino-enamel junction is a little less than 2 μm and this does not change much with age. Midway along the length of the dentinal tubules their diameter is 2.5 to 3 μm (the wider diameter is found in younger teeth). Near the pulp the dentinal tubules are widest: 3 to 4 μm (again, the wider diameters are in the younger teeth).

The *functional diameter* of a tubule, that is that part of the tubule diameter that is patent, allowing movement of fluid and small molecules, is much smaller. Much of the tubule lumen is occupied by a long odontoblastic process. Dentinal tubules also often contain fat droplets, mineral deposits or uncalcified collagen fibers, in addition to tissue fluid.

In some dentinal tubules a delicate, afferent (sensory) nerve axon is present. This axon is not covered by a Schwann cell and it terminates on the odontoblastic process, which is located in the same tubule. If present, a nerve axon does *not* extend as far into the dentinal tubule as the odontoblastic process itself. The presence of an axon inside a dentinal tubule is probably explained by the fact that it became enclosed in the forming dentin, together with the odontoblastic process.

With age, the contents of the dentinal tubules may calcify gradually. This is the case especially near the dentino-enamel and dentino-cementum junctions.

At the beginning of this chapter, we described the possibility of having exposed dentin at the cervix of the tooth. When the dentin has been acutely exposed, the tubules form an open connection between the outside world and the dental pulp, thus causing a painful situation. However, if the contents of the dentinal tubules are calcified, they seal off the remainder of the tubular contents from the outside world. This, in turn, affords protection for the dental pulp, and little pain may be experienced when such dentin is exposed. Certain clinical treatments for painful cervical dentin actually stimulate the calcification of the dentinal tubules, thereby reducing the pain.

Peritubular and Intertubular Dentin

The extracellular matrix of dentin (fibrous matrix, ground substance and the mineral hydroxyapatite) is not completely homogeneous. The dentin immediately around each dentinal tubule *(peritubular dentin)* differs in composition from the rest of the dentin *(intertubular dentin)*.

Peritubular dentin forms a 1 μm thick layer around each tubule.

This layer consists of a very delicate collagenous matrix and a relatively abundant ground substance, and is usually heavily calcified.

In the *intertubular dentin* the collagen fibers are much coarser, and, since they occupy a certain volume that cannot be occupied by hydroxyapatite, intertubular dentin is generally less heavily calcified than peritubular dentin.

During dentin formation, the intertubular dentin is produced first. The protein-producing organelles (granular endoplasmic reticulum, Golgi systems) are all located in the odontoblastic cell body. The secretory granules, which contain the protein precursors of the collagen fibers and the proteins of the ground substance, to which carbohydrates have been added in the Golgi system, are secreted at the secretory end of the odontoblastic *cell body.* Thus, the odontoblastic processes *first* become surrounded by the *intertubular dentin matrix.*

The odontoblastic processes themselves do *not* contain any protein-synthesizing organelles, and their cytoplasm is relatively empty, apart from some microtubules and microfilaments, which give support to these long cell processes.

During calcification of the intertubular dentin, additional matrix materials are released by the odontoblasts on the inside surfaces of the dentinal tubular walls, which still consist of intertubular dentin. The newly released materials form the matrix of the peritubular dentin, which calcifies almost as soon as it is deposited (Fig. 10–8).

The difference in composition between peritubular and intertubular dentin causes these two dentins to behave differently, notably during *decalcification.* When peritubular dentin is decalcified, its delicate fibrous matrix is disrupted completely and is lost. In de-

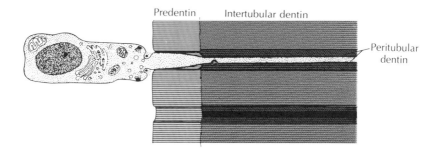

Fig. 10–8.   Diagram of an odontoblast with its cytoplasmic process extending into a dentinal tubule. A second, empty tubule appears below the first. Continued dentin deposition by the odontoblasts (secretory vesicles in the cell body) leads to the formation of more predentin, which calcifies and becomes (intertubular) dentin. During the calcification of the intertubular dentin matrix, additional dentin matrix is deposited on the inside walls of the dentinal tubules. This is peritubular (darkly shaded) dentin, which has a different composition than the intertubular dentin and calcifies almost immediately. The layer of peritubular dentin reduces the diameter of the dentinal tubule substantially.

calcified sections of dentin, only the decalcified matrix of the inter-tubular dentin remains, and as a result, the tubules appear much wider than they are in the nondecalcified tooth. Compare the widths of the dentinal tubules in decalcified histologic sections and in ground sections of dentin and verify this statement (Fig. 10–9).

Clinically, whenever dentin is in contact with a decalcifying agent (even small amounts of acid, such as the acids produced by bacteria in carious dentin, or acids leaked out in the cement of a temporary filling), some peritubular dentin is lost, and the tubules become wider, giving even more access to the dental pulp and causing more pain.

Pain

Pain has been mentioned several times on the preceding pages. It is well known that exposed, healthy dentin, with open dentinal tubules, may be painful. The pain is severe at the dentino-enamel junction, less so in the middle of the dentin, and becomes more severe in the dentin nearest the pulp. The question, why dentin should be so painful, has been asked for a long time. Several answers have been given and some have been proven wrong.

Nerve endings do *not* run along the *entire* lengths of the dentinal tubules, the odontoblastic processes do. Therefore the pain at the dentino-enamel junction might be explained by direct damage to these cell processes; the disturbance would be communicated via the cell membrane to the nerve axons, which terminate on some of the odontoblasts. Such stimuli would be perceived as pain.

Another explanation is that the fluid present in the dentinal tu-bules evaporates when the tubules are exposed. The resulting fluid movement would stress the odontoblasts and stimulate the nerve axons.

Such explanations seem to fit most clinical experiences and are at present the best available for dentin pain.

Other Aspects of Dentin

For a good understanding of dentin in clinical practice, an un-derstanding of the dentinal tubules, as well as the peritubular and intertubular dentin, is most important. However, the following points are of interest and we will discuss them briefly here.

Dentin, Once Deposited, Does Not Undergo Any Remodeling

Throughout life, some dentin deposition continues to take place, but except for the resorption of roots of primary teeth, which leads

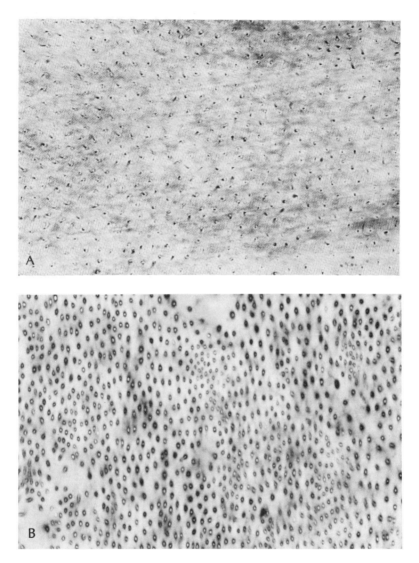

Fig. 10–9.   Cross-sectioned dentinal tubules in a ground section, *A*, a decalcified histologic section, *B*, and an electron micrograph of a decalcified section, *C*. In the ground
section *(A)* the dentinal tubules are narrow, dark, and surrounded by bright "halos" of
well-calcified peritubular dentin. Between the halos, intertubular dentin is present. In the
decalcified section *(B)*, the dentinal tubules appear wider. This is the result of the total
loss of the peritubular dentin layer during decalcification. Only the intertubular dentin
remains. The electron micrograph of a decalcified section *(C)* similarly shows a loss of
peritubular dentin. The arrow indicates the location of the inner wall of the dentinal
tubule, housing the odontoblastic process (not well visible here). The relatively empty
space between tubule and intertubular dentin was occupied by peritubular dentin (P)
before decalcification. The dark cross-banded structures in the intertubular dentin are
Type I collagen fibers. Two narrow side branches extend from the dentinal tubule. Original
magnification *A* and *B*, ×125; *C*, ×14,000. (Courtesy Dr. S. Doty.) (Continued p. 177.)

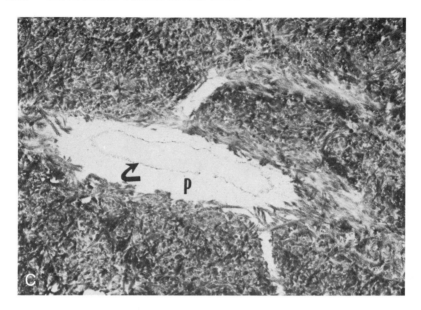

Fig. 10–9 (Cont'd).

to the shedding of those teeth, resorption of dentin is an indication of a pathologic condition. This means that dentin provides us with a record of metabolic events that occurred in the body during dentin deposition.

IMBRICATION LINES (von Ebner). Dentin deposition is not an entirely uniform process. In a given 24-hour period specific changes take place in the rates of secretion and calcification of the dentin matrix. These changes are repeated in successive 24-hour periods. This rhythmic pattern of dentin deposition produces regular bands in the tissue, somewhat like growth rings in a tree cross section. The average layer of dentin produced daily is about 4 μm thick. Each 4 μm of dentin in a ground section is composed of a somewhat lighter (better calcified) and a somewhat darker (less calcified) band. In *decalcified* sections such bands or *imbrication lines* (von Ebner) are visible as well (Fig. 10–10). The dark and light bands differ in composition and degree of calcification of the matrix, reflecting differences in dentin deposition during daytime and nighttime.

CONTOUR LINES (Owen). During periods of illness or other major changes in body metabolism (birth, for example), the dentin deposition may be somewhat affected as well. As a result, a band of dentin of a slightly different composition may be produced. Such a band is usually less well calcified than the adjacent dentin (formed before and after) and shows as a darker band in ground sections of dentin. These bands, which are far less frequently present than im-

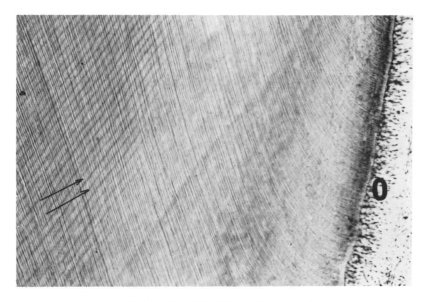

Fig. 10–10.   Imbrication lines in a decalcified histologic section of a young, newly erupted premolar. Odontoblasts (O) line the pulpal surface of the dentin. Their cytoplasmic processes are located within the dentinal tubules, of which the lower part of the S-shaped curve is visible. The imbrication lines appear as very regular, alternately dark and light bands running obliquely from lower left to upper right *(arrows)*. Original magnification ×40.

brication lines, are called *contour lines* (Owen). They follow the contour of what used to be the pulpal surface of the forming dentin at the time of the disturbance or change (Fig. 10–11). Since only the teeth of the primary dentition and the first molars of the secondary dentition are involved in dentin production at the time of birth, a clear *neonatal line* (a pronounced contour line) is present only in the dentin of these teeth.

MAN-MADE CONTOUR LINES. Certain antibiotics, most notably tetracyclines, are chemically bound to matrix components and even more to hydroxyapatite at the *growing surfaces* of bone, cementum, and dentin.

Bone and cementum are well embedded in soft tissues, so that any discoloration of these two tissues, as the result of the binding of tetracycline, remains undetected. Furthermore, bone is constantly remodeled and so, in time, rids itself of the tetracycline. But dentin is permanently marked because the tetracycline remains fixed in this nonremodeling tissue for the life of the tooth. Since the tetracycline attaches itself to the components of the forming dentin, along what is the pulpal surface of the dentin at the time of tetracycline administration, the band of stained dentin has the same shape as a contour line. Tetracycline has a deep golden color, which changes to greyish

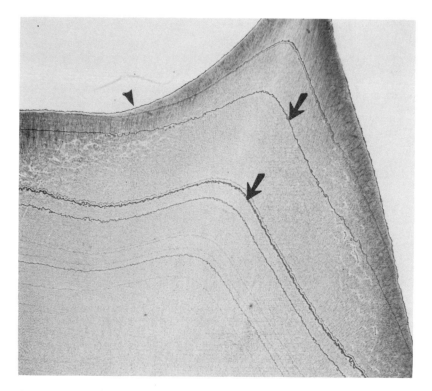

Fig. 10–11. Decalcified, histologic section through the anatomical crown of a human premolar. With the use of a special stain, several dark contour lines (Owen) are shown in the dentin *(arrows)*. Each of these lines represents the position of the odontoblast layer at the time when that particular line was produced. Notice that the contour lines in this plane of section run obliquely toward the dentino-enamel junction *(arrowhead)*. Original magnification × 50.

green with age. Enamel is a transparent tissue. This is especially evident in areas where the enamel layer is thin, as it is near the cervix of the tooth. If stained dentin is located in the crown, a dark band may be visible through the enamel. As a result, the tooth becomes esthetically unattractive. Although it is possible to bleach such teeth somewhat, the tetracycline remains. It cannot be removed.

Not All Dentin Calcifies Perfectly

Occasionally, during dentin matrix calcification, small islands of dentin matrix remain uncalcified. In number and size, these noncalcified regions vary from individual to individual. They are imperfections in calcification, but generally are *not* considered pathologic, since most teeth have them.

Once the imperfections are present, they usually do *not* disappear.

With age, some minerals may diffuse into such areas and become deposited in them. This makes these areas somewhat better, but by no means perfectly, calcified. We distinguish two types of imperfections in dentin calcification:

INTERGLOBULAR DENTIN AREAS. These small islands of noncalcified or imperfectly calcified dentin are located in the crown. They are found mostly along the line between the outer third and the middle third of the dentin width. These areas represent a developmental defect in the process of dentin calcification. The calcification front of regularly calcifying dentin is roughly linear (see Fig. 10–5). Imperfectly calcifying dentin has irregular, spherical or globular islands of calcified dentin along its calcification front. These islands fuse, but not always completely, leaving *interglobular,* uncalcified or poorly calcified dentin areas, with rounded depressions on their outer surfaces, between them.

GRANULAR LAYER (Tomes'). In the most peripheral dentin of the root, multitudes of noncalcified dentin islands are present, appearing as dark grains immediately next to the dentino-cementum junction, in ground sections. These islands have the same shapes as the interglobular dentin areas, but they are considerably smaller (Figs. 10–12 and 10–13). The reason for the imperfect calcification of this layer of dentin remains elusive. The "granules" may represent uncalcified cores of heavy collagen fibers found uniquely in the peripheral root dentin.

Mantle Dentin and Circumpulpal Dentin

Although most dentin is called *circumpulpal* (around the pulp), the *outermost layer* of the *crown* dentin, immediately next to the dentino-enamel junction, is called *mantle dentin.* This layer is about 30 μm thick. It is different from the circumpulpal dentin, because it contains, *in addition* to the normal collagen fibers of the dentin, another group of collagen fibers, which are considerably thicker. These thicker collagen fibers are called *von Korff's* fibers. The normal collagen fibers run parallel to the dentino-enamel junction. The von Korff's fibers run nearly perpendicular to the dentino-enamel junction.

In the section on peritubular and intertubular dentin, we noted that a fibrous matrix of thick collagen fibers is *less* calcified than a matrix with more delicate fibers. The same is true for mantle dentin. It is somewhat less calcified than the circumpulpal dentin because of the presence of the heavy von Korff's fibers. This lesser degree of calcification may explain the spread of caries along the dentino-enamel junction, once this junction is reached by the caries process.

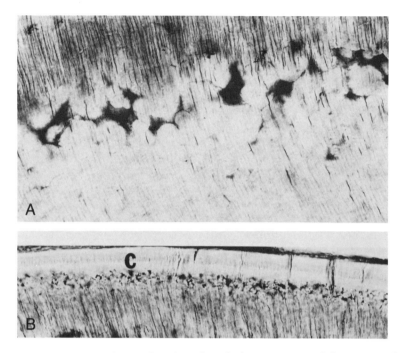

Fig. 10–12.   Horizontal ground sections through the crown, A, and the root, B, of a human tooth. In the crown dentin, interglobular dentin areas are present (dark structures). The granular layer (Tomes') is found in the root dentin, in the most peripheral layer, immediately adjacent to the (acellular) cementum, C. In both sections, the less calcified dentin areas have been stained with a dye, to make them more clearly visible. A, The rounded surfaces of well-calcified dentin globules demarcate the less calcified interglobular dentin areas. The granules of the granular layer (Tomes') have similar shapes, but are considerably smaller. Original magnification × 50.

AGE-RELATED AND PATHOLOGIC CHANGES IN THE PULP

In the pulp certain changes occur with age. Cell death results in a *decrease* in the number of cells. The surviving fibroblasts gradually produce *more fibrous matrix,* with an increased proportion of Type I collagen fibers, at the expense of Type III fibers. *Less ground substance* is produced, and the ground substance contains *less water.* Thus, with age the pulp becomes less cellular and more fibrous, while its actual *size decreases* as a result of further dentin deposition (p. 227).

Dental pulp tissue is somewhat unique, mainly because it is almost completely surrounded by hard tissues. Because of its location, *minor pathologic events,* such as an inflammation, may have far-reaching effects. Inflammation is usually accompanied by a swelling of the affected tissue. Elsewhere in the body this does not lead to complications. However, a dental pulp is not capable of undergoing swelling because the surrounding hard tissues prevent its expansion.

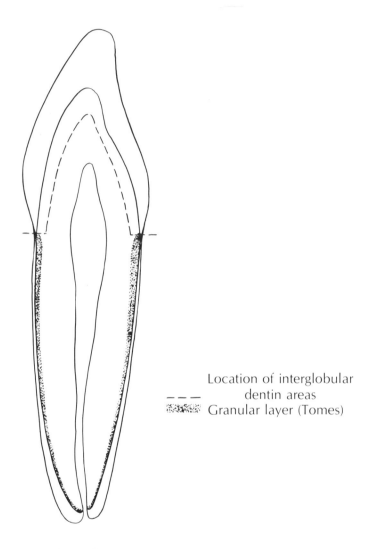

Location of interglobular
dentin areas
Granular layer (Tomes)

Fig. 10–13. Diagram illustrating the principal locations of interglobular dentin areas and the granular layer (Tomes') in a section of human tooth. The interglobular dentin areas generally are located in the crown dentin, along a line between the outer third and middle third of the dentin width (where the dentinal tubules make their first curve of the S-shape). The granular layer is found in the most peripheral dentin of the root only.

Since there is no place to accommodate an increase in dimension of this tissue, it becomes compressed. This can cause extreme pain and almost invariably, it leads to the demise of the inflamed pulp.

Calcified Bodies in the Pulp

Small calcified bodies are present in 25 to 50% of the dental pulps of newly erupted teeth and in over 90% of the dental pulps of older adults. Calcified bodies are variably classified on the basis of their development, histology, and relative location.

Development

Calcified bodies may be formed by one of two possible mechanisms:

EPITHELIO-MESENCHYMAL INTERACTIONS. Small groups of epithelial cells may become isolated from the epithelial root sheath or from the cervical epithelial flaps of multirooted teeth during development. The isolated epithelial cell groups come to lie in the dental papilla, where their interaction with mesenchymal cells leads to the cytodifferentiation of the latter into true odontoblasts. These cells form a small dentin structure within the pulp.

CALCIFIC DEGENERATIONS. Spontaneous calcification may occur of components of the pulp (a collagen fiber, ground substance, cellular debris, a segment of a capillary) any time throughout the life of a tooth. The calcified mass may expand in an irregular fashion by spreading calcification of the surrounding structures, or it may induce pulpal cells to differentiate into osteoblasts, or even odontoblasts. Such cells then produce concentric layers of calcifying matrix on the surface of the calcified mass (no cells enclosed).

DIFFUSE CALCIFICATIONS. These are a variant of calcific degenerations. When a pulp becomes seriously degenerated, it may undergo calcification in a large number of locations, rather than in one or a few. These tiny bodies resemble the calcific degenerations, except for their size and number (Fig. 10–14).

Histology

Calcified bodies in the pulp may be composed of dentin, irregularly calcified tissue or a combination of both. In the customary classification a calcified body that contains tubular dentin is called a "true" *denticle.* Usually the calcified bodies that form as the result of an epithelio-mesenchymal interaction, are initially true denticles (Fig. 10–15).

Irregularly calcified tissue usually does not bear much resemblance to any known tissue in the human body. It is found in diffuse calcifications and in the cores of calcific degenerations. In the customary classification the latter are called "false" denticles or *pulp stones* (Fig. 10–16).

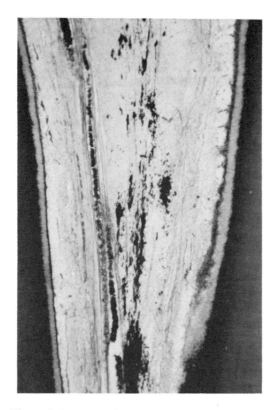

Fig. 10–14.   Diffuse calcification in the root pulp of a human primary tooth. Dark, tiny areas of diffuse calcification are visible. Most appear to be related to existing structures such as collagen fibers and blood vessels. This tooth was in an advanced state of resorption, due to the eruption of its secondary successor. This was the apparent cause for the advanced degeneration of the pulp tissue, and diffuse calcification resulted. Original magnification × 12.5.

Location

Calcified bodies may be located anywhere in the pulp. They usually begin to form as *loose* bodies in the pulp tissue. However, because they continue to increase in size, and because the dental pulp continues to decrease in size with age, the calcified bodies may become *attached* to, or even *embedded* in the dentin walls.

AGE-RELATED AND PATHOLOGIC CHANGES IN DENTIN

As we stated before, dentin production continues throughout the functional life of the tooth. All dentin formed *before* the completion of the apical foramen is considered primary dentin.

SECONDARY DENTIN. Once the apical foramen is com-

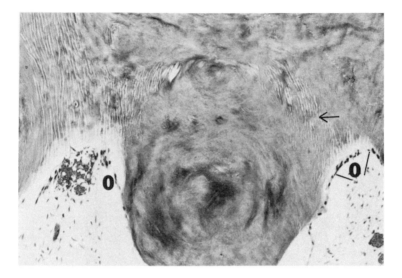

Fig. 10–15.   Large true denticle in a histologic section through the root pulp of a human tooth. Some irregular dentinal tubules *(arrow)* are visible inside the denticle, and odontoblasts (O) line those parts of the denticle which contain the dentinal tubules. Original magnification ×50.

pleted, dentin formation continues, but at a considerably slower rate. This dentin is *secondary dentin.*

Morphologically, secondary dentin may be recognized by an abrupt *change* in the *course* of the dentinal tubules, at the transition between primary and secondary dentin. Also, there is a slight *reduction* in the *number* of dentinal tubules that can be explained only by the cell death of some of the odontoblasts, at the completion of the primary dentin. Finally, the secondary dentin *matrix* is somewhat *more calcified* than the primary dentin matrix (Fig. 10–17).

Secondary dentin is not formed evenly along all dentin walls of the pulp. It is formed mostly on those dentin surfaces that are underneath functionally loaded surfaces of the tooth, such as the lingual surfaces of incisors and canines.

REACTIVE DENTIN. This type of dentin is also frequently, and inappropriately, called reparative dentin. However, it does not really repair anything. Reactive dentin is formed fast and in localized regions, involving only the areas underneath those dentinal tubules that are exposed to some external insult. The insult may be caries, a cavity preparation, or dentin exposure resulting from excessive wear of the enamel.

In all these cases a localized group of odontoblasts related to the

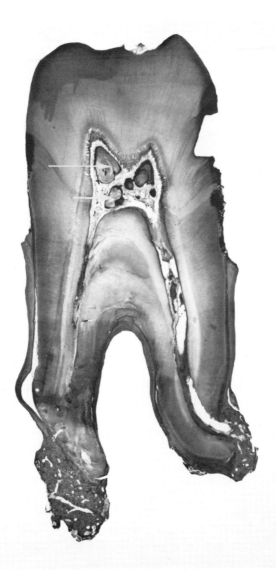

Fig. 10–16.   Several pulp stones are present in this decalcified histologic section of a molar tooth of an older individual. Notice the extensive caries at the cervix and an old cavity on the right side. Some of the denticles have a regular, lamellar appearance *(arrows)*. Others have an irregular appearance (and are darker in this section). Original magnification ×1.

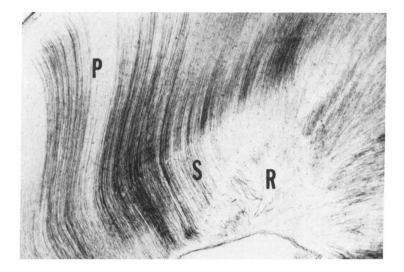

Fig. 10–17. Primary (P), secondary (S), and reactive (R) dentin in a ground section of a human tooth. The difference between primary and secondary dentin is primarily due to the slight change in the course of the dentinal tubules, as they pass from the primary into the secondary dentin, and to a somewhat higher degree of calcification of the secondary dentin (lighter in ground section). The reactive dentin is associated with wear of the cusps, which has exposed part of the dentin (not visible in this photograph). The dentinal tubules in the reactive dentin are irregular and fewer in number than in primary and secondary dentin. Original magnification × 10.

tubules that are affected by the insult may perish. If odontoblasts perish, neighboring, undifferentiated mesenchymal cells move to the affected dentin and become odontoblasts. These cells produce a small, localized path of reactive dentin.

The new tissue has irregular dentinal tubules and occasionally no tubules at all. Sometimes odontoblasts become trapped in this dentin.

The dentinal tubules, which run between the dentino-enamel junction and this new patch of reactive dentin, usually no longer contain any odontoblastic processes. These processes were lost when the odontoblasts themselves perished. During the preparation of a ground section such empty tubules tend to fill up with air. Because of the presence of air in a band of dentinal tubules, such a band appears dark in the section and is called a *dead tract* (Fig. 10–18).

SCLEROTIC (TRANSPARENT) DENTIN. Even during completion of the primary dentin, some groups of odontoblasts may perish and their dentinal tubules may be filled with mineral deposits. With age, this process continues and a number of tubules will become obliterated with mineral, especially in the root dentin and in the peripheral dentin. As long as dentinal tubules have organic contents

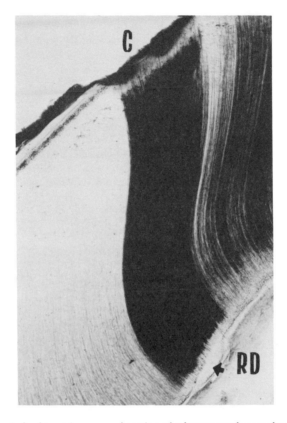

Fig. 10–18.   A dead tract in a ground section of a human tooth near the cervix. The S-shaped tubules of the dead tract were filled with air during histologic processing. As a result, they appear dark in ground section. On one end of the dead tract, a carious lesion is present (C). On the other end, a light patch of reactive dentin (RD) may be seen. The reactive dentin is localized in the area of the insult only. Original magnification × 10.

(odontoblastic process, other uncalcified matter), the tubules will be visible in a ground section because the light rays that pass through the section, are deflected by the organic contents. This enables us to see the tubules and it makes the dentin an opaque tissue.

However, when the tubules are filled with mineral, the light rays pass relatively straight through the section, without deflection, making it a *transparent* tissue. We call this *transparent* or *sclerotic* dentin. Turnover of the ground substance in such tissue is much more difficult and slower than in normal dentin. For this reason sclerotic dentin will become more brittle with time.

Transparent or sclerotic dentin is also formed adjacent to carious dentin. During the caries attack, the dentin is locally decalcified by the action of the acid produced by the bacteria. The minerals dissolved during this decalcification precipitate in adjacent dentinal tubules, which are already empty (a dead tract). As those tubules are filled with mineral, the tissue becomes locally transparent.

SELECTED READING LIST

Arwill, T., et al.: Ultrastructure of nerves in the dentinal–pulp border zone after sensory and autonomic nerve transection in the cat. Acta Odont. Scand., 31:273, 1973.

Bishop, M.A.: A fine-structural investigation of the extent of perineural investment of the nerve supply to the pulp in rat molar teeth. Arch. Oral Biol., 27:225, 1982.

Bradford, E.W.: Microanatomy and histochemistry of dentin. In Structural and Chemical Organization of Teeth. Vol. II. Edited by A.E.W. Miles. New York, Academic Press, 1967.

Brännström, M., and Johnson, G.: Effect of various conditioners and cleaning agents on prepared dentin surfaces. A scanning electron microscopic investigation. J. Prosthet. Dent., 31:422, 1974.

Calle, A.: Intercellular junctions between human odontoblasts. Acta Anat., 122:138, 1985.

Farnoush, A.: Mast cells in human dental pulp. J. Endodont., 10:250, 1984.

Fearnhead, R.W.: Innervation of dental tissue. In Structural and Chemical Organization of Teeth. Vol. 1. Edited by A.E.W. Miles. New York, Academic Press, 1967.

Finn, S.B. (ed.): Biology of the Dental Pulp Organ. A Symposium. Birmingham, University of Alabama Press, 1968.

Frank, R.M., Wiedemann, P., and Fellinger, E.: Ultrastructure of lymphatic capillaries in the human dental pulp. Cell Tissue Res., 178:229, 1977.

Furseth, R.: The structure of peripheral root dentin in young human premolars. Scand. J. Dent. Res., 82:557, 1974.

Gvozdenovic-Sedlecki, S., Qvist, V., and Hansen, H.P.: Histologic variations in the pulp of intact premolars from young individuals. Scand. J. Dent. Res., 81:433, 1973.

Holland, G.R.: Non-myelinated nerve fibres and their terminals in the sub-odontoblastic plexus of the feline dental pulp. J. Anat., 130:457, 1980.

Holland, G.R., and Robinson, P.P.: The number and size of axons at the apex of the cat's canine tooth. Anat. Rec., 205:215, 1983.

Johansen, E., Ultrastructure of dentine. In Structural and Chemical Organization of Teeth. Vol. II. Edited by A.E.W. Miles. New York, Academic Press, 1967.

Johnson, G., and Brännström, M.: The sensitivity of dentin. Changes in relation to conditions at exposed tubule apertures. Acta Odont. Scand., 32:29, 1974.

Kawasaki, K., Tanaka, S., and Ishikawa, T.: On the daily incremental lines in human dentine. Arch. Oral Biol., 24:939, 1979.

Köling, A., and Rask-Andersen, H.: Membrane junctions in the subodontoblastic region. Acta Odont. Scand., 41:99, 1983.

Moss-Salentijn, L., and Hendricks-Klyvert, M.: Calcified structures in human dental pulps. A review. J. Endod., 14:184, 1988.

Ogilvie, A.L., and Ingle, J.I.: An Atlas of Pulpal and Periapical Biology. Philadelphia, Lea & Febiger, 1965.

Osborn, J.W.: A mechanistic view of dentinogenesis and its relation to the curvatures of the processes of the odontoblasts. Arch. Oral Biol., 12:295, 1967.

Philippas, G.G., and Applebaum, E.: Age factor in secondary dentin formation. J. Dent. Res., 45:778, 1966.

Rapp, R., El-Labban, N.G., Kramer, I.R.H., and Wood, D.: Ultrastructure of fenestrated capillaries in human dental pulps. Arch. Oral Biol., 22:317, 1977.

Selvig, K.A.: Ultrastructural changes in human dentine exposed to a weak acid. Arch. Oral Biol., 13:719, 1968.

Shimauchi, K., et al.: A scanning electron microscope study of intratubular dentin fibers. J. Nihon Univ. Sch. Dent., *15*:113, 1973.

Sigal, M.J., Aubin, J.E., Ten Cate, A.R., and Pitaru, S.: The odontoblast process extends to the dentinoenamel junction: An immunocytochemical study of rat dentine. J. Histochem. Cytochem., *32*:872, 1984.

Siskin, M.: *The Biology of the Human Dental Pulp.* St. Louis, The C.V. Mosby Co., 1973.

Skinner, H.C.W.: Tetracycline and mineralized tissues. Review and perspectives. Yale J. Biol. Med., *48*:377, 1975.

Symons, N.B.B.: The microanatomy and histochemistry of dentinogenesis. In *Structural and Chemical Organization of Teeth. Vol. I.* Edited by A.E.W. Miles. New York, Academic Press, 1967.

Takuma, S.: Ultrastructure of dentinogenesis. In *Structural and Chemical Organization of Teeth. Vol. I.* Edited by A.E.W. Miles. New York, Academic Press, 1967.

Thylstrup, A., Leach, S.A., and Qvist, V. (eds.): *Dentine and Dentine Reactions in the Oral Cavity.* Oxford, IRL Press, 1987.

Tsukada, K.: Ultrastructure of the relationship between odontoblast processes and nerve fibres in dentinal tubules of rat molar teeth. Arch. Oral Biol., *32*:87, 1987.

Vasiliadis, L., Darling, A.I., and Levers, B.G.H.: The histology of sclerotic human root dentine. Arch. Oral Biol., *28*:693, 1983.

Wigglesworth, D.J., Longmore, G.A., Kuc, I.M., and Murdoch, C.: Early dentinogenesis in mice: von Korff fibres and their possible significance. A preliminary study by light and electron microscopy. Acta Anat., *127*:151, 1986.

11

Enamel

Enamel covers the anatomical crowns of the teeth. It is the hardest tissue found in the human body. This hardness results from its high degree of calcification. The mineral hydroxyapatite accounts for 96% of the total weight of enamel, compared with 70% of the total weight in dentin and 45% of the total weight in bone. Water comprises 3% of the enamel weight.

The epithelially produced enamel matrix is composed of glyco-protein (specifically *enamelin*). It represents only about 1% of the total weight of mature enamel and it is intimately related to the hydroxyapatite mineral. When the mineral is removed from enamel by decalcification, the enamel matrix is lost along with it and an empty space is left. Because of this, enamel usually is studied with the light microscope in ground sections, rather than in sections of routinely decalcified teeth.

If any enamel matrix remains in a routinely decalcified section, you may be assured that this matrix was incompletely calcified before the tooth was placed in the fixating agent. This may be the case in developing teeth, in which some of the enamel matrix has not yet been removed during enamel maturation. In mature teeth, the presence of enamel matrix in a histologic section indicates that a disturbance occurred during enamel maturation.

One may become acquainted with the structure of enamel by using an old method to study it:

Place a newly extracted tooth in 12 ml of a 10% solution of hydrochloric acid. At the end of 30 hours in this acid, the enamel is partially decalcified and quite soft. Remove a small portion of this softened tissue with a needle or brush and place it on a microscopic glass slide. Now carefully tease out this mass thinly with fine needles. Place a drop of saline solution on this preparation and cover it with a small cover glass. The preparation may be stained by allowing a histologic stain to run beneath the cover glass by capillary action.

When you study this material with the light microscope, you will notice that the enamel has been separated into what seem to be fine fibers. Actually, these are the cores of the structural units of the enamel tissue. The units of enamel, *enamel prisms* or *rods*, are highly calcified rods, containing little enamel matrix, separated from each other by thin, noncalcified sheaths of enamel matrix, the *prism sheaths.*

CLINICALLY IMPORTANT FEATURES OF ENAMEL

GROOVES OR FISSURES IN THE OCCLUSAL SURFACES OF MOLARS AND PREMOLARS. During tooth development, the enamel-forming cells, the ameloblasts, move from the dentino-enamel junction outward. Since these cells usually are located on *convex* surfaces, this means that they move from a smaller area to a larger one. However, the areas between adjacent cusps of molars and premolars are *concave*, and the ameloblasts on those surfaces have the same problems as do the odontoblasts during dentin production: they soon suffer from crowding.

In the deeper parts of these concave surfaces, ameloblasts occasionally "back into each other" and may become strangulated. The result is cell death of the affected ameloblasts and incomplete maturation of the enamel matrix, which is produced by these cells.

This leads to the presence of a "weak spot" in the tooth's defense against caries. The incompletely calcified areas are readily attacked by caries. The situation is further complicated by the fact that the presence of remnants of the enamel organ leave a deep, narrow groove (narrower than the thickness of a dental probe in most cases) in the occlusal surface. Food remnants and bacteria are caught and retained in such grooves, and they are hard to remove, even with careful toothbrushing (Fig. 11–1).

These grooves and fissures are real trouble spots, where caries can easily develop. Some prevention of these problems may result from the application of a protective coating (a *sealant*), which covers the grooves of the occlusal surfaces for some time.

ORIENTATION OF ENAMEL PRISMS. As a rule, all enamel prisms run from the dentino-enamel junction to the outer enamel surface, across the entire width of the enamel. This means that the *length* of an enamel prism depends on its location. Near the cusps, or near the incisal edges, the prisms are long (3 to 4 mm); near the cervix of the tooth, where the enamel becomes knife-edged, the prisms are almost negligible in length.

The average *diameter* of an enamel prism is about 5.5 μm, but this diameter varies slightly. Near the outer enamel surface the diameter of the prisms is about 1.3 times larger than their diameter near the dentino-enamel junction.

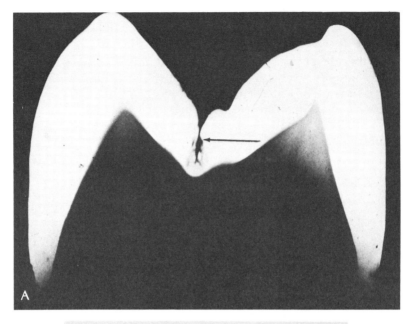

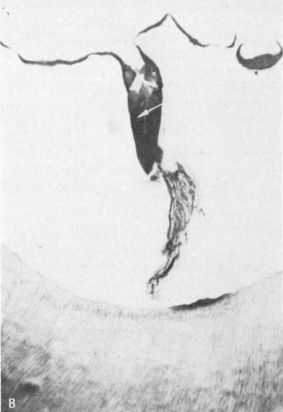

Fig. 11–1. Legend on facing page.

236

As an easy rule of thumb, it should be remembered that enamel prisms run toward the outer enamel surface, like the spokes of a wheel, *perpendicular* to the outer surface, or more precisely, to its tangents. Near the cervix, the prisms are oriented more apically (Fig. 11–2). Most prisms are *wavy* near the dentino-enamel junction, but they are relatively straight near the enamel surface.

The course of the enamel prisms is complicated in the enamel of a cusp or incisal edge. Here the prisms are twisted around each other, and when studied in ground section, single prisms are difficult to follow from the dentino-enamel junction to the outer surface. Such enamel is called *gnarled* enamel.

Knowledge of the course of the prisms is important clinically, because isolated enamel prisms, or parts of prisms, are extremely brittle and break easily. The strength of intact enamel is attributable, to a large degree, to its support by the underlying dentin. When cutting through enamel during a cavity preparation, *no enamel prisms should be left unsupported by dentin.* If a prism, or a part of a prism, is undercut at the edge of a cavity preparation, it will break off easily, making the margin of the restoration defective and leaky.

The designs of cavity preparations in restorative dentistry take the course of the enamel prisms into account. Since it is nearly impossible to avoid undermining groups of enamel prisms in gnarled enamel at a cusp or incisal edge, the margins of restorations are better placed in non-gnarled enamel.

DIFFERENTIAL ETCHING PATTERNS IN ENAMEL. In recent years the introduction of several new materials has brought about exciting changes, particularly in the practice of orthodontics, as well as preventive and restorative dentistry. Application of sealants on occlusal surfaces protects these surfaces against caries for limited periods of time. Orthodontic brackets are "bonded" directly to tooth surfaces and restorative materials are bonded directly to the walls of cavity preparations.

If such materials were to be applied directly to untreated enamel, they would detach easily, since they are unable to hold onto the smooth enamel surface. The enamel surface has to be "primed" first

---

Fig. 11–1. *A,* A radiograph of a ground section through a premolar shows the presence of a deep occlusal fissure (*arrow*). The entrance to this is too narrow for a dental probe. The enamel around the deep end of the fissure is incompletely calcified. × 1. *B,* The contents of the fissure in a decalcified section of the tooth shown in *A.* What looked like an empty groove on the radiograph is in fact filled with organic debris and bacteria (*arrow*). Some partially calcified enamel matrix is visible as well. Original magnification × 5.

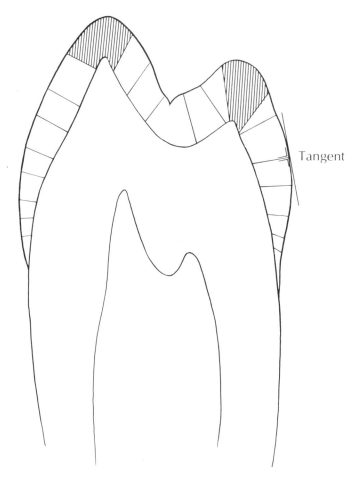

Tangent

Fig. 11–2.   Diagram indicating the general orientations of enamel prisms as lines within the enamel cap. Generally, all prisms run from the dentino-enamel junction perpendicularly to the tangent of the enamel surface. The areas of gnarled enamel at the cusps, where enamel prisms have a more complicated course, are hatched.

and this is done by *etching* it for a brief period of time. The concept of etching depends on the different chemical compositions of enamel prisms and prism sheaths.

Etching is done by the application of an acid to the tooth surface. The acid penetrates for a short distance (about 30 μm) into the enamel. Initially, the acid probably moves more easily through the uncalcified prism sheaths, attacking the mineral at the peripheries of the prisms and leaving the prism cores behind. This gives the treated enamel surface a rougher texture.

In some areas the prism sheaths seem to be relatively impermeable to the acid. Here the acid attacks the prism cores preferentially, leaving a honeycomb-like pattern of prism sheaths behind. This too makes the enamel surface rougher. It makes, therefore, no difference which part of the enamel tissue is etched away, as long as there is a differential etching pattern, which leaves the enamel surface rougher (Figs. 11–3 and 11–4).

The sealants and bonding materials form little spurs in the spaces where the enamel has been etched away. Such spurs hold these materials firmly attached to the tooth surface.

In all primary teeth and about 70% of all secondary teeth, parts of the outer layer of enamel have no prism structure. Such areas of *prismless enamel* are composed of evenly calcified enamel matrix and may be 30 to 50 μm thick. Etching of a homogeneous, prismless layer will not appreciably roughen the enamel surface, since most etching procedures depend on the different compositions of prisms and prism sheaths and do not affect the enamel to a level deeper than 30 μm. The etching and the subsequent attachment of sealants and bonding materials may be less successful in such cases.

ENAMEL PRISMS AND PRISM SHEATHS

You have learned already that the structural units of enamel are *enamel prisms*: rod-like structures running from the dentino-enamel junction to the outer enamel surface. Their lengths are determined by the local enamel thickness, while their *average* diameters (an

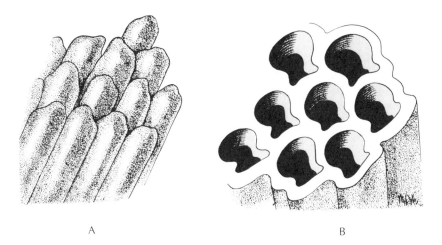

A   B

Fig. 11–3. Diagram showing, in strong magnification and with exaggeration, the effects of acid etching on enamel. The acid may preferentially attack, to a certain depth, the prism sheaths and peripheries, leaving the prism cores behind, *A*. Or, the prism cores may be etched away to a certain depth, leaving a honeycomb of prism peripheries and sheaths behind, *B*.

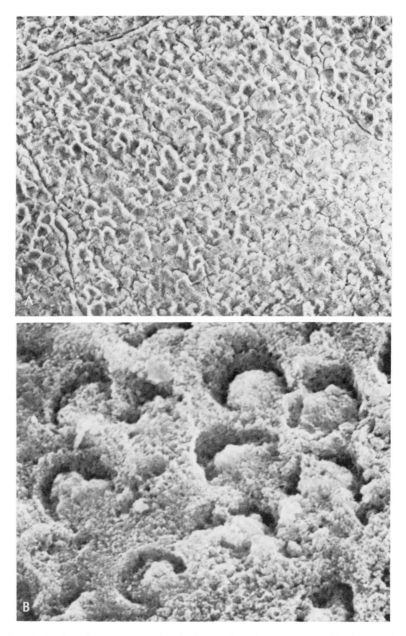

Fig. 11–4.   Actual appearance of etched enamel surfaces, as seen with the scanning electron microscope. *A*, Survey of an etched enamel surface. The etching pattern in the top half of the photograph differs from the pattern in the bottom half. Original magnification ×1000. *B*, Detail from the bottom half of the area shown in *A*. In this part of the etched surface, the prism cores have been left preferentially. Most etching has occurred in the horseshoe-shaped depressions, which correspond with the prism sheaths around the "heads" of the enamel prisms (this chapter). Original magnification ×5000.

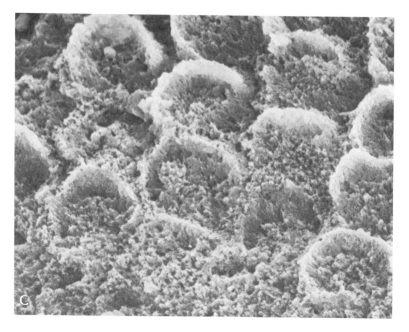

Fig. 11–4. (Cont'd). C, Detail from the top half of the area shown in A. In this part of the etched surface, the prism peripheries have been left preferentially, resulting in a rough honeycomb-like pattern. Original magnification ×5000. (Courtesy Dr. A. J. Gwinnett.)

average of the very different dimensions of widths and heights) are 5.5 μm. Neighboring enamel prisms are separated from each other by 0.1 to 0.2 μm wide *prism sheaths.*

The distinction between enamel prisms and prism sheaths is based primarily on their relative amounts of enamel matrix and their relative degrees of calcification. In the prisms the hydroxyapatite occupies nearly all available space, leaving little for the matrix components. In contrast, the prism sheaths consist almost exclusively of enamel matrix, with little or no hydroxyapatite present.

In cross section the prisms in human enamel most frequently have a keyhole shape. The rounded heads of these keyholes are pointed toward the occlusal/incisal ends of the teeth, while their tails are pointed cervically.

The rows of prisms are stacked fairly neatly, with the tails of one prism layer interlocked with the rounded heads of a second layer of prisms, which is located below the first layer, and touching the tops of the rounded heads of a third prism layer, which is located below the second one (Fig. 11–5, A). The prism sheaths are distinctly visible around the rounded heads of the prisms, but they become blurred, or even absent around the thinner tails of the prisms.

The small crystals of the mineral salt (*hydroxyapatite crystallites*)

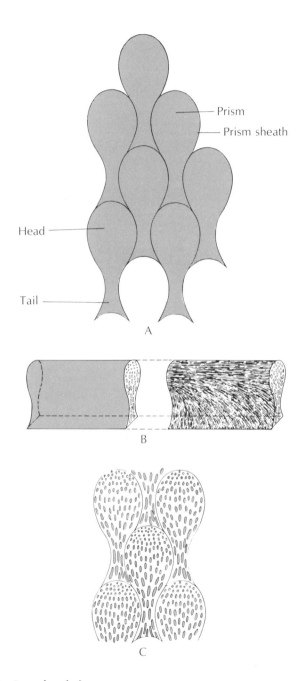

Fig. 11–5.   Legend on facing page.

in enamel are unusual in that they are about 4 times larger, in all dimensions, than the hydroxyapatite crystallites in bone, dentin or cementum. These hydroxyapatite crystallites run within each enamel prism with their *long axes parallel* to the long axis of the prism in the rounded *head* area, but *perpendicular* to the long axis of the prism in the *tail* area (Fig. 11–5, B, C). In the area between the head and the tail of one enamel prism, there is a gradual change in the orientation of the hydroxyapatite crystallites.

Prism sheaths are most pronounced where they separate two groups of hydroxyapatite crystallites, running at nearly right angles to each other: one group in the top of the rounded head of one prism and the other group in the bottom of the tail of the prism directly above the first one.

DEVELOPMENT OF ENAMEL PRISMS. The average diameter of an enamel-producing cell (ameloblast) is about 4 μm, comparable to the average *width* (*not diameter*) of an enamel prism. There are approximately as many ameloblasts during development as there are enamel prisms in the fully formed tooth. The ameloblasts are hexagonal in cross section. (This provides a highly efficient packing system, comparable to the structure of a honeycomb.) Most enamel prisms are keyhole-shaped in cross section. When the outlines of cross-sectioned ameloblasts and enamel prisms are superimposed, there is an *uneven overlap* (Fig. 11–6).

The specific shape of an enamel prism and the peculiar relationship between prisms and ameloblasts are the result of the particular shape of the *Tomes' process* of a *human ameloblast*. The Tomes' process is shovel-shaped, concave on one surface, with a wide, hexagonal base and a thin, horseshoe-shaped, knife-edge tip (Fig. 11–7).

During enamel formation, two groups of matrix proteins: *amelogenins and enamelins*, are released from the *concave* surface of

---

Fig. 11–5. *A*, Idealized cross sections through enamel prisms, showing the keyhole-shaped outlines of the individual prisms. The prisms are stacked together in an intricate, interlocking pattern. *B*, Three-dimensional diagram of an enamel prism. The prism runs from left to right, from the dentino-enamel junction to the outer enamel surface. A section is left out, to indicate that the prism at this magnification would be considerably longer than the page. The rounded head of the enamel prism faces the cuspal/incisal region of the tooth, while the thin tail region faces the cervix of the tooth. Inside the prism, the orientation of the long, thin, needle-like hydroxyapatite crystallites is indicated. In the head region of the prism, the crystallites run parallel to the long axis of the prism. In the tail region, they run perpendicular to the long axis of the prism. *C*, The orientation of the hydroxyapatite crystallites is shown in this diagram of several cross sectioned enamel prisms. In the head regions, the hydroxyapatite crystallites are cut transversely; while in the tail regions, the crystallites are cut along their lengths.

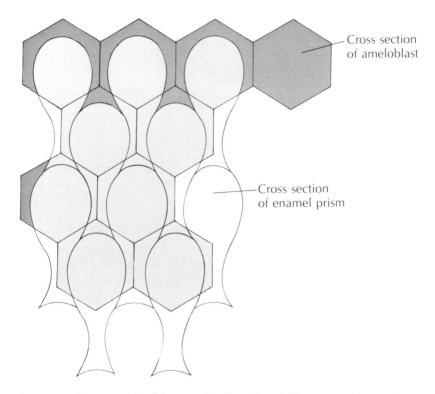

Cross section
of ameloblast

Cross section
of enamel prism

Fig. 11–6. The cross sectional, hexagonal outlines of ameloblasts are superimposed over the cross sectional, keyhole-shaped outlines of the enamel prisms produced by the ameloblasts. Notice the ratio of ameloblasts:prisms = 1:1.

Tomes' process. The amelogenins are randomly dispersed, but the enamelins, highly ordered structural proteins that serve as templates for the hydroxyapatite crystallites, are deposited in an oriented fashion. The crystallites become oriented similarly, with their long axes perpendicular to the cell membrane of the Tomes' process.

There is an abrupt change in the orientation of the crystallites, where there is an abrupt change in the orientation of the cell membrane of the Tomes' process: at its thin, horseshoe-shaped edge. As a result of this abrupt change in the crystallite orientation, an interface without crystallites remains between the two groups of crystallites. This interface is the future prism sheath at the rounded head of the enamel prism (Fig. 11–8).

When the enamel is formed initially, it contains a relatively large amount of matrix and a small amount of mineral. The mineral crystallites are very thin. With further calcification (maturation) of the enamel, some components, specifically amelogenins, are removed. This allows the existing crystallites to increase in thickness and in width, but not in length or in number. Thus, the original widths of

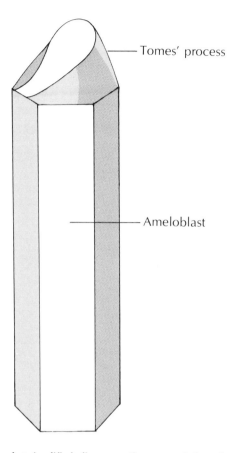

Tomes' process

Ameloblast

Fig. 11–7. Somewhat simplified, diagrammatic representation of an ameloblast in three dimensions. The ameloblast has a tall, columnar cell body, hexagonal in cross section. At its secretory end, a shovel-shaped Tomes' process is present with a thin, horseshoe-shaped, knife-edged tip. The light area of the Tomes' process in this diagram is slightly concave.

the areas without crystallites, the prism sheaths, remain about the same, with only a minimal reduction compared with its original dimensions.

Finally, areas of *prismless enamel* are found frequently near the dentino-enamel junction and near the outer surface of the enamel. Their presence may be explained by the *absence* of distinct Tomes' processes at the times these layers of enamel were deposited. Near the dentino-enamel junction, the ameloblasts may not immediately form a Tomes' process after they have differentiated and have begun depositing enamel matrix. At or near the completion of their secretory activities, the ameloblasts lose their Tomes' processes again. The cell membranes of ameloblasts without Tomes' processes form a smooth surface. All hydroxyapatite crystallites are deposited per-

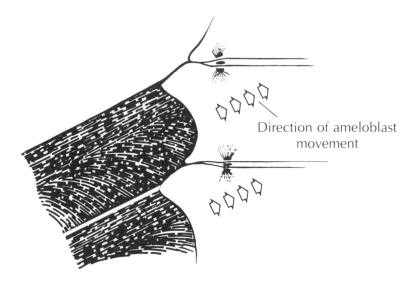

Direction of ameloblast
movement

Fig. 11–8. Illustration of the formation of enamel prisms, during enamel deposition by the ameloblasts. The ameloblasts are located to the right. They move outward, in the direction indicated by the arrows, during their secretory activities. In the newly deposited enamel matrix, the hydroxyapatite crystallites (black) are oriented perpendicularly to the membrane of the Tomes' process. Where the process makes its sharp knife-edge (see Fig. 11–7), the crystallites run at right angles to each other. Between these two groups of crystallites, the prism sheath (white line) is located.

pendicularly to this surface and parallel to each other. No sharp interfaces, and thus no prisms or prism sheaths are formed in this way.

CURVATURES OF ENAMEL PRISMS. In the introduction of this chapter we noted that enamel prisms do not run entirely straight from the dentino-enamel junction to the outer enamel surface.

The prisms are curved predominantly in the *inner third* of the thickness of enamel (nearest the dentino-enamel junction). These curves can be demonstrated clearly on an extracted tooth which has been broken in half *lengthwise.* Near the dentino-enamel junction the fracture surface is not flat, but wavy. Since these waves are visible with the unaided eye, each wave must consist of *groups* of enamel prisms, not single ones.

These waves are produced by groups of enamel prisms curving *above* the level of the fracture plane, *alternating* with groups of prisms that curve *below* the level of the fracture plane. Thus, the first groups make convexities and the second groups make concavities relative to the fracture plane of the tooth. In the transition areas between two groups, other groups of prisms run more or less straight, at the *level* of the fracture plane (Fig. 11–9).

If one were to make a ground section of a tooth, the groups of prisms in the transition areas would be cut along the long axes of these prisms in the section. The other two groups would be cut either obliquely or in cross section. The prisms that curved above the fracture plane would first run out of this section, toward the viewer, and then back into the section, away from the viewer, when the enamel is scanned from the dentino-enamel junction toward the outer surface. The prisms that curved below the fracture plane would first run into the section and later out of the section, under the same conditions (Fig. 11–10).

Such alternatively longitudinally and transversely sectioned groups of enamel prisms are called *Hunter-Schreger bands.* These bands are only visible if a tooth is sectioned along its longitudinal axis, because the waves of the enamel prisms are oriented predominantly in a horizontal plane (Fig. 11–11).

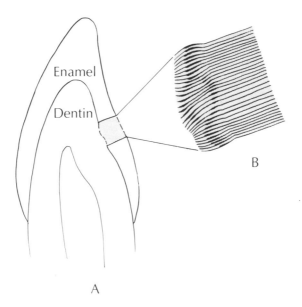

Fig. 11–9.   Diagram of a tooth, broken in half lengthwise. The fracture surface is not smooth, but as shown in insert B, the surface is very wavy near the dentino-enamel junction. Groups of prisms curve upward above the general plane of the fracture surface, or downward, below this plane. In this picture, two groups of upward curving prisms are shown, on either side of a group of downward curving prisms, B. In the transition areas, between upward and downward curving prisms, groups of prisms run more or less within the general plane of the fracture surface. Similarly, in the outer two thirds of the enamel width, all prisms run more or less smoothly within this plane.

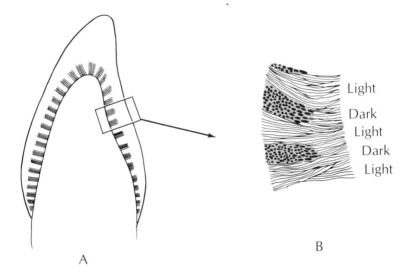

Fig. 11–10. In a smoothly ground section of a tooth, the surface of the section is no longer wavy, as it is in a fractured tooth. Groups of prisms, curving either upward or downward, relative to the fracture plane, are both partially cross sectioned, near the dentino-enamel junction, *B*. Only in the outer enamel and in the transitional regions, between upward and downward curving groups of prisms, the prisms are cut lengthwise. As a result, when a longitudinal ground section is viewed with incident light (not light transmitted through the section), the cross-sectioned enamel prisms reflect less light and appear dark, while the longitudinally sectioned prisms reflect more light and appear light.

OTHER FEATURES OF ENAMEL

We have purposely stressed the *clinical* importance of understanding the differences in composition between enamel prisms and prism sheaths and the course of the enamel prisms. However, since enamel is a complicated tissue, with several additional points of interest, some of these will be discussed briefly.

Enamel, once deposited, is not remodeled. Since enamel-forming cells, or ameloblasts, are lost shortly after the emergence of the tooth in the oral cavity, no additional enamel is formed after this event. Thus, the crown of a tooth does *not* increase further in size, and enamel is incapable of structural repair. Only physico-chemical changes such as decalcification (in caries) and to a lesser degree recalcification (halting and even partially reversing the caries process) are possible. Any imperfections in the enamel, produced during enamel formation, remain present in this tissue throughout the functional life of the tooth.

CROSS-STRIATIONS OF ENAMEL PRISMS. In a ground section of enamel, especially after some decalcification, alternately light and dark cross striations are visible in the enamel prisms. These cross striations are 4 to 8 μm apart and they are comparable with

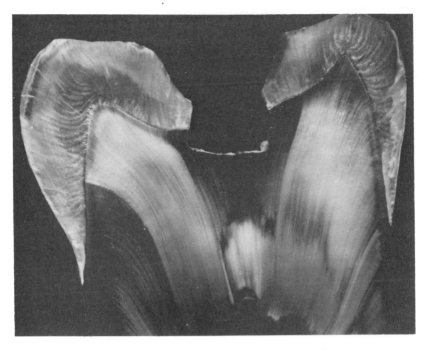

Fig. 11–11.   Hunter-Schreger bands appear as alternately light and dark bands of enamel prisms, running from the dentino-enamel junction to about one half of the width of the enamel cap, in a longitudinal ground section of a human molar, viewed with incident and reflected light. Original magnification × 2.

the imbrication lines (von Ebner) in the dentin, in that they are probably produced as the result of rhythmic variations in enamel deposition during successive 24-hour periods (Fig. 11–12).

The enamel matrix in the light striations may differ somewhat from the matrix in the dark striations: the light striations may be a little better calcified than the dark striations.

INCREMENTAL LINES (RETZIUS). If, during enamel formation, the organism is under some stress (disease, birth), the enamel deposited at that time may show some irregularities in its calcification and a disruption in the course of the enamel prisms, resulting in *incremental lines* (Fig. 11–13).

In ground sections, such incremental lines, which correspond with the contour lines (Owen) in the dentin, usually appear dark as the result of their relatively lesser degree of calcification and a correspondingly larger amount of enamel matrix. Frequently, adjacent to such a dark line, a lighter line of well calcified enamel may be present (perhaps overcompensation during recovery).

The course of the enamel prisms is usually disturbed in an incremental line. The prisms may have a zig-zag orientation, and in some

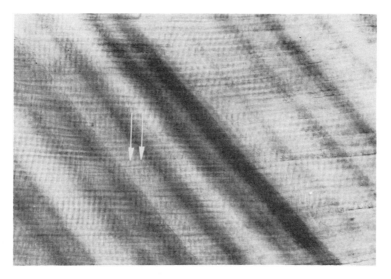

Fig. 11–12. Enamel prisms, running from left to right, with vertical cross striations (*arrows*). The large, dark bands, running obliquely across the photograph, are incremental lines (Retzius). Notice that the cross striations are more distinct in these incremental lines. In a longitudinal section of a tooth, the incremental lines characteristically run at an angle to both the enamel prisms and the cross striations. Original magnification × 125.

cases they may even lose their sharp distinction completely and prismless enamel may locally replace them.

An incremental line marks the position of the ameloblasts at the time of the stress. The width of the line corresponds with the length of time the organism was under stress. For example: if the birth process is difficult and prolonged, a broad and distinct incremental line develops in the enamel formed at the time. This is known as a *neonatal line.*

A neonatal line is found in all teeth where enamel is formed at the time of birth: all teeth of the primary dentition and the first molars of the secondary dentition. Occasionally, the line is not clear, but the differences between enamel formed prenatally and enamel formed postnatally may be striking. Usually the prenatally formed enamel is regular and highly calcified, whereas the postnatally formed enamel is somewhat irregular and less calcified. However, in some teeth this may be reversed. Clearly, it depends on the quality of intrauterine life, compared with the quality of life after birth, which may be variable for different individuals.

Near the cervix of the tooth, large numbers of regularly spaced incremental lines may be found in the enamel. Their regular spacing seems to suggest that something other than disease may be involved in the production of those lines. Because of the pattern of deposition

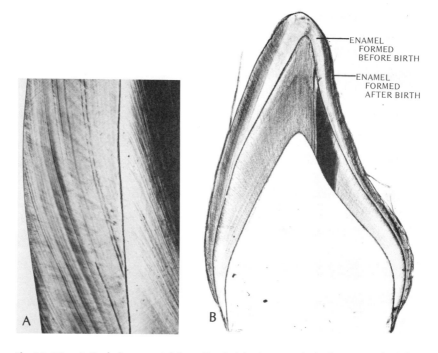

ENAMEL
FORMED
BEFORE BIRTH

ENAMEL
FORMED
AFTER BIRTH

A

B

Fig. 11–13. *A,* Dark, incremental lines (Retzius) in the enamel of a human tooth. If the tooth is cut lengthwise, as is the case in this ground section, the incremental lines run from the dentino-enamel junction obliquely outward, in the direction of the incisal edge or cusps (located at the top of the picture). In a cross section through a tooth, the incremental lines run parallel with the dentino-enamel junction and with the outer enamel surface. Original magnification × 12.5. *B,* Ground section of the anatomical crown of a primary incisor tooth. The enamel formed before birth is light and better calcified than the enamel formed after birth. Several incremental lines are present in the darker postnatal enamel. Notice also the fainter corrésponding contour lines (Owen) in the dentin. Original magnification × 2.

of enamel, the lines in the cervical area run obliquely from the dentino-enamel junction to the outside surface of the enamel.

External manifestations of these lines are visible as grooves running horizontally, parallel to each other, all around the enamel surface in newly erupted teeth. Between adjacent grooves the enamel is slightly ridged, which results in a series of transversely oriented wrinkles or delicate waves on the crown surface. These grooves and ridges are known as *perikymata*. Except in protected areas, the perikymata are rapidly worn down during the function of the teeth.

In contrast with the situation in dentin, the antibiotic *tetracycline* does *not* form distinct incremental lines in enamel, owing to the differences in the nature of enamel and dentin matrices and the differences in the way these matrices calcify. In high doses tetracycline may temporarily disturb the ameloblasts, and this may lead to defects in the enamel being formed at that time. Such defects may take up some of the tetracycline.

DENTINO-ENAMEL JUNCTION AND ENAMEL SPINDLES. The dentino-enamel junction is frequently *scalloped* rather than smooth. The rounded, convex sides of such a scalloped surface are always facing the dentin, while the concavities are facing the enamel. It is not clear precisely what causes this scalloping. It must happen during tooth development, in the brief period between the breakdown of the smooth basal lamina between odontoblasts and preameloblasts, and the first deposition of dentin and enamel. Once the first layers of dentin and enamel are laid down, these two hard tissues preserve the existing morphology of the dentino-enamel junction (Fig. 11–14).

The scalloping of the dentino-enamel junction takes place at a time when a great deal of motion is taking place in this region. You will remember that, following the breakdown of the basal lamina, cell processes of both odontobasts and preameloblasts extend across the former border making contact with each other.

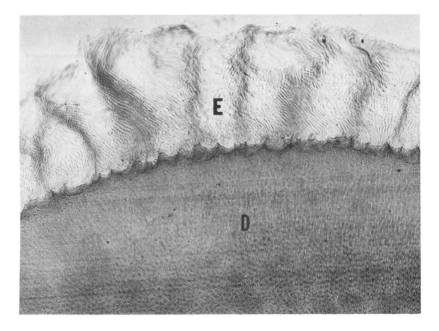

Fig. 11–14. Scalloped dentino-enamel junction in a decalcified cross section of a developing tooth. The not yet fully calcified enamel matrix (E) is preserved, showing the wavy course of the enamel prisms, in different directions at different vertical levels. The concavities of the dentino-enamel junction face the enamel, while the rounded, convex sides face the dentin (D). Notice the relative proportions of the enamel prism diameters and the sizes of the concavities of the dentino-enamel junction. Original magnification ×125.

The processes themselves are not responsible for the scalloping of the junction. The concavities of this scalloped surface are broad, corresponding to a large number of enamel prisms and thus, at an earlier time, to large numbers of odontoblasts and ameloblasts.

Some of the odontoblastic processes are not withdrawn rapidly enough, following their interactions with the preameloblastic cell processes. The first deposited enamel surrounds such processes, leaving a few small defects in the enamel, in the form of short, blind-ending tubules. Since they are frequently spindle-shaped, these structures are called *spindles.*

They are recognizable as short extensions of some of the dentinal tubules, *crossing* the dentino-enamel junction. Their course is independent of the course of the enamel prisms. The contents of a spindle have not been adequately studied so far. Most probably a spindle contains the tip of an odontoblastic process, or it may be empty, apart from some tissue fluid.

The scalloping of the dentino-enamel junction is most pronounced near the tips of cusps and incisal edges. Similarly, the largest numbers of spindles are found in these regions. Toward the cervix of the tooth the dentino-enamel junction becomes smooth, and the dentino-cementum junction in the root similarly continues in a smooth fashion.

TUFTS AND LAMELLAE. Tufts and lamellae are normal features in enamel, consisting of characteristically shaped defects of calcification.

Tufts are found in the inner third layer of enamel, the same layer in which the course of the enamel prisms is curved. Tufts consist of non-calcified parts of enamel prisms and widened prism sheaths, appearing dark in ground sections. In a horizontal ground section through the crown of a tooth, tufts resemble bundles of grass, which become fragmented further away from the dentino-enamel junction. Each "leaf" in such a bundle is located at a different vertical level within the section. The leaves all originate from one vertical line along the dentino-enamel junction, and since a vertical line in a horizontal projection is represented by a point, all leaves of the tuft seem to originate at that same point in a horizontal section.

The appearance of a bundle of grass leaves, all fanning out in different directions, is caused by the fact that enamel prisms at different vertical levels *curve* in different directions (see the section on Hunter-Schreger bands in this chapter). The uncalcified parts of the prisms follow the same course as the surrounding calcified prisms at their particular vertical level (Fig. 11–15).

When you are viewing a tuft with the microscope, notice that you are able to focus on only one vertical level of the ground section at any time. Thus, only the "leaf of grass" of the tuft, which is located

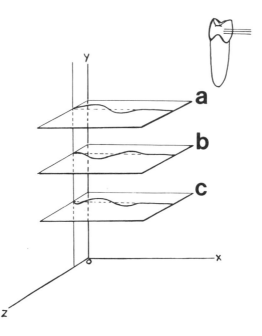

Fig. 11–15. Diagram showing the different courses of enamel prisms and tuft components at three vertical levels (a, b, c) in the enamel. The locations of these are indicated by the three lines in the diagram in the upper right hand corner. Plane YOZ in the diagram represents the plane of the dentino-enamel junction.

at that particular level, will be clearly in focus. The other leaves of the tuft are less clear and out of focus (Fig. 11–16).

Focusing up and down with the microscope will enable you to bring different levels of the tuft in focus consecutively, giving you a three-dimensional appreciation of this structure.

It is not clear what causes the formation of tufts. The suggestion has been made that, within certain tension planes, internal stress in the developing tissue prevents parts of prisms from calcifying. What produces this internal stress has not been resolved. Perhaps the ameloblasts themselves, moving backward in different directions, at dif-

Fig. 11–16. Tufts in a horizontal ground section of a human tooth. The dark tufts run from the dentino-enamel junction to approximately one third of the enamel width. *A, B,* and *C,* show different planes of focus (which means different vertical levels) of the same section. Different "leaves" of each tuft are in focus in the different photographs, illustrating the different courses of enamel prisms in these different vertical levels. Original magnification × 50.

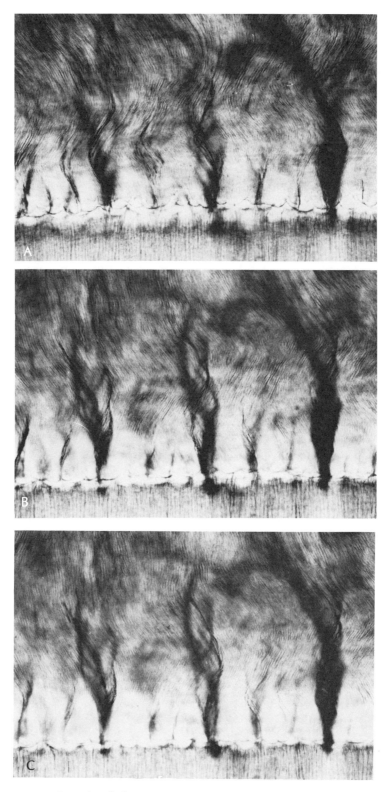

Fig. 11–16. Legend on facing page.

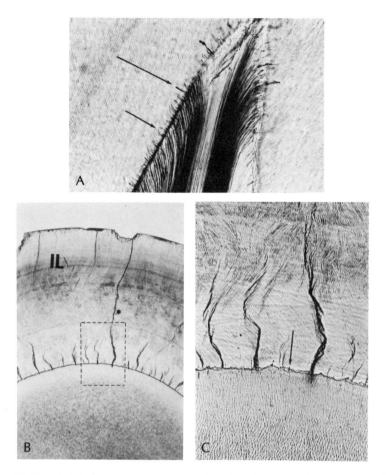

Fig. 11–17. *A,* Spindles (*arrows*) in a ground section of the cuspal region of a molar tooth. In such regions, spindles are particularly abundant. Notice the different shapes in the spindles. All are blind-ending continuations of dentinal tubules across the dentino-enamel junction. Some, however, are just simple extensions, while others have enlarged, club-shaped ends. Original magnification × 50. *B* and enlarged boxed area, *C,* A lamella (*asterisk*), several tufts, and a spindle in a horizontal ground section through a human tooth. Compare the different dimensions and shapes of these three structures. The lamella extends all the way across the enamel width. The tufts do not extend beyond one third of the enamel width. The spindle is visible only in C (*arrow*). Two dark incremental lines (Retzius) are visible (IL), running parallel to the dentino-enamel junction and to the enamel surface. Original magnification *B,* × 12.5; boxed area *C,* × 50.

ferent times and at different vertical levels (remember the different curvatures of the enamel prisms), produce these tension planes.

Lamellae also originate at the dentino-enamel junction, but these structures run across the entire width of the enamel. Lamellae are uncalcified vertical sheets of organic material. They may have the same height as the anatomical crown, but more frequently they are about half as high, running from the cervix of the tooth occlusally (Fig. 11–17).

Lamellae may form in at least three different ways, producing noncalcified organic sheets of different compositions.

1. LAMELLAE CONSISTING OF UNCALCIFIED ENAMEL MATRIX. These lamellae are similar to tufts in appearance and in the way they form. However, while tufts are limited to the inner third of the enamel, lamellae run through the entire enamel width. This type of lamella develops while enamel is being deposited by the ameloblasts. They probably represent a tension plane in which entire prisms, as well as large parts of prisms failed to calcify.

2. LAMELLAE CONSISTING OF CELLULAR DEBRIS OF THE ENAMEL ORGAN. During tooth development, and prior to the emergence of the tooth into the oral cavity, the developing, or just completed, enamel may fracture. What causes such fractures is not clear. The fracture becomes filled with cells of the enamel organ and other organic matter. The result is an organic sheet, or lamella, interrupting the continuity of the calcified enamel.

The preceding two types of lamellae were lamellae formed *during tooth development.* The third type of lamellae is produced *after the eruption* of the tooth.

3. LAMELLAE CONSISTING OF ORGANIC DEBRIS FROM THE ORAL CAVITY. Following the eruption of the tooth, its enamel cap may suffer fractures. These fractures become filled with salivary proteins and cellular debris from the oral cavity, which form the organic substance of this type of lamellae. These lamellae may become more frequent with age, because of the possibility of fractures that may occur as the result of uneven loading of the teeth during function.

SELECTED READING LIST

Boyde, A.: The structure of developing mammalian dental enamel. In *Tooth Enamel.* Edited by M.V. Stack and R.W. Fearnhead. Bristol, John Wright and Sons, 1965.

Crabb, H.S.M., and Darling, A.I.: *The Pattern of Progressive Mineralization of Human Dental Enamel.* New York, Pergamon Press, 1962.

Dean, M.C.: Growth layers and incremental markings in hard tissues; a review of the literature and some preliminary observations about enamel structure in *Paranthropus boisei.* J. Human Evol., *16*:157, 1987.

Fearnhead, R.W., and Stack, M.V. (eds.): *Tooth Enamel II.* Bristol, John Wright and Sons, 1971.

Fearnhead, R.W., and Suga, S. (eds.): *Tooth Enamel IV.* Amsterdam, Elsevier Science Publ., 1984.

Frank, R.M., and Nalbandian, J.: Ultrastructure of amelogenesis. In *Structural and Chemical Organization of Teeth. Vol. I.* Edited by A.E.W. Miles. New York, Academic Press, 1967.

Garant, P.R., and Nalbandian, J.: Observations on the ultrastructure of ameloblasts with special reference to the Golgi complex and related components. J. Ultrastruct. Res., *23*:427, 1968.

Gustafson, A.-G.: A morphologic investigation of certain variations in the structure and mineralisation of human dental enamel. Odont. Tidsskr., *67*:361, 1959.

Gustafson, G., and Gustafson, A.-G.: Microanatomy and histochemistry of enamel. In *Structural and Chemical Organization of Teeth. Vol. II.* Edited by A.E.W. Miles. New York, Academic Press, 1967.

Gwinnett, A.J.: The ultrastructure of the "prismless" enamel of the deciduous teeth. Arch. Oral Biol., *11*:1109, 1966.

Gwinnett, A.J.: The ultrastructure of the "prismless" enamel of permanent human teeth. Arch. Oral Biol., *12*:381, 1967.

Gwinnett, A.J.: Histologic changes in human enamel following treatment with acidic adhesive conditioning agents. Arch. Oral Biol., *16*:731, 1971.

Gwinnett, A.J.: Structural changes in enamel and dentin of fractured anterior teeth after acid conditioning in vitro. JADA, *86*:117, 1973.

Helmcke, J.-G.: Ultrastructure of enamel. In *Structural and Chemical Organization of Teeth. Vol. II.* Edited by A.E.W. Miles. New York, Academic Press, 1967.

Hodson, J.J.: An investigation into the microscopic structure of the common forms of enamel lamellae with special reference to their origin and contents. Oral Surg. Oral Med. Oral Pathol., *6*:305, 1953.

Marshall, G.W., Olson, L.M., and Lee, C.V.: SEM investigation of the variability of enamel surfaces after stimulated clinical acid etching for pit and fissure sealants. J. Dent. Res., *54*:1222, 1975.

Meckel, A.H.: Structure of mature human dental enamel as observed by electron microscopy. Arch. Oral Biol., *10*:775, 1965.

Meckel, A.H., Griebstein, W.J., and Neal, R.J.: Ultrastructure of fully calcified human dental enamel. In *Tooth Enamel.* Edited by M.V. Stack and R.W. Fearnhead. Bristol, John Wright and Sons, 1965.

Osborn, J.W.: The three dimensional morphology of the tufts in human enamel. Acta Anat., *73*:481, 1969.

Osborn, J.W.: Variations in structure and development of enamel. Oral Sci. Rev., *3*:3, 1973.

Risnes, S.: Rationale for consistency in the use of enamel surface terms: perikymata and imbrications. Scand. J. Dent. Res., *92*:1, 1984.

Robinson, C., Weatherall, J.A., and Höhling, H.J.: Formation and mineralization of dental enamel. Trends Biochem. Sci., *8*:284, 1983.

Rönnholm, E.: An electron microscopic study of the amelogenesis in human teeth. I. The fine structure of the ameloblasts. J. Ultrastruct. Res., *6*:229, 1962.

Rönnholm, E.: An electron microscopic study of the amelogenesis in human teeth. II. The development of the enamel crystallites. J. Ultrastruct. Res., *6*:249, 1962.

Rönnholm, E.: The structure of the organic stroma of human enamel during amelogenesis. J. Ultrastruct. Res., *6*:368, 1962.

Sasaki, T., and Higashi, S.: Scanning and transmission electron microscopy of developing enamel surfaces in the kitten tooth germs. J. Electron Microsc., *32*:163, 1983.

Stack, M.V., and Fearnhead, R.W. (eds.): *Tooth Enamel.* Bristol. John Wright and Sons, 1965.

Tyler, J.E.: A scanning electron microscopic study of factors influencing etch patterns of human enamel. Arch. Oral Biol., *21*:765, 1976.

Warshawsky, H., et al.: The development of enamel structure in rat incisors, as compared to the teeth of monkey and man. Anat. Rec., *200*:371, 1981.

Whittaker, D.K.: Structural variations in the surface zone of human tooth enamel observed by scanning electron microscopy. Arch. Oral Biol., *27*:383, 1982.

12

Cementum and Alveolar Bone

Cementum and alveolar bone are two of the three tissues that are responsible for the attachment of the teeth to the bones of the jaws. Cementum covers the dentin of the anatomical roots. The alveolar bone forms the bony sockets (*alveoli*), which are continuous with the jawbone. The third tissue is the periodontal ligament. It is located between cementum and alveolar bone and it will be the topic of Chapter 13.

Cementum, periodontal ligament, and the inner layer of bone of the tooth socket are formed during development by cells of the dental sac. These in turn are derived from neural crest cells.

Clinically, both cementum and alveolar bone are needed for the attachment of a functioning tooth, somewhat like the two towers of a suspension bridge. If one of the two is missing, the bridge cannot exist.

If *cementum* is absent, as is the case when the root of a primary tooth is resorbed during the eruption of its secondary successor, the tooth becomes loose. Fortunately, most of the time the resorption of cementum is a localized process, so that some surfaces of the root remain covered with cementum, enabling the tooth to continue functioning. In addition, periods of repair alternate with active episodes of resorption. During such periods a small amount of cementum fills in some of the resorption cavities providing a new, but usually temporary attachment for the tooth. This lasts until the next wave of resorptions.

If *alveolar bone* is absent, as in cases of severe periodontal disease, the teeth become loose and useless for chewing functions.

Under normal conditions, both cementum and bone are not exposed to the oral cavity, but are covered with other tissues. A small part of the cementum surface may, however, be uncovered, when the gingiva recedes as the result of passive eruption. Since cementum is thin near the cervix, and since this tissue is much softer (it contains less mineral) than enamel, the cementum may soon be worn away (toothbrushing) and dentin may become exposed. The uncovered cementum is also extremely susceptible to caries and exceptionally good oral hygiene should be recommended in such cases.

Both cementum and alveolar bone are *calcified connective tissues.* Each has the three components commonly found in connective tissues (Table 12–1).

In both tissues the fibrous matrix is the dominant component. Both tissues are calcified, which means that hydroxyapatite is present in their fibrous matrix and ground substance. Of the three calcified tissues of the tooth, cementum is most comparable to bone, both in appearance and in composition.

Fibrous Matrix

An interesting feature in cementum and alveolar bone is that these tissues contain *2 groups of collagen fibers* (Figs. 12–1 and 12–2):

1. Collagen fibers of the *cementum or bone* tissue itself. These collagen fibers are produced by either cementoblasts or osteoblasts as the components of the fibrous matrices of these tissues. They run generally parallel to the dentino-cementum junction and to the cementum and bone surfaces, more or less perpendicular to the course of the second group of collagen fibers:

2. Collagen fibers of the *periodontal ligament.* These fibers attach *into* the cementum and alveolar bone. They run into these tissues at an angle that is nearly 90 degrees. These fibers are coarse (somewhat coarser still on the alveolar bone side than on the cementum side), and they do not become completely calcified during the calcification of the surrounding hard tissue. Since the cores of these fibers remain uncalcified, they remain separately visible, inside the calcified bone or cementum. Inserting collagen fibers which remain visible inside a calcified tissue are called *Sharpey's fibers.*

Sharpey's fibers first develop during root formation, when the fibers of the periodontal ligament are synthesized at the same time as the first cementum and alveolar bone are deposited. Gradually,

Table 12–1.   **Components of Cementum and Alveolar Bone**

	Cementum	Alveolar Bone
1. Cells	Cementoblasts Cementocytes (Cementoclasts)	Osteoblasts Osteocytes (Osteoclasts)
2. Fibrous matrix	Collagen fibers (Type I)	Collagen fibers (Type I)
3. Ground substance	Proteoglycans and glycoproteins; similar to the ground sub- stance in bone	Proteoglycans and glycoproteins

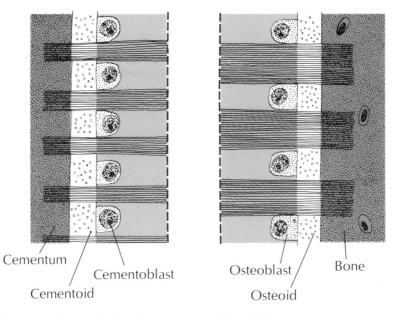

Cementum

Cementoblast

Cementoid

Osteoblast

Osteoid

Bone

Fig. 12–1.   Diagram showing the cementum and alveolar bone on either side of a peri-odontal ligament. Collagen fibers of the periodontal ligament insert into cementum with one end and into bone with the other. More and thinner fiber bundles insert into the cementum than into the alveolar bone. Cementoblasts and osteoblasts line those areas of the cementum and bone surfaces which are located between the inserting fiber bundles. The most recently formed bone and cementum (respectively osteoid and cementoid) layers are noncalcified.

these hard tissues are deposited *around* the ends of the periodontal ligament fibers, embedding them and fixing them in place.

CEMENTUM

Development of Cementum

Cementum can be deposited *only* after the epithelial root sheath has broken down, allowing cells of the dental sac to move to the surface of the root dentin. Upon calcification of the root dentin, the dental sac cells differentiate into *cementoblasts* and start depositing cementum on the *calcified* root dentin surface.

Actually, little cementum is formed until the tooth reaches its functional position in the oral cavity. At that time two thirds of the total length of the root has been formed. The root surface is covered with a layer of cementoblasts, which are producing cementum. Only a thin layer of mostly uncalcified cementum is actually present at that time.

Cementoblasts deposit cementum in a manner similar to the way

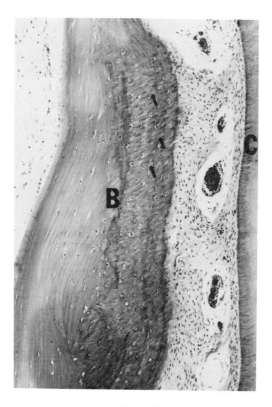

Fig. 12–2. The cores of the thicker collagen fibers, which insert into cementum and alveolar bone, remain uncalcified (*arrows*). As a result, they stain less darkly than the surrounding calcified tissues and remain visible as light "streaks" (Sharpey's fibers) in bone (B) and cementum (C). Original magnification × 40.

in which osteoblasts produce bone. They secrete the proteins, the proteoglycans and glycoproteins of the cementum matrix, while they are moving slowly away from the dentino-cementum junction. Once the layer of uncalcified cementum (or *cementoid*) has reached a certain thickness, the earliest formed matrix begins to calcify. From the dentino-cementum junction outward, we encounter first calcified cementum, next a strip of cementoid, and finally a layer of cementoblasts.

Mature Cementum

The root surface of a fully formed tooth is covered with a cementum layer of uneven thickness and composition.

The cervical half of the root is covered with a thin layer of cementum. At the cervix this cementum may be only 10 μm thick. Although cementoblasts line the surface of the root throughout the functional life of the tooth, little additional deposition of cementum occurs on the cervical half.

In contrast, on the apical half of the root, cementum deposition continues throughout the life of the tooth. Most of this cementum deposition takes place near the apex, where the cementum may reach a thickness of 100 to 150 μm. If the cementum deposition here is excessive, the apical end of the root becomes club-shaped. This is visible in radiographs, especially of teeth that are no longer in functional occlusal contact, because their antagonist (tooth in opposite jaw) has been lost.

These club-shaped root tips do not give the patients any problems unless extraction of the teeth becomes necessary. In such cases the bony sockets may have to be fractured before the tooth can be removed.

The cementum covering the cervical half to two thirds of the root differs from the cementum covering the apical third of the root, in that the former does not contain any embedded *cementocytes* (comparable to osteocytes), while the latter does (Fig. 12–3).

The cervical cementum is therefore called *acellular* (or primary, because it forms first in time). The more apically located cementum is called *cellular* (or secondary, because it forms at a later time than primary cementum). All cellular cementum is formed after the tooth has reached functional occlusion. It is not clear which factor(s) may be responsible for the switch from acellular to cellular cementum production.

During the functional life of a tooth, the width of the *acellular* cementum does *not* increase dramatically. Relatively few cementoblasts continue to line this cementum. They are located *between* the inserting fibers of the periodontal ligament, which are numerous and particularly fine in acellular cementum, leaving only a limited cementum surface available for the cementoblasts. These cells seem to have a role in the maintenance of the existing tissue and only a minor role in new tissue production.

Cellular cementum frequently overlaps acellular cementum on the middle third of the root surface (Fig. 12–4). It contains *cementocytes*, enclosed within cementocytic *lacunae.* These lacunae resemble osteocytic lacunae, with this exception: the cementocytic *canaliculi* have a preferential orientation toward the periodontal ligament (Fig. 12–5). The periodontal ligament is the only source of nutrition for the cementocytes, which receive this nutrition via their canaliculi. This is true for all cementocytes except those near the apical foramen, who receive nutrition from the pulpal blood vessels as well.

The *cementoblasts,* which line the cellular cementum, interspersed between the inserting periodontal ligament fibers, have a secretory role. New cementum is deposited throughout life. As is the

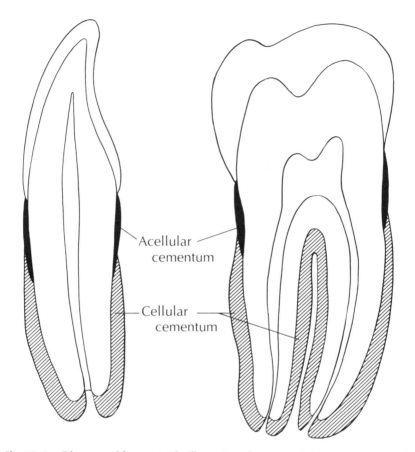

Fig. 12–3. Diagrams of human teeth, illustrating what parts of the roots are covered with acellular cementum (darkly shaded) or cellular cementum (hatched). The middle of the root may be covered with acellular cementum, overlapped by a layer of cellular cementum. Acellular cementum increases very little in thickness with age. Continuous, slow appositional growth takes place on the cellular cementum surfaces.

case with bone deposition, cementum deposition takes place at intervals. When the layer of cementoblasts pauses, a highly calcified layer of cementum is produced. This is an *arrest line*. As in bone, the arrest lines in cementum are smooth (Fig. 12–6).

Reversal lines may be present in cementum, although they are far less abundant than in bone. Cementum undergoes mainly apposition and it does *not* undergo any significant remodeling. However, cementum is not resistant against resorption and an occasional reversal line may be found in nearly all teeth. This means that, at some time during the tooth's presence in the jaw, the conditions were right for cementum resorption, for example, extreme orthodontic movement

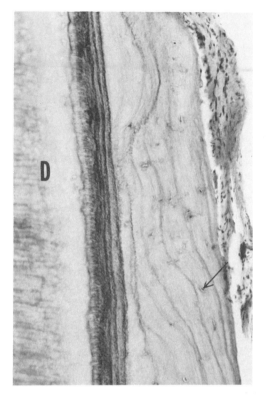

Fig. 12–4.   Histologic section, halfway down the length of a dental root. Darkly staining, acellular cementum covers the root dentin (D) and is, in turn, covered by a thick layer of cellular cementum. The dark lines in both types of cementum are arrest lines, comparable to arrest lines in bone. Several cementocytic lacunae, with enclosed cementocytes, are visible in the cellular cementum (*arrow*). Original magnification × 50.

of teeth, trauma, or dental roots that came too close together (Fig. 12–7).

In such circumstances some resorption (by "cementoclasts," similar in appearance and function to osteoclasts) may occur. When resorption ceases, a highly calcified line forms in the cementum. This line is not smooth, but scalloped, reflecting the final outlines of the resorption cavities. When new cementum is again deposited on this surface, a scalloped reversal line remains, providing us with evidence that resorption did occur.

Since cementum does not undergo any consistent remodeling, this tissue generally becomes thicker with time. This causes some problems for the cementocytes, which are located in the deepest layers of cementum, near the dentino-cementum junction. Most *osteocytes* are no further than 200 μm removed from the nearest blood vessel, and are extensively interconnected, via canaliculi, with each other

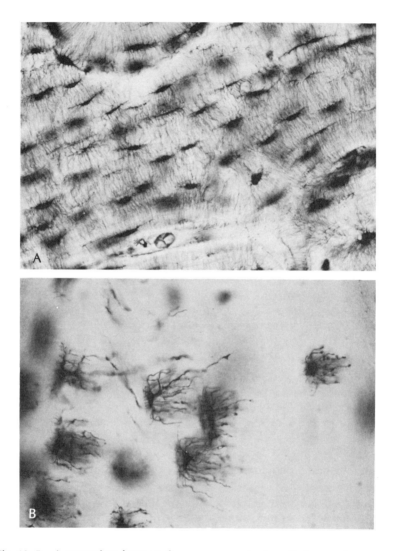

Fig. 12–5. A comparison between the appearance of osteocytic lacunae in a ground section of lamellar bone (with some parallel lamellae and some osteons), shown in A, and cementocytic lacunae in a ground section of cellular cementum, shown in B. The comparison shows that, at the same magnification, the osteocytic lacunae are grouped much closer together than the cementocytic lacunae. The ostecytic lacunae seem to be arranged more orderly. The small canaliculi, which house the osteocytic cell processes, are oriented in all directions. The cementocytic lacunae, which house the cementocytic cell processes, are oriented preferentially toward the periodontal ligament. Original magnification A and B ×125.

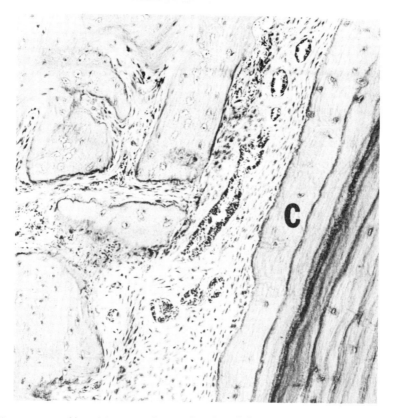

Fig. 12–6.   Darkly staining, smooth arrest lines in cellular cementum (C). This cementum is deposited slowly, throughout life, with long rest intervals. Cementoblasts line the surface of the cementum. Original magnification × 50.

and with the vascular spaces in and around the bone. The *cementocytes*, in contrast, tend to be further away from the nearest blood vessels and from each other, and, although their canaliculi are interconnected, the connections are not as numerous as those between osteocytes. All this causes the deepest cementocytes to be slowly deprived of their nourishments and respiratory gases, and these cells perish. It is, therefore, quite normal to find the lacunae near the dentino-cementum junction empty.

Cementicles

Abnormal, calcified bodies are occasionally found in the periodontal ligament at some distance from the root surface. These structures are called *cementicles.* It is not completely clear why they form. Generally cementicles seem to form first on cellular debris, such as the epithelial root sheath remnants (cell rests of Malassez). In their

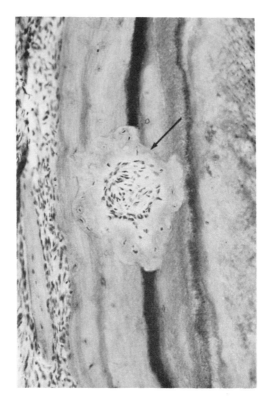

Fig. 12–7.   Scalloped reversal line (*arrow*), interrupting the regular pattern of arrest lines in cellular cementum. The reversal lines represent the final outlines of earlier resorption cavities, which have subsequently been filled (still partially) with repair tissue (cellular cementum). While resorption of cementum is not common in functional teeth, some resorption does occur and most teeth have one or more reversal lines in the cementum. Original magnification × 50.

appearance, cementicles resemble most the regularly growing pulp stones in the dental pulp.

The cementicles may be completely free inside the periodontal ligament. In that case they are called *free* cementicles. Continued cementum deposition on the root surface, as well as on the cementicle's surface, combined with a possible motion of the tooth toward the cementicle, may cause the latter to become *attached* to and eventually *embedded* in the cementum layer on the root.

ALVEOLAR BONE

We have already noted that the alveolar bone, which comprises the sockets in which the roots of the teeth are suspended, is continuous with the bone of the jaws. There is no sharp line of division, and we can only designate bone *arbitrarily* as *alveolar bone* versus *basal bone* of the jaw.

This arbitrary decision is in fact based on clinical experience, especially the cases in which a human being loses all teeth or in which an individual never forms teeth. In the first case we speak of an *edentulous* patient, a candidate for full dentures. In the second case we speak of a totally *anodontic* patient, also a candidate for full dentures.

Following tooth extractions, all alveolar bone gradually is lost in an edentulous patient. This loss is the result of bone resorption, which continues until only the basal bone remains. In the anodontic patient the alveolar bone is never formed.

From these examples it should be clear that alveolar bone depends for its existence entirely on the presence of dental roots (Fig. 12–8). In practice, it also means that full dentures should be checked regularly because they will become looser with the years as more and more alveolar bone (upon which the denture rests) is resorbed.

Gross Appearance of Alveolar Bone

When alveolar bone is inspected with the unaided eye on radiographs (see Chap. 5) or in sectioned bone specimens, the following observations can be made (Fig. 12–9).

1. The cortex of the basal bone of the jaw continues as the *cortical plate* of the alveolar bone. We distinguish an *outer cortical plate*, the cortical plate facing the lips and cheeks, and an *inner cortical plate,* the cortical plate facing the tongue or palate. These cortical plates consist of compact, lamellar bone.

2. The actual bone socket around the root is another layer of relatively compact bone. It is called the *cribriform plate.* This gross anatomical term indicates that there are numerous small openings in this bone plate, allowing blood vessels and nerves in the bone and in the periodontal ligament to communicate freely. The cribriform plate is also sometimes called the *lamina dura.* This is a radiologic term, which indicates that this part of the alveolar bone usually shows up as a light line on radiographs. This, in turn, can lead to the *incorrect* impression that this plate is more calcified than the surrounding bone, making it "harder" (lamina dura literally means hard plate). In fact, the lamina dura is *not* more calcified than the surrounding alveolar bone. The particular radiologic appearance of the lamina dura is caused by the geometry of the bone plate, rather than by its degree of calcification. Finally, a third name for this bone is *alveolar bone proper*, which simply indicates that this bone constitutes the actual bone socket. In these chapters, we will use the term cribriform plate.

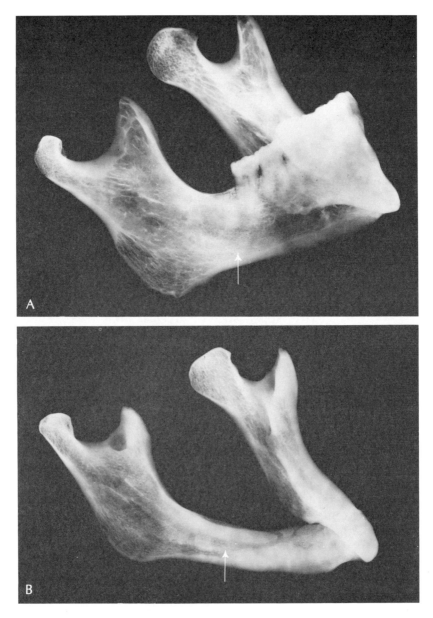

Fig. 12–8.   Contact radiographs of a lower jaw, with most teeth present, *A*, and of a lower jaw without teeth, *B*. The jaws were placed with one surface, indicated with an arrow, flat against the x-ray film. Comparison of the two images reveals how much of the bone is basal bone. In *A*, both basal and alveolar bone are present; while in *B*, no alveolar bone is left. The existence of alveolar bone is related to the presence of teeth.

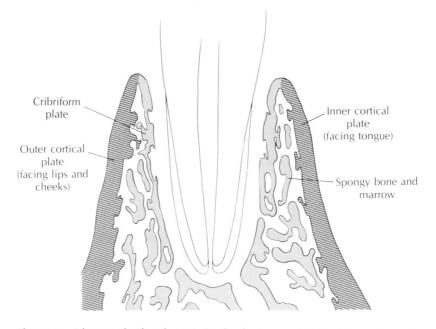

Cribriform plate

Outer cortical plate (facing lips and cheeks)

Inner cortical plate (facing tongue)

Spongy bone and marrow

Fig. 12–9. Diagram of a dental root in its alveolar bone socket. The intervening periodontal ligament is not shown. The alveolar bone may be subdivided into a thin cribriform plate (alveolar bone proper), which forms the inside wall of the socket; thick, compact plates of cortical bone, on the surfaces of the jaw; and intervening spongy bone. The spaces between the bone trabeculae of the spongy bone are filled with marrow. In young individuals, this bone marrow serves as a reservoir for blood cell development (one of many). In older individuals, the marrow consists largely of fat.

3. Between the cortical plates and the cribriform plate *spongy bone* may be present. Spongy bone consists of a sparse number of bone trabeculae running inside bone marrow. In young individuals, this bone marrow is red marrow, involved in blood cell production. With age, it turns into predominantly fatty, yellow marrow.

Of these three gross components, the *essential* one is the *cribriform plate.* The outer cortical plates and the spongy bone may or may not be present. Their role is confined to the support and the streamlining of the cribriform plate (Fig. 12–10, A). If a tooth leans toward lips or cheeks, the spongy bone on that side of the tooth is absent and the outer cortical plate is of minimal thickness and fused to the cribriform plate.

The cribriform plate forms separate sockets (*alveoli*) around the roots of the various teeth. Between the socket of one tooth and the socket(s) of its neighbor, an *interdental septum* is present. This septum consists of the cribriform plates of both teeth, between which some spongy bone may or may not be present (Fig. 12–10, B).

Similarly, the sockets of two roots of a multi-rooted tooth are sep-

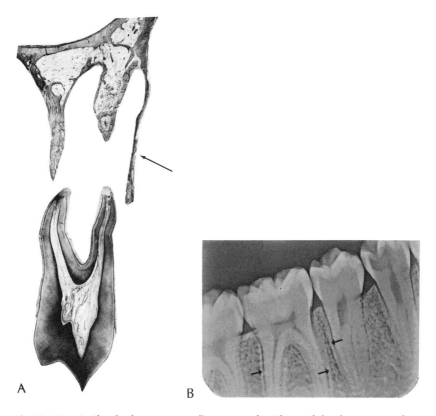

A   B

Fig. 12–10.   *A,* Alveolar bone, surrounding a premolar. The tooth has been removed to show the anatomy of the socket more clearly. Only a thin cribriform plate (alveolar bone proper) surrounds the roots, at the side marked with an arrow (facing the cheeks). On the opposite side of the tooth, all three components of alveolar bone (cribriform plate, spongy bone, and a thick, inner cortical plate) are present. The interradicular septum, between the sockets of the individual roots, is composed of two cribriform plates and an intervening layer of spongy bone. Original magnification × 1. *B,* Xeroradiograph of teeth in their alveolar bone sockets. Between adjacent sockets, an interdental septum is visible. The septum is composed of two cribriform plates (*arrows*) and an intervening layer of spongy bone. An interdental septum is comparable in structure to an interradicular septum.

arated from each other by an *interradicular septum* (radix means root). This septum consists of the cribriform plates of both roots and, possibly, some spongy bone (Fig. 12–10, A).

Development of Alveolar Bone

Alveolar bone is formed almost entirely during the eruption of the teeth. Prior to that stage, in the period when dentin and enamel are deposited, the tooth germs are located in a wide bony groove. This is initially a *common* bony groove for all primary and secondary teeth. Only in late fetal life are small bone septa formed between the different primary teeth (see Fig. 9–22). At that time each primary tooth lies in a separate bony compartment together with its secondary successor. Bony separations between primary teeth and their secondary successors are formed much later, when the primary teeth erupt (see Fig. 9–26).

Also during this eruption, most alveolar bone of a primary tooth is formed by the deposition of new bone at the rim of the bony groove. This bone grows in an *occlusal* direction, along with the erupting tooth, but when the tooth has reached functional occlusion, the rim, or *alveolar crest* of the bone socket remains located slightly more apically than the cervix of the tooth.

The formation of a bony socket around the root of a primary tooth divides the common space in which the primary tooth and its secondary successor were housed before. The secondary successor now comes to lie in a separate *bony crypt,* which has a small occlusal opening, containing the remnants of the successional lamina. One wall of this crypt serves also as part of the bony socket of the primary tooth (see Fig. 9–26, B).

With the eruption of the secondary tooth, this common wall is broken down first, and subsequently the secondary tooth erupts through the bony socket of its predecessor. The socket is remodeled extensively to accommodate the (often larger) dimensions of the secondary tooth (Fig. 12–11).

Mature Bone Socket

The cribriform plate of the bone socket follows rather precisely the outline of the root surface, which it surrounds. A narrow space, with the thickness of a fraction of a millimeter, is left between the bone and the root. This space is occupied by the periodontal ligament.

Alveolar bone is composed of *lamellar bone.* The outer and inner compact plates are *compact, lamellar bone,* with a few osteons. The spongy bone between cribriform plate and cortical plates is *spongy, lamellar bone.* The trabeculae consist of parallel lamellae of bone, without osteons. The trabeculae of the spongy bone are oriented in two principal directions, parallel with and perpendicular to the net direction of the functional loading patterns of this bone.

The cribriform plate itself consists of two layers of bone tissue: (1) compact, lamellar bone, with an occasional osteon, and (2) a layer of so-called *bundle bone,* which faces the periodontal ligament. The second bone layer is of variable thickness, but always thick enough to anchor the fibers of the periodontal ligament, which insert into this bone layer. The inserting fibers remain visible as *Sharpey's fibers*

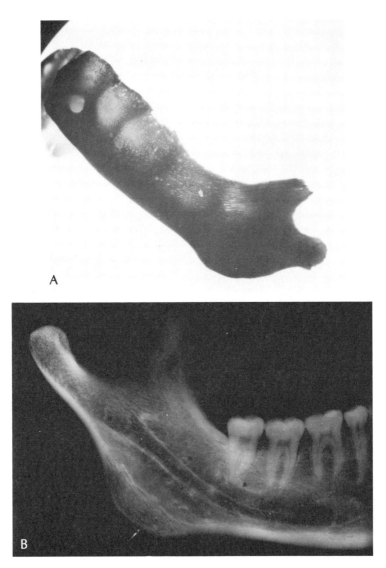

Fig. 12–11. *A*, The lower jaw of a human fetus, stained with a dye and photographed in transmitted light. No alveolar bone is present as yet in this structure, composed largely of spongy, woven bone. The bony compartments around each of the primary teeth (with their secondary successors) are visible as lighter areas. This is because there is less bone in those areas and the transmitted light passes more easily through them. Original magnification ×5. *B*, Contact radiograph (original magnification ×1) of the molar region of an adult jaw. The secondary dentition has erupted completely. A second premolar and three molars are visible. The alveolar bone, which surrounds those teeth, has developed largely by bone apposition, in an occlusal direction, on the rims of the original bony crypts. In addition, substantial growth has enlarged this part of the jaw to allow enough space for the individual teeth.

inside the bone, and they dominate its appearance so much that they are responsible for the name bundle bone (Fig. 12–12).

Remodeling of the Bony Socket

In addition to a small amount of functional, active eruption, the fully erupted teeth may undergo some movements in a horizontal direction. The most common movement is called *mesial drift*. This is a slight movement of all teeth toward the front of the oral cavity. This movement occurs at a slow rate, since it depends mostly on wear at the contact points between adjacent teeth. Nevertheless, this movement is frequently substantial enough to make a difference in the appearance of the walls of the bony sockets.

If a tooth moves in a certain direction, part of the bone (in the path of the movement) has to be removed to make room for the advancing tooth. In that part of the bony socket you may see osteoclasts inside resorption lacunae (Fig. 12–13). The bone to be broken down first is the bundle bone. The breakdown may result in the detachment of the periodontal fibers, which insert in the bone. How-

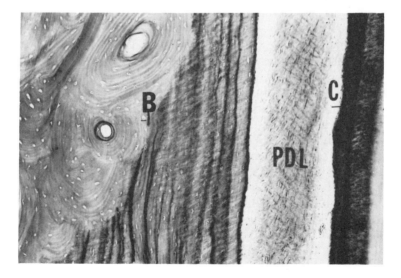

Fig. 12–12.   Histologic section through the cribriform plate (alveolar bone proper), which surrounds a tooth. The periodontal ligament (PDL) and the darkly staining cementum (C) on the root surface are to the right of the photograph. The bone (B) of the cribriform plate is to the left. Its two layers are clearly visible: the lightly staining compact lamellar bone (to the far left) and the darkly staining bundle bone with several (vertical) arrest lines. The bundle bone was named for the large number of Sharpey's fibers (light streaks, running obliquely, nearly horizontally) inside the bone matrix. Original magnification ×40.

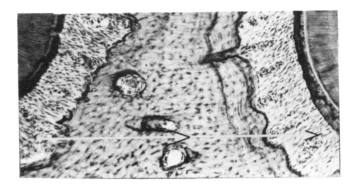

Fig. 12–13. Cross section through the roots of two adjacent primate teeth with an intervening interdental septum, close to the alveolar crest, where the septum is very thin. Consequently, the two cribriform plates are very thin (consisting only of bundle bone), and they are fused together, without an intervening spongy bone layer. The teeth have been moved orthodontically, toward the right hand side (*arrow*). As a result, many resorption cavities are present on the left side of the septum, which is in the path of the moving tooth, while massive new bone deposition (two arrest lines are visible) has taken place on the opposite side of the septum. Original magnification ×40.

ever, since the bone resorption is localized, the tooth usually does not become loose.

Occasionally the resorption may extend into the lamellar bone. When enough resorption has taken place, new bone fills in some of the resorption cavities. The new bone re-anchors the fibers of the periodontal ligament, and this bone becomes the new bundle bone.

The side of the bony socket, from which the tooth moves away, does not undergo bone resorption, but rather bone deposition to fill in the distance over which the tooth has moved. In this way the width of the space between the bony socket and the root is kept about the same.

The new bone is deposited around the fibers of the periodontal ligament, and thus it too is of the bundle bone variety. This increases the width of the bundle bone layer at the deposition side. However, continuous bone *remodeling* rapidly removes some of the deeper layers of the bundle bone (the *older* bundle bone) and replaces it with lamellar bone and osteons.

The same remodeling patterns in the bone socket allow the teeth to be moved *orthodontically*. If done properly, orthodontic treatment is always accompanied by bone remodeling, which enables the alveolar bone to accommodate to the new conditions. Most orthodontic movements are tipping movements, leading to corresponding bone remodeling patterns (Fig. 12–14), because orthodontic forces generally can only be applied to the clinical crown of the tooth. The

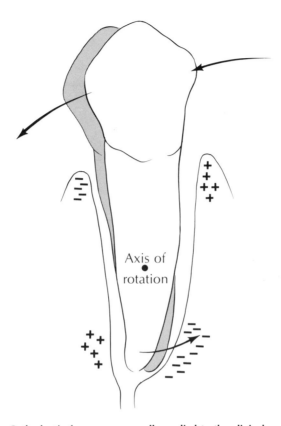

Fig. 12–14. Orthodontic forces are generally applied to the clinical crown of a tooth, resulting in a tipping movement, with the axis of rotation about midway down the length of the dental root. The alveolar bone reacts to this movement by resorption (−) and deposition (+) in the indicated areas.

tooth responds by tipping around an axis of rotation located midway down the length of the root.

In addition to bone remodeling to accommodate tooth movements, normal bone remodeling takes place throughout life. The orientation of the bone trabeculae in the spongy bone reflects the loading patterns of the jaw. These patterns are remarkably constant. However, if the loading conditions are altered, the bone trabeculae must undergo some remodeling to adjust to the new conditions. Finally, throughout the body bone remodeling takes place to adjust constantly to the circulating levels of calcium and phosphate ions, which are the building blocks of hydroxyapatite, but are also necessary ions for many vital functions.

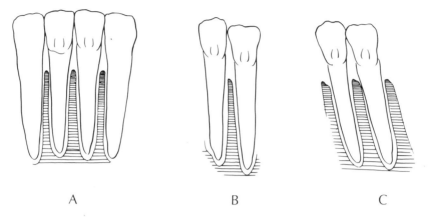

A   B   C

Fig. 12–15.   Under most normal conditions, the tops of the interdental septa, the alveolar crests, are rounded or pointed evenly, A. However, if two adjacent teeth have erupted to unequal vertical positions, B, or if several teeth are slanted, C, the alveolar crests may be slanted as well. A slanted alveolar crest is an important diagnostic sign for the presence of periodontal disease around the tooth at the deep end of the slant. However, when a slanted alveolar crest is noted on a radiograph, the examples shown in this figure should be remembered and checked, to eliminate the possibility of such normal anatomical variations.

Shape of the Alveolar Crest

The radiographic image of the top of the interdental septum is used frequently as an indicator of periodontal health or disease. However, some factors may influence the shape of this structure, even in the absence of a pathologic condition.

On dental radiographs the top of the interdental septum, or alveolar crest, is normally rounded or pointed evenly. This is the case when the cervices of the two adjacent teeth are at the same vertical level. If one tooth is on a considerably lower level and is less erupted, or if both teeth are strongly slanted, the alveolar crest will reflect such positional relationships by being slanted as well. Since slanting is also frequently an indication of periodontal disease, affecting the tooth adjacent to the lowest point of the slanted surface, careful note should be taken of the relationship between the two teeth and of their orientation before you decide whether this is a pathologic condition (Fig. 12–15).

SELECTED READING LIST

Cho, M.-I., and Garant, P.R.: Ultrastructural evidence of directed cell migration during initial cementoblast differentiation in root formation. J. Periodont. Res., *23*:268, 1988.

Furseth, R.: The fine structure of acellular cementum in young human premolars. Scand. J. Dent. Res., *82*:437, 1974.

Giansanti, J.A.: The pattern and width of the collagen bundles in bone and cementum. Oral Surg. Oral Med. Oral Pathol., *30*:508, 1970.

Ismail, A.S., and Weber, D.F.: Light and scanning electron microscopic observations of the canalicular system in human cellular cementum. Anat. Rec., *222*:121, 1988.

Jones, S.J., and Boyde, A.: A study of human root cementum surfaces as prepared for and examined by electron microscope. Z. Zellforsch., *130*:318, 1972.

Marks, S.C., and Cahill, D.R.: Ultrastructure of alveolar bone during tooth eruption in the dog. Am. J. Anat., *177*:427, 1986.

Melcher, A.H., and Bowen, W.H.: *Biology of the Periodontium.* New York, Academic Press, 1969.

Owens, P.D.A.: A light microscopic study of the development of the roots of premolar teeth in dogs. Arch. Oral Biol., *19*:525, 1974.

Ritchey, B., and Orban, B.: Crests of the interdental alveolar septa. Dent. Radiogr. Photogr., *27*:37, 1954.

Scott, J.: The development, structure and function of the alveolar bone. Dent. Pract. Dent. Rec., *19*:19, 1968.

Ten Cate, A.R.: Formation of supporting bone in association with periodontal ligament organization in the mouse. Arch. Oral Biol., *20*:137, 1975.

Updegrave, W.J.: Normal radiographic anatomy. Dent. Radiogr. Photogr., *31*:57, 1957.

13

Periodontal Ligament

Caries and periodontal disease are the two diseases most frequently encountered in dental practice. With the introduction of fluorides and sealants, caries is preventable to a large degree, if not totally. Teeth that are protected against caries now may fall victim to periodontal disease in the future. An understanding of the anatomy and physiology of the periodontal ligament and the dentogingival junction is particularly important in dental practice. We will discuss the periodontal ligament in this chapter and the dentogingival junction in Chapter 14.

The periodontal ligament is a sheet of tendon-like tissue that ties the tooth to the alveolar bone, to the neighboring teeth and to the gingiva. We mentioned in Chapter 12 that the three tissues responsible for attaching the teeth to the jaw bone (cementum, alveolar bone, and the periodontal ligament) may be compared with a suspension bridge. If bone and cementum function as the "towers," the periodontal ligament functions as the complex of cables of the bridge. Neither the towers nor the cables may be removed if the bridge is to remain intact.

If either cementum or alveolar bone are lost, the attachment of the tooth fails. Similarly, if the fibers of the periodontal ligament are broken down, for instance by bacterially produced enzymes in periodontal disease, the tooth is lost. A healthy periodontal ligament is yet another key to the survival of the tooth.

The periodontal ligament is approximately 0.20 mm wide. This width allows it to serve as a compliant interface between 2 rigid calcified tissues (bone and cementum), somewhat like a padding, which reduces the stress on the alveolar bone during function.

There is some variation in the width of the periodontal ligament depending largely on the amount of *use* a tooth gets. The greater the use of a tooth, the wider the ligament. Most movements of a functionally loaded tooth are *tipping* movements (see Fig. 12–14). The ligament is wider, where the root moves most (near the cervix and near the apex) and narrower where the root moves least (near the axis of rotation in the middle of the root).

280

When a tooth is subjected to less motion, for example because of wear of its cusps, or because of the loss of its antagonist, the width of the ligament is reduced. Thus, the periodontal ligaments in older people are frequently narrower than those of younger people for this reason.

TISSUE COMPONENTS OF THE PERIODONTAL LIGAMENT

The periodontal ligament is a product of the cells of the dental sac. These cells, in turn, are derived from neural crest cells. It is a specialized *connective tissue* resembling both in function and in certain aspects of its histologic appearance, a tendon. The periodontal ligament consists of three components commonly found in connective tissues: (1) *cells* (fibroblasts and other cell types, normally found in connective tissue proper and necessary for the maintenance and protection of this tissue), (2) *fibrous matrix* (collagen fibers, mostly Type I, with a smaller amount of Type III collagen; delicate oxytalan fibers), and (3) *ground substance* (proteoglycans and glycoproteins similar to those found in connective tissue proper).

The dominant feature of the periodontal ligament is a series of thick collagen fiber bundles, running between the root cementum and the alveolar bone. These are called *principal fiber bundles.* They are surrounded by a network of loose connective tissue, containing blood vessels and nerves. In histologic sections the principal fiber bundles and the areas of loose connective tissue (*interstitial areas*) alternate with each other (Fig. 13–1).

Cells

The cells responsible for the production of the fibrous matrix and ground substance of the periodontal ligament are the *fibroblasts.* These are active cells, continuously engaged in secretory activities. The periodontal ligament has a fast turnover rate, probably even faster than that of the lamina propria of the oral mucosa.

New fibrous matrix and ground substance are produced at about the same rate at which the old fibrous matrix and ground substance are broken down. The cells responsible for this breakdown and subsequent digestion of the waste materials appear to be the same fibroblasts that are responsible for their production. Thus, the fibroblasts in the periodontal ligament are actively engaged in both secretory and digestive activities. Many fibroblasts have been observed with phagocytic vacuoles, containing fragments of collagen fibers.

Fibroblasts are found both within the principal fiber bundles and in the interstitial areas. Those located in the fiber bundles have the

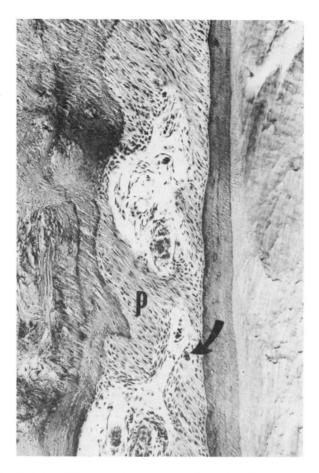

Fig. 13–1. Periodontal ligament of a primate tooth, sectioned lengthwise. The dense, highly organized, collagenous, principal fiber bundles (P) resemble tendon tissue. They alternate with interstitial areas consisting of loose connective tissue. These areas contain the blood vessels and nerves of the periodontal ligament. The arrow points at a small clump of epithelial cells. This is a remnant of the epithelial root sheath. Original magnification ×40.

same, typical "squeezed" appearance as fibroblasts in tendons (Fig. 13–2). In cross sections such fibroblasts are star-shaped, with their cell bodies, containing little more than a nucleus and a few organelles, squeezed in a cornered space between three or more collagen fibers; and their cytoplasmic extensions squeezed in the narrower spaces between two adjacent fibers.

In the interstitial areas, a more diverse group of cells is found. The interstitial areas contain blood vessels and nerves (pp. 287–290), as well as fibroblasts and occasionally other cells, which are commonly found in connective tissue proper (see Chap. 4).

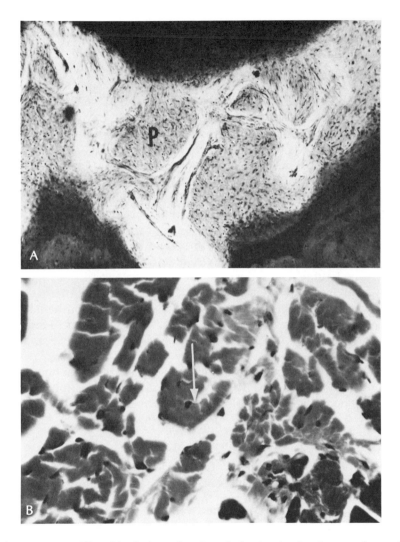

Fig. 13–2. *A,* Oblique histologic section through the tip of a dental root and several principal fiber bundles (P) of the periodontal ligament (periapical fibers). In this near-cross section, the principal fiber bundles are demonstrably rounded bundles, while the (lighter) interstitial areas form a network surrounding the bundles. Nuclei of fibroblasts are visible as dark dots in both fiber bundles and interstitial areas. Original magnification ×40. *B,* A higher magnification of a cross section through collagen fibers in mature tendon tissue. The collagen fibers, seen in cross section (grey), have shrunk, leaving many artificial open spaces between them. The dark dots, squeezed between the fibers, are nuclei of fibroblasts. Some thin cell processes extend between adjacent collagen fibers (*arrow*). Original magnification ×160.

Cementoblasts, occasional cementoclasts, osteoblasts, and osteo-clasts are physically located inside the periodontal ligament, al-though they belong, strictly speaking, to the cementum and alveolar bone. The cementoblasts and osteoblasts line all of the cementum and bone surfaces that are left between the fibers of the periodontal ligament, which insert in these hard tissues.

Osteoclasts require the proximity of the blood vessels in the in-terstitial areas, and the bone next to these areas is, more often than not, the first to be resorbed.

Finally, in the periodontal ligaments of newly erupted teeth, small clusters and cords of epithelial cells may be found parallel to, but some distance from, the root surface. These are the *epithelial rem-nants* (Malassez) of the root sheath. Three-dimensionally, these cell groups form an irregular network, that surrounds the root and is continuous at several points with the gingival attachment epithelium (see Chap. 14).

The epithelial cells in those remnants are alive, but minimally active, although there is some evidence that they may be involved in prostaglandin production. Under appropriate conditions they can be stimulated to divide and proliferate. The epithelial remnants are surrounded by a basal lamina, which separates the epithelial cells from the surrounding connective tissues. No clearly defined function has been attributed to these cell groups and cell death slowly reduces their numbers.

The presence of epithelial remnants has been held responsible for some pathologic conditions such as cementicle formation and cyst development, but adequate proof for this is not available.

Fibrous Matrix

The dominant components of the periodontal ligament are its col-lagen fibers. These fibers all insert into the cementum covering the anatomical root and run from there into the lamina propria of the gingiva, the periosteum of the outer cortical plate of the alveolar bone, the cementum of a neighboring tooth, or most importantly, into the cribriform plate of the alveolar bone.

The fibers inserting into the alveolar bone are somewhat coarser than the ones inserting into the cementum. The 2 groups of fibers meet midway, across the width of the periodontal ligament, where they are interconnected with each other.

The collagen fiber bundles may be classified into two distinct groups (Figs. 13–3, 13–4):

FIBER BUNDLES THAT DO *NOT* INSERT IN ALVEOLAR BONE:

1. *Gingival Fibers.* These fibers run from the most cervical ce-

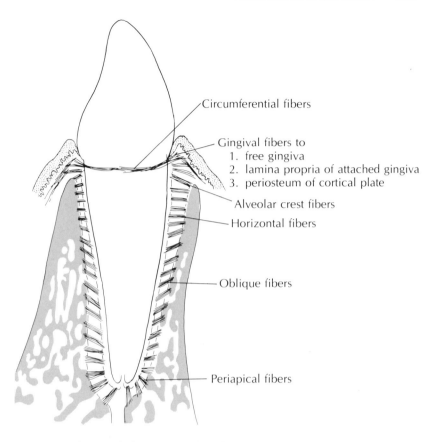

Circumferential fibers

Gingival fibers to
1. free gingiva
2. lamina propria of attached gingiva
3. periosteum of cortical plate

Alveolar crest fibers

Horizontal fibers

Oblique fibers

Periapical fibers

Fig. 13–3. Diagram of a human tooth (lingual side to the left, side facing lips and cheeks to the right). The various principal fiber groups are indicated. Circumferential fibers are shown in three dimensions. They insert in the most cervical cementum, run partially around the dental root, and insert either in the gingival lamina propria or in the bone of the alveolar crest. All other fiber groups are shown in only two dimensions (as if they are sectioned). About two thirds of the length of the root is suspended by oblique fibers.

mentum into the gingiva (lamina propria). Some may actually run *over* the alveolar crest into the lamina propria of the attached gingiva and into the periosteum of the cortical plates.

2. *Circumferential Fibers.* These fibers originate in the most cervical cementum and run horizontally around and parallel to part of the root. Most fibers then insert into the lamina propria of the gingiva; a few may insert into the alveolar crest.

3. *Transseptal Fibers.* These fibers run from the cementum of one tooth, over the top of the interdental septum, into the cementum of the next tooth.

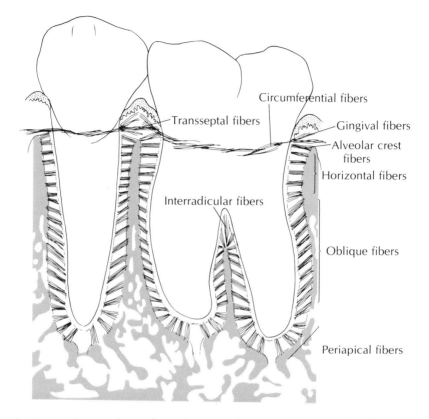

Fig. 13–4. Diagram of two adjacent human teeth, separated by an interdental septum. Compared with Figure 13–3, two additional fiber groups are visible in this view. Transseptal fibers run from one tooth to the next over the interdental septum. Interradicular fibers run from the tip of the interradicular septum in a radiating pattern into the furcation areas between the roots.

FIBER BUNDLES THAT INSERT IN THE ALVEOLAR BONE:

1. *Alveolar Crest Fibers.* These fibers run from the cementum of the tooth, in an apically slanted direction, to the alveolar crest.

2. *Horizontal Fibers.* These fibers run, in a horizontal direction, from the cementum covering the cervical third of the root toward the alveolar bone.

3. *Oblique Fibers.* These fibers run from the cementum covering the apical two thirds of the root, in an occlusally slanted direction toward the alveolar bone.

4. *Periapical Fibers.* These fibers run, in a radiating fashion, from the cementum of the apex toward the alveolar bone.

5. *Interradicular Fibers* (in *multirooted* teeth *only*). These fibers

run from the cementum in the furcation area (the concave area where the bases of the roots meet), converging toward the top of the inter-radicular septum of the alveolar bone.

It is clear from the foregoing list that the periodontal fibers, which insert into the cementum all along the root of the tooth, tie the tooth to *all* surrounding structures.

The most important mechanical role of the principal fiber bundles is to transform the compressive loading on the tooth during chewing into evenly distributed tension on the alveolar bone. Since bone is particularly resistant to *tensile* loading (see Chap. 5), this is an effective mechanical arrangement.

The orientations of the fiber bundles are varied, giving the tooth optimal resistance to all types of loading. For example, the oblique fibers resist occlusal loading; the circumferential fibers resist rotational movements of the tooth; the alveolar crest fibers and the periapical fibers resist the pull of the tooth from the socket.

The transseptal fibers connect all teeth and are responsible for the maintenance of the uninterrupted dental arch. Once a single tooth has been lost, the integrity of the dental arch is disturbed, and the remaining segments behave as independent units.

A delicate network of *oxytalan* fibers is also present within the periodontal ligament. Some of these fibers run parallel to the root surface; others insert into the cementum. While the function of these fibers is not clear, they appear to serve as a supporting network for the blood vessels in the periodontal ligament.

Blood Vessels

A tooth, its periodontal ligament, and its alveolar bone have a common blood supply. Each tooth and its periodontium are supplied by one common artery, which runs as a branch from the main arterial supply in the jaw toward the apical foramen of the tooth (Fig. 13–5). Before it enters this foramen, the artery gives off a group of small branches to the alveolar bone, and a second group of branches that supply the periodontal ligament all around the tooth. The remaining artery branches once more into a few arterioles, which finally enter the pulp through the apical foramen (Fig. 13–6).

The blood vessels supplying the pulp tissue have no further connection with the other blood vessels outside the tooth. This means that if the arteriolar supply to the dental pulp is blocked, the pulp no longer receives any vascular supply and perishes.

The arterioles supplying the alveolar bone, on the other hand, have many connections with each other, and if one blood vessel is blocked or cut, others take over its functions. The arterioles supplying the periodontal ligament are also richly interconnected with each other.

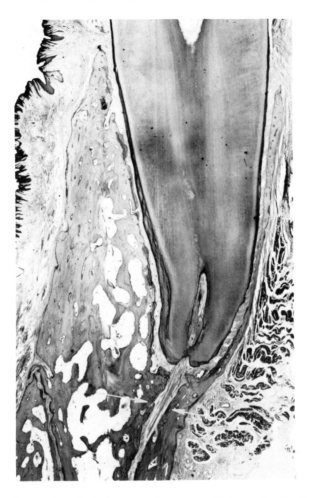

Fig. 13–5. Section through the bony canal (*arrows*), which contains the blood vessels and nerves supplying a single tooth and its surrounding tissues. Original magnification ×10.

All these vessels run inside the netlike structure of the interstitial areas. The blood vessels lie closer to the surface of the alveolar bone than to the cementum surface.

The vascular networks of periodontal ligament and alveolar bone form numerous connections with each other. The connecting blood vessels cross the cribriform plate via the many small openings that give the cribriform plate its name.

Venous drainage pathways roughly parallel the arterial supply pathways. A particularly extensive venous network is present in the periodontal ligament surrounding the apex of the tooth.

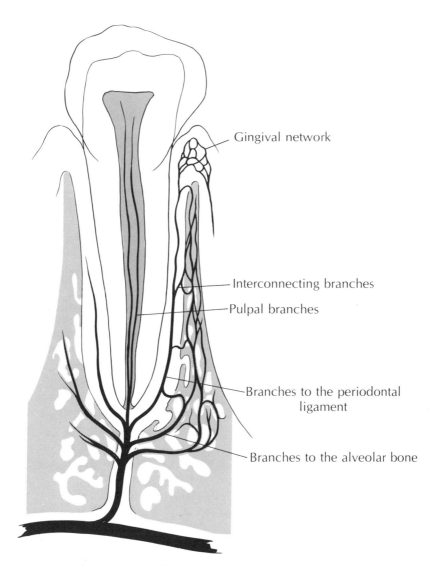

Gingival network

Interconnecting branches

Pulpal branches

Branches to the periodontal ligament

Branches to the alveolar bone

Fig. 13–6.   Diagram showing schematically the pattern of the vascular (arterial) supply to a human tooth and surrounding tissues. A single artery branches off the main arterial supply of the jaw (*bottom*). From this artery, several branches supply the alveolar bone all around the socket. In addition, several branches supply the periodontal ligament all around the root. Finally, the remaining artery subdivides into a few pulpal branches, which enter the tooth through the apical foramen. Notice the numerous interconnecting branches between blood vessels of the periodontal ligament and the alveolar bone. A particularly extensive vascular network is present in the gingiva. It is formed by interconnecting branches of the gingival blood vessels, periodontal blood vessels and alveolar bone blood vessels.

Nerves

The periodontal ligament contains two types of nerves: (1) autonomic, sympathetic nerve fibers, which run parallel with the blood vessels and regulate the blood flow in the microvascular beds; and (2) afferent, sensory nerves, which are mostly myelinated branches of the second and third divisions of the fifth cranial nerve (trigeminal nerve). The periodontal ligament is extremely richly supplied with these afferent fibers. Two types of nerve endings are found: (1) *free*, uncovered nerve endings, and (2) *encapsulated* nerve endings.

The free nerve endings appear to be responsible for pain sensation, while the encapsulated endings register pressure changes. The encapsulated endings are far less complicated structures than the ones found in the skin and in the oral mucosa. However, their large numbers are responsible for the delicate perceptive abilities of the periodontal ligament.

You may test the fine perceptive ability of the ligament by placing a thin piece of paper between the occlusal surfaces of your teeth. Notice how aware you are of its presence. This should be remembered when a restoration is finished. If the "bite" is too high, the patient is certainly sensitive to this. Follow the indications of the patients when correcting the problem. The patient's perception may be more precise than your own observations, in this case.

DEVELOPMENT OF THE PERIODONTAL LIGAMENT

During the early stages of tooth development, the enamel organ is surrounded by the neural crest-derived dental sac.

As a result of the expansive growth of the enamel organ, the surrounding dental sac tissue becomes stretched. This produces a preferential orientation of the cells and collagen fibers in the dental sac along the lines of tension, *parallel to the outer surface* of the *enamel organ.* This situation persists until the root begins to develop and the tooth is erupting.

At that time, the dental sac cells closest to the root surface, as well as those closest to the bone surface, differentiate into fibroblasts. They arrange themselves in rows oriented at nearly right angles to the surfaces of the root and the bone, and start producing collagen fibers, which are deposited between the fibroblast rows, in a direction parallel to these rows. The fibers become anchored in cementum and bone by the appositional growth of those two tissues.

The formation of these two groups of fibers: root-related and bone-related, marks the earliest stage in the development of the periodontal fiber bundles.

As the two fiber groups grow toward each other, they meet ap-

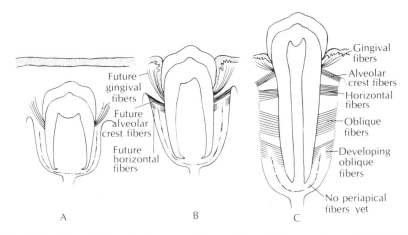

Fig. 13–7.   Stages in the development of the periodontal ligament of a tooth: *A,* Early, during active, prefunctional eruption. *B,* During emergence of the tooth into the oral cavity. *C,* Upon reaching functional occlusion. A single, interrupted line, parallel to the surface of the root, and running around the developing apex, reflects the orientation of the dental sac fibers. Those are gradually replaced, in a direction from cervix to apex, by the principal fiber bundles, which are characteristic for a functioning tooth.

proximately midway between tooth and bone. Here, connections are established between them in an *intermediate plexus.* As soon as the connections have been made, the fiber bundles are completed and the tooth is attached to the bone. The earliest fiber bundles to be formed are the gingival fibers. Development of the other fiber bundles proceeds gradually in an apical direction (Fig. 13–7).

Initially, almost all fiber bundles have an oblique orientation, similar to the orientation of the later formed oblique fiber group. They run from the developing root in an occlusal direction, toward the bone (Fig. 13–7). With further eruption of the tooth, this orientation is changed by the altered position of the tooth, relative to the bone. This change is most striking for the alveolar crest fibers, which become slanted in an opposite direction, and less striking for the horizontal fibers, which change only from an oblique to a horizontal direction. The oblique fiber group is established toward the end of the eruptive period, and these fibers keep their oblique orientation. The periapical fibers, of course, are the last to be formed.

SELECTED READING LIST

Freeman, E., and Ten Cate, A.R.: Development of the periodontium: An electron microscopic study. J. Periodontol., *42:*387, 1971.

Fullmer, H.M.: Connective tissue components of the periodontium. In *Structural and Chemical Organization of Teeth. Vol. II.* Edited by A.E.W. Miles. New York, Academic Press, 1967.

Grant, D., and Bernick, S.: Formation of the periodontal ligament. J. Periodontol., *43*:17, 1972.

Hindle, M.O.: The intermediate plexus of the periodontal membrane. In *The Mechanisms of Tooth Support.* Edited by D.J. Anderson. Bristol, John Wright and Sons, 1967.

Levy, B.M., Dreizen, S., and Bernick, S.: *The Marmoset Periodontium in Health and Disease.* Basel, S. Karger, 1972.

Listgarten, M.A.: Intracellular collagen fibrils in the periodontal ligament of the mouse, rat, hamster, guinea pig and rabbit. J. Periodont. Res., *8*:335, 1973.

Melcher, A.H., and Bowen, W.H.: *Biology of the Periodontium.* New York, Academic Press, 1969.

Severson, J.A., Moffett, B.C., Kokich, V., and Selipsky, H.: A histologic study of age changes in the adult human periodontal joint (ligament). J. Periodontol., *49*:189, 1978.

Sims, M.R.: Oxytalan-vascular relationships observed in histologic examination of the periodontal ligaments of man and mouse. Arch. Oral Biol., *20*:713, 1975.

Sims, M.R.: Oxytalan meshwork associations observed histologically in the periodontium of the mouse mandible. Arch. Oral Biol., *22*:605, 1977.

Spouge, J.D.: A new look at the rests of Malassez. A review of their embryologic origin, anatomy, and possible role in periodontal health and disease. J. Periodontol., *51*:437, 1980.

Ten Cate, A.R., and Deporter, D.A.: The role of the fibroblast in collagen turnover in the functioning periodontal ligament of the mouse. Arch. Oral Biol., *91*:339, 1974.

Tonna, E.A.: Histological age changes associated with mouse parodontal tissues. J. Gerontol., *28*:1, 1973.

Weekes, W.T., and Sims, M.R.: The vasculature of the rat molar periodontal ligament. J. Periodont. Res., *21*:186, 1986.

14

Dentogingival Junction

The dentogingival junction is the junction between the gingival epithelium and the tooth surface. The particular nature of this junction makes it a rather vulnerable structure which is fairly easily disturbed. Once the dentogingival junction *is* disturbed, for instance by the presence of dental plaque or calculus, the underlying connective tissue and the periodontium (bone, cementum and periodontal ligament) are readily invaded by microorganisms, and periodontal disease may result. If not checked, this disease may ultimately lead to the demise of the tooth. The microorganisms and their products destroy the periodontal ligament's fibers and cause resorption of the alveolar bone.

A healthy dentogingival junction is therefore the key to a healthy periodontium, which in turn is an important factor in the life expectancy of a tooth.

In this chapter the *development* of the component parts of the dentogingival junction: the gingiva and the cervical area of the tooth, will be described, as will the *mature morphology* of this junction.

DEVELOPMENT OF THE JUNCTIONAL EPITHELIUM OF THE GINGIVA

1. PERIOD PRIOR TO THE TOOTH'S EMERGENCE INTO THE ORAL CAVITY. Following the completion of enamel formation, the remnant of the enamel organ, the reduced enamel epithelium, continues to cover the anatomical crown of the tooth. The ameloblasts are still lying next to the incompletely calcified outermost layer of the enamel. A basal lamina separates these ameloblasts from the enamel.

2. PERIOD OF TOOTH EMERGENCE. During tooth eruption, the reduced enamel epithelium consists of a thin, nonkeratinized, stratified squamous epithelium. The inner layer of this epithelium, the former ameloblast layer, is separated from the enamel surface by a basal lamina. This basal lamina is continuous at the tooth cervix

with the basal lamina, which separates the outer epithelial cells of this same epithelium from the surrounding connective tissue.

The epithelial cells of the reduced enamel epithelium probably assist in the eruption process by producing enzymes that break down the connective tissue between them and the oral epithelium. As the tooth approaches the oral epithelium, the outer basal lamina of the reduced enamel epithelium fuses with the basal lamina of the oral epithelium, an event that is followed by a fusion of the epithelia themselves. The epithelial cells, which are located in the center of this fused mass, disintegrate, and this establishes an opening through which the crown emerges into the oral cavity (Fig. 14–1, A, B).

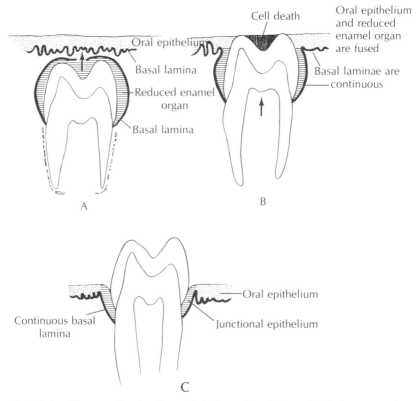

Fig. 14–1. Diagrams showing the epithelial covering of the anatomical crown surface prior to the tooth's emergence in the oral cavity, *A*; during the tooth's emergence into the oral cavity, *B*; and following the tooth's emergence into the oral cavity, *C*. Prior to emergence, the reduced enamel organ (shaded with horizontal lines) approaches the oral epithelium (stippled) and is subsequently fused with it. Cell death occurs in the center of the fused epithelium, *B*. This results in the development of an opening through which the tooth emerges. The first junctional epithelium of the dentogingival junction is the most cervical part of the reduced enamel organ, *C*.

3. PERIOD FOLLOWING THE TOOTH'S EMERGENCE INTO THE ORAL CAVITY. As the tooth erupts further, more and more enamel is uncovered. However, when functional occlusion is reached, a small strip of reduced enamel epithelium, *including the former ameloblasts,* still covers the most cervical enamel (Fig. 14–1, C).

This epithelium, which is fused with the oral epithelium, constitutes the first *junctional epithelium* of the dentogingival junction. Secondarily, some time after the tooth has reached functional occlusion, epithelial proliferation in the basal layer of the fused epithelium results in the replacement of all the older cells of the reduced enamel epithelium, *including* the ameloblasts, which formed the first attachment to the tooth surface. The newly proliferated cells now establish the *definitive junctional epithelium.* A basal lamina separates the new junctional epithelial cells from the tooth surface.

DEVELOPMENT OF THE CERVIX OF THE TOOTH

The cervix of the tooth marks the borderline between anatomical crown and anatomical root. Theoretically, this border should be a fine line, where enamel and cementum meet in an edge-to-edge relationship. In practice, the *cemento-enamel junction* is frequently less than perfect.

In many instances, a strip of cementum overlaps the most cervical enamel. In other cases, the enamel and cementum do not meet, leaving a strip of dentin uncovered along the tooth cervix (Fig. 14–2). There is a great deal of variation in the cemento-enamel relationship. Generally, the pattern of overlap is found in the greatest number of teeth. Incisors and canines have a greater incidence of uncovered cervical dentin than do molar teeth. Different relationships may even be present along the cervix of a single tooth.

The various types of cemento-enamel relationships can only be understood when the development of this region is reviewed (see Chap. 9). There are several distinct differences in the development of anatomical crown and root:

1. The anatomical crown is shaped by a *complex* epithelial enamel organ, consisting of four distinct layers. The anatomical root is shaped by the epithelial root sheath, consisting *only* of a continuation of outer and inner enamel epithelium.

2. Following the induction of the odontoblasts, the inner enamel epithelial cells in the enamel organ *themselves* differentiate into enamel-producing cells, the ameloblasts. The cells of the epithelial root sheath do not appear to have any further function after the shaping of the root and the induction of the root odontoblasts.

3. Following all of its activities, the remnant of the enamel organ, the reduced enamel epithelium, must continue to *cover* the enamel

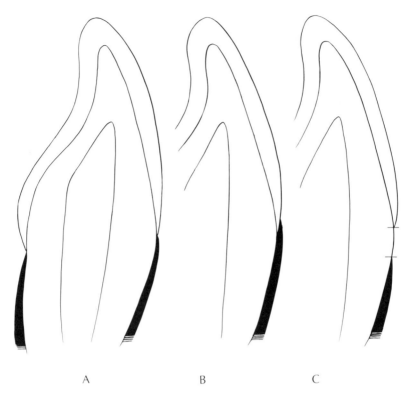

Fig. 14–2. Diagram showing three possible relationships between enamel (blank) and cementum (black) at the cervix of the tooth. *A,* Edge-to-edge relationship. *B,* Cementum overlaps a narrow strip of enamel. *C,* Cementum and enamel do not meet, leaving a narrow strip of exposed dentin.

surface until the anatomical crown emerges (partially) into the oral cavity. If the reduced enamel epithelium falls apart *before* eruption is completed, the enamel surface, exposed to the surrounding connective tissues, is soon covered by a layer of cementum, produced by newly differentiated cementoblasts. Occasionally, when a tooth fails to erupt, this is precisely what happens. The cementum-covered crown of such an *impacted* tooth becomes eventually attached to the surrounding bony crypt walls. In *contrast,* the epithelial root sheath *must* fall apart in order for the cementoblasts to differentiate and move to the root surface, to begin producing cementum.

The last-mentioned point is critical to the development of the cemento-enamel junction. If the anatomical crown retains its epithelial cover while the anatomical root loses its epithelial cover, a perfect edge-to-edge relationship between enamel and cementum is established.

However, in many cases, the most cervical part of the reduced enamel epithelium breaks down along with the epithelial root sheath. In such cases, cementoblasts cover the exposed strip of cervical enamel with cementum, creating an overlap of cementum over enamel.

Rather less frequently, the most cervical part of the root sheath continues to exist intact, together with the reduced enamel epithelium. In such cases cementoblasts are not able to move in, underneath this epithelium, and no cementum is deposited. This leaves a narrow strip of uncovered dentin at the cervix.

Following eruption, the *first* junctional epithelium of the dentogingival junction consists of whatever part of reduced enamel epithelium still covers the tooth surface. In both the edge-to-edge cemento-enamel junction and the overlap junction the first junctional epithelium is in contact with the most cervical, noncementum-covered *enamel* only.

When a strip of the epithelial root sheath continues to exist, it becomes part of the first junctional epithelium. In such cases the first junctional epithelium is in contact with *both* the most cervical enamel and the strip of uncovered dentin.

MORPHOLOGY OF THE DENTOGINGIVAL JUNCTION

The fully developed dentogingival junction is an extension of the gingiva, which folds over the crest of the free gingiva and then faces the surface of the tooth. We will call *all* gingival epithelium, which faces the tooth, *dentogingival epithelium.* It consists of nonkeratinized, stratified squamous epithelium. It is subdivided into *sulcular epithelium*, which is located more occlusally, at the level of the free gingiva, and *junctional epithelium,* which is located more cervically and closely adheres to the tooth surface.

The sulcular epithelium stands away from the tooth surface, leaving a shallow groove (sulcus), all around the tooth, between epithelium and tooth surface. The floor of this 0.5 mm deep sulcus is at about the same level as the free gingival groove on the outside (keratinized) surface of the gingiva. Thus, the gingival wall of the sulcus is formed by free gingiva.

When the depth of the sulcus is probed clinically, the probe frequently is pushed down, far beyond the floor of the anatomical sulcus, through the entire junctional epithelium. In doing this, we create our own clinical sulcus by tearing the epithelium itself. This is possible because the attachments between different epithelial cells are disrupted more easily than the attachments between epithelial cells and the tooth surface (Fig. 14–3).

The *junctional epithelium* forms hemidesmosomal contacts with the basal lamina, which it has deposited on the enamel surface. The physical nature of this attachment is therefore similar to the nature

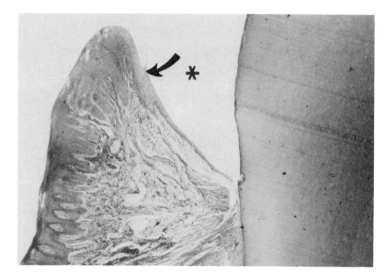

Fig. 14–3. The dentogingival junction in a decalcified histologic section of a human tooth. No enamel is visible; it was formerly located in the space marked with an asterisk, but was lost during decalcification. The epithelium of the gingiva, which faces the space, is dentogingival epithelium. The floor of the gingival sulcus is indicated (*arrow*). The epithelium above it is sulcular epithelium, while the epithelium below it is junctional epithelium. The interface between junctional epithelium and underlying connective tissue is smooth. Several gingival fiber bundles are visible in this section. Some run into the free gingiva, others run into the lamina propria of the attached gingiva. Original magnification × 12.5.

of the attachment between an epithelium and the underlying connective tissue (Fig. 14–4).

Since the junctional epithelium faces the tooth surface on one side and connective tissue on the other side, it is sandwiched between two basal laminae, which are continuous with each other, around the most cervical edge of the junctional epithelium.

Cell renewal takes place in the basal cells of the epithelium, where it faces the connective tissue, and the most cervical cells as well. The newly proliferated cells move slowly in an occlusal direction, toward the oral cavity, where the older cells are sloughed off.

Mechanically the dentogingival attachment is strong. The basal lamina adheres to the tooth surface and the junctional epithelial cells adhere to the basal lamina. This adhesion is enhanced by capillary action, which keeps these structures together, rather like two glass plates with a thin film of liquid between them.

The junctional epithelial cells are relatively undifferentiated cells. They are engaged in cell divisions and in making attachments to each other and to the basal laminae. However, they do not provide

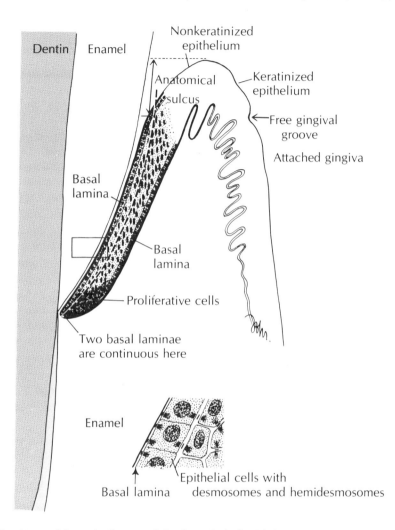

Fig. 14–4. Schematic diagram of the dentogingival epithelium. The nature of the attachment between junctional epithelium and tooth surface is shown in more detail in the insert. A basal lamina adheres to the tooth surface, while the junctional epithelial cells, in turn, form hemidesmosomal attachments on the basal lamina. The free gingival groove and the floor of the anatomical sulcus are at the same vertical level. Careless clinical probing may lead to the establishment of a "clinical sulcus" (which will, under normal conditions, heal rapidly) along the broken line indicated in this diagram.

a good protective barrier to protect the underlying tissues, as would be the case in well differentiated stratified squamous epithelia.

With age, the junctional epithelium may recede apically and migrate onto the root surface, exposing more of the crown of the tooth. This is the process of *passive eruption*. The dentogingival junction is formed initially by the junctional epithelium and the enamel surface. With age it becomes a junction between this epithelium and both enamel *and* cementum surfaces. Ultimately, the junction may become located *entirely* on the cementum surface.

Gingival recession may be sped up by an inflammation of the gingiva. Inflammation is generally brought about by microorganisms in the dental plaque, whose toxins easily pass through the "leaky" junctional epithelium to the connective tissues. Clinically, an inflamed gingiva becomes swollen and red. Histologically, *large numbers* of inflammatory cells are present in the gingival connective tissue. (Even in healthy gingivae *some* lymphocytes are usually present underneath the junctional epithelium.)

The inflammation process leads to the breakdown of the dentogingival attachment and a real deepening of the gingival sulcus. Apical downward proliferation of the cervical-most epithelial cells follows, and the entire attachment is displaced apically. Once substantial apical proliferation has taken place, treatment frequently must include periodontal surgery, removing much of the free gingiva to reduce the depth of the gingival sulcus.

INVESTMENTS OF THE TOOTH SURFACE

The dentogingival attachment is frequently complicated by the presence of a thin *cuticle,* located between the surface of the tooth and the basal lamina, associated with the junctional epithelial cells. The dental cuticle is composed of proteins. It is first formed during late eruption, probably by the reduced ameloblasts.

If a newly erupted tooth is placed in 10% solution of hydrochloric acid, a delicate membrane floats off the surface in approximately $2\frac{1}{2}$ hours. This membrane is called *Nasmyth's membrane,* and it consists of a thin dental cuticle with some cells of the reduced enamel organ adhering to it.

With age, the dental cuticle slowly increases in thickness. With a light microscope, it is best seen in a section through the dentogingival junction of an older person, in which it may exceed a thickness of 1.0 μm (Fig. 14–5).

BLOOD VESSELS

The *gingiva* around the neck of a tooth receives an especially rich vascular supply. The gingival vascular network is formed by interconnecting blood vessels from three different sources: the periodontal ligament, the alveolar bone, and the periosteum of the cortical plates (see Fig. 13–6). The periosteum, in turn, is supplied by branches of the blood vessels of the bone and of the muscles, that attach to the bone surface.

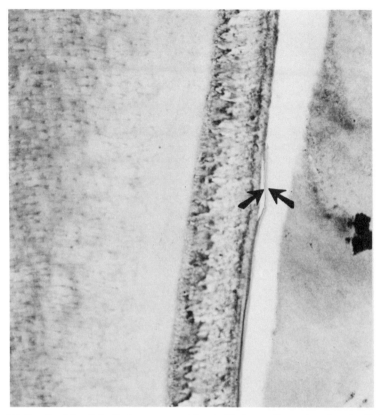

Fig. 14–5.   Dental cuticle (*between arrows*) located between the root surface (acellular cementum) to the left and plaque to the right. Original magnification ×50.

Venous drainage pathways roughly parallel the arterial supply pathways. An extensive venous network is present in the gingiva around the neck of the tooth.

This extensive blood vessel supply should be remembered when you deal clinically with this critically important region of the gingiva and the dentogingival junction.

SELECTED READING LIST

Armitage, G.C., and Christie, T.M.: Structural changes in exposed human cementum. I. Light microscopic observations. J. Periodont. Res., *8*:343, 1973.

Armitage, G.C., and Christie, T.M.: Structural changes in exposed human cementum. II. Electron microscopic observations. J. Periodont. Res., *8*:356, 1973.

Brady, J.M., and Woody, R.D.: Scanning microscopy of cervical erosion. JADA, *94*:726, 1977.

Kobayashi, K., Rose, G.C., and Mahan, C.J.: Ultrastructure of the dentoepithelial junction. J. Periodont. Res., *11*:313, 1976.

Listgarten, M.A.: Structure of surface coatings on teeth: a review. J. Periodontol., *47*:139, 1976.

Löe, H.: The structure and physiology of the dentogingival junction. In *Structural and Chemical Organization of Teeth. Vol. II.* Edited by A.E.W. Miles. New York, Academic Press, 1967.

Newman, H.N.: The pre-eruptive portion of the human enamel integument. J. Dent., *3*:110, 1975.

Nyvad, B., Fejerskov, O., and Josephsen, K.: Organic structures of developmental origin in human surface enamel. Scand. J. Dent. Res., *96*:288, 1988.

Schroeder, H.E., and Listgarten, M.A.: *Fine Structure of the Developing Epithelial Attachment of Human Teeth.* Basel, S. Karger, 1971.

Schroeder, H.E., and Scherle, W.F.: Cemento-enamel junction—revisited. J. Periodont. Res., *23*:53, 1988.

Stern, I.B.: Current concepts of the dentogingival junction: the epithelial and connective tissue attachments to the tooth. J. Periodontol., *52*:465, 1981.

Taylor, A.C., and Campbell, M.M.: Reattachment of gingival epithelium to the tooth. J. Periodontol., *43*:281, 1972.

Weekes, W.T., and Sims, M.R.: The vasculature of the rat molar gingival crevice. J. Periodont. Res., *21*:177, 1986.

Appendix I

Use of the Microscope

One of the most important aspects of studying histology is the art of making careful observations with the microscope. Here are a few guidelines for the use of the light microscope (Fig. A–1).

1. Make sure that the lenses in the *eyepiece, objectives* and *condenser* are clean at all times. To prevent scratching of these valuable lenses, use special lens paper for cleaning.

2. Place a glass slide on the microscopic *stage* and clamp it into place.

3. Turn on the *light source* at the base of the microscope.

4. Select the objective lens with the lowest power of magnification. Looking through the eyepiece, inspect the slide. Turn first the *coarse adjustment,* then the *fine adjustment,* until the image is clear (focused).

5. Now, turn the lever of the *iris diaphragm,* until almost all the light is *blocked.*

6. With the diaphragm in this closed position, turn the *condenser adjustment* until you see (through the eyepiece) a sharp edge between the diaphragm's shadow and the central light area. This means that the light beam passing through your slide is also *focused* properly.

7. Remove your eyepiece and look directly down into the *body tube* of the microscope. Now, slowly *open the diaphragm,* just until you see, at the base of the tube, a clear light field, from which the edge of the diaphragm's shadow has disappeared. Do *not* open the diaphragm any further, or you will lose some of the light, that should be passing through the specimen on the stage.

8. *Replace the eyepiece* and hold a sheet of white paper over it. The light, which comes through the body tube and out of the eyepiece, will make a sharp light dot on the paper, when you hold it about ⅓ to ½ inch away from the eyepiece.

This *should be the position* of your eye during the use of the microscope.

The microscope is now optimally adjusted for study.

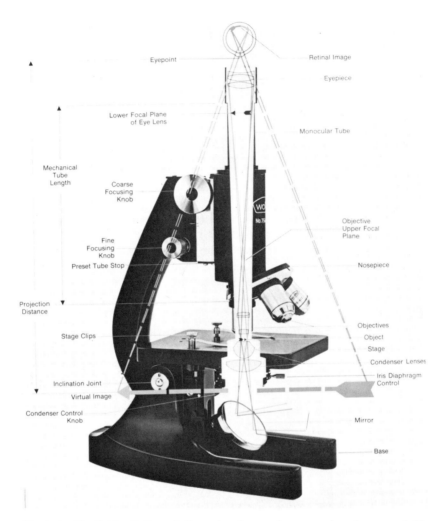

Fig. A–1. The light path through the various lenses of a monocular microscope (with only one eyepiece) is shown. The light beam may come directly from a light source at the base of the microscope or it may be reflected by a mirror, as is shown here. The various parts of the microscope are clearly indicated on this photograph/diagram. From the base upward: condenser lenses, with condenser adjustment (control knob) and the lever (control) of the iris diaphragm; the stage with the object (illustrated here by an arrow). The object usually is mounted on a glass slide, which in turn is clamped firmly to the stage by stage clips. There are several objectives (lenses), for different magnifications, mounted in a revolving nosepiece. The entire tube of the microscope may be moved up and down by coarse adjustment and fine adjustment (focusing knobs). The approximately correct position of the eye, relative to the lenses in the eyepiece, is demonstrated. (The Wolfe microscope, path of the light, kindly supplied by Carolina Biological Supply Company, Burlington, North Carolina.)

Appendix II

Histologic Technique

The light microscope, in its simplest form, was first developed around 1600 A.D. The instrument has undergone many refinements since.

The Englishman Robert Hooke and the Dutchman Anthony van Leeuwenhoek were among the earliest microscopists, who with great curiosity looked at a variety of microscopic structures and described them meticulously. This took place in the seventeenth century. Their ingenuity and accuracy of description made the scientific world at that time familiar with structures such as the eyes of a fly, chips of plants, wood and cork, sand and the various microorganisms that could be found in drops of fresh water. Van Leeuwenhoek also made some original microscopic observations on the components of dental plaque and small segments of elephants' teeth.

It soon became clear that any object studied with the microscope had to be thin, so as to allow the light to pass through it. To illustrate this point, try to make a thin section of a plant leaf. When you study such a handcut section by light microscopy, you will find that only in the thin areas of the section is any structure visible.

Also remember your experiment (Chap. 3), in which you studied whole cells from your own oral mucosa. Few details could be seen in those cells. If you could have cut the cells in half, stained them and made them transparent, you would have seen many more details. It has been found that ideally, for light microscopic purposes, we need sections that are thinner than the diameters of individual cells.

In the nineteenth century, a great many improvements were made in the optics of the light microscope and, simultaneously, improvements were made in the preparation of the specimens. Machines (microtomes) were developed to cut rather thin sections, and the microscopists began to use a number of stains (originally dyes from cloth dying industries) to highlight and identify various components of cells and tissues. The discipline of *histology* was now established as an independent branch of the morphologic sciences.

ROUTINE HISTOLOGIC PROCEDURES

On the following pages, you will find a simple description of the basic steps in specimen preparation, as used at present for simple light microscopy.

Fixation

A tissue to be studied microscopically may be taken from a living individual (*biopsy*) or from an individual who has recently died (*necropsy*). Soon after death, the process of tissue breakdown begins (as the result of lysosomal enzyme release). It is therefore important to take a necropsy specimen at the earliest possible time, so that the tissues still resemble the living state.

Every histologic specimen needs *fixation*. Fixation is a process in which the structures of tissues and cells are preserved, as much as possible, in the position they occupy during life. While there are several modes of fixation, depending on subsequent treatments of the tissue or the preference of the histologist, the standard fixative for most routine histologic work is a 10% formaldehyde solution. Fixation time varies from 24 hours to several days, depending on the size of the specimen. Other frequently used fixation methods include the use of 70 to 90% alcohol and, for temporary fixation, the freezer.

Embedding

In order to make sections thin enough, the specimen, which is rather soft, has to be hardened, usually by embedding it in *paraffin*. The process of embedding is done in such a way that all the water inside and outside the various tissue components is *replaced* with paraffin. Since water and paraffin do not mix, this cannot be done by placing the specimen in melted paraffin immediately after fixation. Intermediate steps are required.

After fixation the specimen is "run through" an *alcohol series*, a series of alcohol solutions of increasing strengths: 50%, 70%, 96%, and 100%. The total length of time that a specimen spends in the alcohol series varies from ½ day to 2 days. Alcohol replaces water in the tissues, and by the time the tissues are in the 100% alcohol, no water remains in them. In the next steps, the alcohol is gradually replaced with xylene, which in turn is replaced with warm, melted paraffin.

When all xylene is replaced with paraffin, the paraffin is cooled and allowed to harden in a block around the specimen. This paraffin block is mounted in a holder and placed in a microtome.

Sectioning

The hardness of paraffin is well suited to make sections 5 to 10 μm thick. During the sectioning process the sections may become slightly folded and they are stretched in a warm water bath, following which sections are "glued" to glass slides. If nothing else is done to these sections, it will be very hard to see any detail under the microscope, owing to the presence of the paraffin, the opacity and the absence of color of the tissue.

Therefore, the paraffin must be removed and the tissue rendered transparent in xylene. This is followed by a reversed alcohol series: 100%, 96%, 70%, and 50% alcohol. A section, thus treated, reveals more of the structure of the tissues, but it still does so in a rather unsatisfactory way. The section must be *stained.*

Staining

While many different stains are available for numerous purposes of histologic study, one of the most commonly used stains is the combination of hematoxylin and eosin (*H & E*). The components of this stain react chemically with the tissue components. The acid components of the tissue are selectively stained with hematoxylin, while the alkaline components are selectively stained with eosin.

Hematoxylin-stained components are purplish blue: all nuclei of cells, some components of cartilage ground substance, granules in the granular layer of cells of keratinized, stratified squamous epithelium. Eosin-stained components are pink: protein-rich structures such as the cytoplasm of some cells and collagen fibers, bone matrix.

Mounting

Finally, the sections are covered with an extremely thin *cover glass*, but not until the water of the stains, in which the sections had been submerged, is replaced, this time with a *mounting medium.* At present, most mounting media are synthetic and they do not mix with water.

Once again, the sections are run through an alcohol series (70%, 96%, 100%) and xylene. They are then covered with a drop of mounting medium. A thin cover glass is now gently placed over the medium. The result is a section in mounting medium, sandwiched between two glass slides.

Why is a mounting medium used?

1. To prevent the section from coming into contact with the air. This would cause a fast fading of the histologic stain.

2. To protect the section itself against any physical harm.

3. To make the section truly transparent, which facilitates its study.

DECALCIFICATION OF CALCIFIED TISSUES

An additional step has to be added to this histologic procedure when hard (calcified) tissues, such as dental tissues or bone, are present in the specimen. In that case, *immediately after fixation,* the specimen must be *decalcified.* The process of decalcification of a hard tissue is essential if one wants to make thin paraffin sections. Calcium salts are much harder than paraffin, and their presence in paraffin-embedded specimens may cause substantial disruptions of the sections and damage to the microtome knives. Usually a mildly acid solution is used for decalcification. When all the calcium salts have been removed, the acid is washed from the specimen, and the specimen is then treated according to the usual histologic technique, already described.

GROUND SECTIONS OF UNDECALCIFIED HARD TISSUES

A second, commonly used, technique to make sections of calcified tissues is the preparation of *ground sections.* This is sometimes a technique of choice, because the removal of calcium salts from the calcified tissues may bring about certain changes in the remainder of these tissues, which may be undesirable. In fact, in a highly cal-cified tissue, such as dental enamel, there is so little ground sub-stance present that it is completely washed away during the process of decalcification. To study enamel with the light microscope, one depends almost exclusively on unstained, undecalcified ground sec-tions (20 to 50 μm thick).

The technique of making ground sections is as follows, with the tooth taken as an example:

1. Fixation (formaldehyde solution, 10%).

2. A gross cut is made through the tooth with a fast rotating dia-mond wheel, under running water.

3. The cut surface of the tooth is polished with progressively finer grades of sandpaper.

4. A second cut is made, parallel to the first one, with the diamond wheel.

5. The resulting thick slab of tooth is now mounted, polished surface down, on a glass slide, with the use of mounting medium.

6. Now, the unpolished surface of the section is ground on *rough* sandpaper. When the slab is as thin as you want it, and as thin as physically possible (you should be able to read newsprint through

it), polishing is completed with progressively finer grades of sand-paper.

7. After thorough washing and drying, a cover glass is mounted over the ground section, in a manner similar to the one used for paraffin sections, using mounting medium. This medium renders the section more transparent and allows it to be studied microscopically, even though it is considerably thicker than a paraffin section.

Appendix III

Interpretation of Sectioned Structures

In histologic sections, we frequently study structures whose dimensions exceed the thickness of the sections themselves, or are located near the section plane and have been cut through. In studying histologic sections, one has to keep this problem in mind constantly. In Figures A–2 and A–3, it is shown how some structures in a histologic section should be interpreted for their three-dimensional appreciation. We show first how some simple structures theoretically would appear in a variety of cuts. Then we show the appearance of structures that could be found in histologic sections, in some of their typical cut profiles.

Finally, in Figure A–4 a series of tracings is shown, representing horizontal cuts through an enamel organ. These tracings have been stacked to make a computer-aided three-dimensional reconstruction showing the original shape of the enamel organ, before it was sectioned histologically.

SELECTED READING LIST

Möllring, F.K.: *Microscopy from the Very Beginning.* Oberkochen (West Germany), Carl Zeiss, Microscopy Department.

Thompson, S.W.: *Selected Histochemical and Histopathological Methods.* Springfield, IL, Charles C Thomas, 1966.

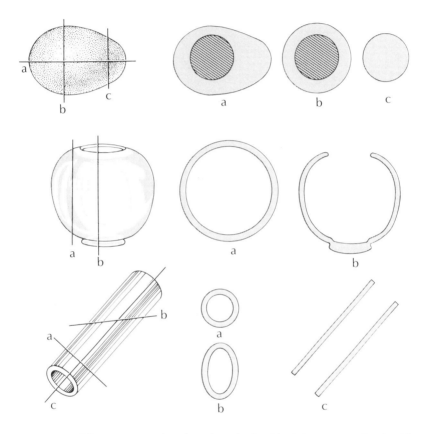

Fig. A–2.   Possible appearance of sections through a hard-boiled egg (*top*), a bowl (*middle*) and a short, cylindrical tube (*bottom*). The intact structures are shown to the left. On each, planes of sections (marked with a, b, or c) are indicated. The sections through the egg are easily tested at home. The sections through the bowl and tube are self-explanatory. Try to think of possible sections through other structures (an orange, for example). In histology, it is important to be able to interpret a structure from its sectioned appearance.

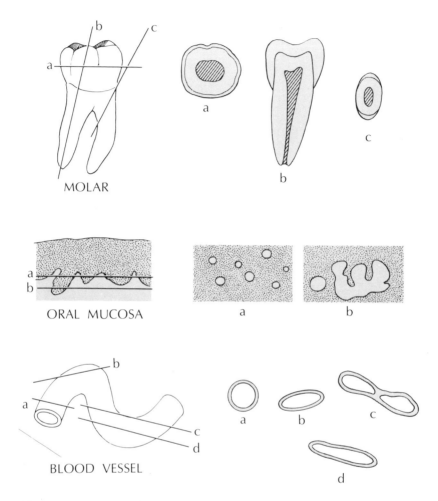

Fig. A–3. Appearance of sections through a molar tooth (*top*), a small piece of oral mucosa (*middle*), and a blood vessel (*bottom*). Section *a* through the anatomical crown of a molar consists of a central core of pulp, surrounded by dentin and a thin, peripheral layer of enamel. Section *b* passes through the entire length of a tooth and one of its roots. Section *c* consists of a central core of pulp, a layer of dentin, and a peripheral layer of cementum. The cementum at the top and bottom of the section is wider than the actual cementum width because of the obliqueness of the section. The horizontal cuts through the oral mucosa both have been made at the level of the interface between epithelium and connective tissue. Section *a* passes largely through the epithelium and only the cross sections through the rounded tops of the connective tissue papillae are included. Section *b* passes through a large area of connective tissue, while the lower parts of some taller epithelial rete pegs are included in the section as well. Finally, various sections through an irregularly curving blood vessel are shown: *a*, a true cross section; *b*, an oblique section, but close to a cross section; *d*, also an oblique section, but closer to a longitudinal section; and *c*, a typical section through a curving blood vessel, looping into and out of the section.

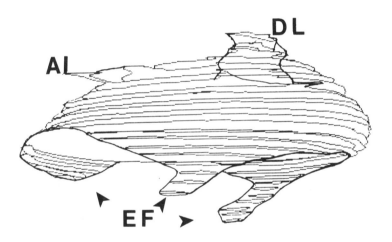

Fig. A–4.   Computer-aided three-dimensional graphic reconstruction from tracings of serial horizontal sections through the enamel organ of a primary maxillary molar. The enamel organ is in the bell stage of development. AL = Accessory lamina; DL = Attachment to dental lamina; EF = The three epithelial flaps subdividing the cervical opening.

Index

Page number in italics refer to figures. Page numbers followed by a "t" refer to tables.

organization of peripheral nerve, 119, *122*
pathways of nervous system, 115, *116*
periodontal ligament, 282, *288*, 290
pulp, 209-210, *210*
salivary glands, 67
teeth, 204
Neural crest, 143-144, *144*
Neural crest cell(s), 144
Neural groove, 143, *144*
Neural plate, 143, *144*
Neural tube, 143, *144*
Neurectoderm, 143
Neuron(s), 115, *117*, 118
Neurotransmitter substance(s), 118, *118*
Neutrophil(s). *See* Polymorphonuclear leukocyte(s)
Non-epithelial resident cell(s), 43-44, *43*
Nongranular leukocyte(s), *129*, 130-131
Nonkeratinized epithelium, 31, 35, 40, *41-42*
Nose, embryologic development of, 148-149, *150*
Nuclear envelope, 15
Nucleolus, 15
Nucleus, of cells, 10, *10*, 14-15

Oblique fiber(s), 286, 291
Odontoblast(s), as polarized cells, 178, 179
 cytodifferentiation during root development, 184-185, *185*
 cytodifferentiation of, 175, *176-178*, 178-179
 dentin, *217*
 dentin and enamel formation and, 179, *180*, 181, *181*
 development of cervix of tooth, 295
 in pulp, *206*, 207
 innervation and vascularization and, 192
 pulp, 209-210
Odontoblastic cell body(ies), 217
Odontoblastic process, 181
Oral cavity, clinical emergence of teeth in, 202t
 embryonic development of, 136, *137*, 138-156, *139*, *140*, *142-144*, 145t, *146-155*
 observation exercise, 3-6, *4*
 organization of, 6-7
 pigmentation in, 44
Oral cavity proper, 3
Oral epithelium, basal layer of, 36
 basement membrane, 45-46, *47*
 blood supply for, 45, *46*
 functions of, 31, 33
 inflammatory cells, 44

interface with lamina propria, 44-45, *45*, *46*
keratinized epithelium, 35, 38, *39*, 40
Langerhans cells, 44
layers in stratified squamous epithelia, 35-38, *37*
melanocytes, 43-44, *43*
Merkel cells, 44
microscopic examination of, 33, 35, *36*
non-epithelial resident cells, 43-44, *43*
nonkeratinized epithelium, 35, 40, *41-42*
orthokeratinized epithelium, 35, 38, *39*, 40
parakeratinized epithelium, 35, 40, *42*
prickle cell layer of, 36, *37*
structure of, 30, *30*, *54*
turnover times of, 33
Oral mucosa, connective tissue of, 30-31, *30*, 54-66, *54-56*, *58*, *60*, *63*, *64*, 66t
 definition of, 5
 epithelium of, 30-31, *30*, 33-52, *34*, *36*, *37*, *41-43*, *45-50*, *52*, *54*
 observation exercise, 27-29
 sensory receptors in, 121, *123*, 124
 structure of, *28*, 30-32, *30*, *32*
 types of, 28, *29*, 31-32, *32*, 72, 73t-75t
Organ(s), 6
Organ system(s), 6
Organelle(s), 10, *10*
Organism(s), 6
Organization of body, 6-7
Oropharyngeal membrane, 143, 146, *148*
Orthodontic treatment, 276-277, *277*
Orthokeratinized epithelium, 35, 38, *39*, 40
Osmosis, 127
Ossification, endochondral, 84, *85*, 94-96, *97-98*, 99
 intramembranous, 84, *85*
Ossification center(s), 96, *98*
Osteoblast(s), 83-85, *86*, 87, 88, *88-89*, 90, *91*, 92, 284
Osteoclast(s), 20, 83, 92, *93*, *94*, 200, 265, 284
Osteocyte(s), 83, 85, 86-87, *86*, 90, 265, 267
Osteocytic lacuna(e), *266*
Osteoid seam, 86, *86*, 87
Osteon(s), 90, *91*
Outer enamel epithelium(a), 167, 169, *172*, 184, 189
Ovulation, 138
Ovum, 138, *139*
Oxytalan fiber(s), 59, 207, 281, 287